MEDICAL
Speech-Language Pathology
Across the Care Continuum
An Introduction

MEDICAL
Speech-Language Pathology
Across the Care Continuum
An Introduction

Care
Transitions

Clinical
Reasoning

Clinical
Practice
Settings

Neuroimaging

Pharmacology

Alex F. Johnson, PhD, CCC-SLP
Barbara H. Jacobson, PhD, CCC-SLP
Megan E. Schliep, PhD, CCC-SLP, MPH
Bridget J. Perry, PhD, CCC-SLP

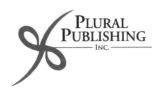

PLURAL
PUBLISHING
INC.

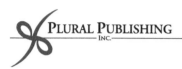

9177 Aero Drive, Suite B
San Diego, CA 92123

e-mail: information@pluralpublishing.com
Website: https://www.pluralpublishing.com

Typeset in 11/13 Garamond by Flanagan's Publishing Services, Inc.
Printed in the United States of America by Integrated Books International

Library of Congress Cataloging-in-Publication Data:
Names: Johnson, Alex F., editor. | Jacobson, Barbara Holcomb, editor. | Schliep, Megan E., editor. | Perry, Bridget J., editor.
Title: Medical speech-language pathology across the care continuum : an introduction / editors, Alex F. Johnson, Barbara H. Jacobson, Megan E. Schliep, Bridget J. Perry.
Description: San Diego, CA : Plural Publishing, Inc., [2024] | Includes bibliographical references and index.
Identifiers: LCCN 2022046690 (print) | LCCN 2022046691 (ebook) | ISBN 9781635502688 (paperback) | ISBN 1635502683 (paperback) | ISBN 9781635504521 (ebook)
Subjects: MESH: Speech-Language Pathology
Classification: LCC RC423 (print) | LCC RC423 (ebook) | NLM WL 21 | DDC 616.85/507--dc23/eng/20221128
LC record available at https://lccn.loc.gov/2022046690
LC ebook record available at https://lccn.loc.gov/2022046691

CONTENTS

PREFACE

W here does one begin to learn about the nature and practice of medical speech-language pathology? Most graduate programs have specialty courses that explore the various disorders commonly seen across health settings. Students leave these courses with a deep understanding of the classifications, diagnosis, and treatment principles for dysphagia, aphasia, dementia, traumatic brain injury, voice disorders, and motor speech disorders. This core information forms the foundation for the clinician to use as they begin practice.

As a new clinician enters the medical setting, they quickly discover that patients are seen across a continuum of care that is not organized around speech-language pathology concerns. Patients exhibit characteristics of multiple disorders. Efficiency in delivering care is an immediate concern because of time demands that are ever present. Each of the settings along the continuum presents with unique priorities that shape the role and the practice characteristics of the speech-language pathologist. As part of their clinical preparation, students have typically not spent focused practicum time in all the different health settings. New medical procedures and medications, unfamiliar to the clinician, may impact communication and swallowing. Thus, the new clinician may feel unprepared, even though they are equipped with state-of-the-art speech-language pathology information and background.

Several universities are beginning to offer courses and seminars in medical speech-language pathology with a goal of preparing new clinicians to enter practice with an awareness of these issues. In talking with colleagues who teach these courses, we discovered that there was no text designed to supplement the core disorder- focused material and to integrate that within the context of medical speech-language pathology practice. That is the purpose of this text.

This book is designed to address the integration of SLP knowledge with practice setting specific issues. The settings covered include acute care settings, rehabilitation, outpatient settings, skilled nursing facilities, and home care. The application of skills, knowledge, and clinical process in each of these settings is highlighted. In addition to the setting-specific foci, we have included two chapters of a more in-depth nature. The first focuses on medications and their effect on communication and swallowing. The second is designed to enhance understanding of neuroimaging and its implications for clinical care. Both areas are critically important in health care settings yet are rarely represented in a thorough manner in graduate preparation. Finally, several cases have been developed. Students and faculty can use these cases to explore application of both clinical and setting-specific principles as a primer for practice in "the real world."

As authors and editors of this content, our hope is that the book can serve as a core text in courses in medical speech-language pathology. The book may also be useful for those speech-language pathologists transitioning from a school-based or private practice setting into health care. We welcome feedback and suggestions for future editions.

We also are happy to acknowledge those who have contributed to this work, including our own students and colleagues at Vanderbilt University and at MGH Institute of Health Professions. Additionally, special appreciation is offered to Megan Wilcox, Zachary Smith, and Rachel Pittman, all who have made significant contributions to this work.

Alex Johnson
Barbara Jacobson
Megan Schliep
Bridget Perry

ABOUT THE EDITORS

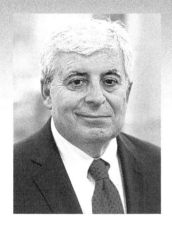

Alex F. Johnson, PhD, CCC-SLP, ASHA Honors, served as Provost at the MGH Institute (Boston, Massachusetts) for 14 years. Prior to that he served as department chair at Wayne State University. In 1998, Johnson launched the Division of Speech-Language Sciences and Disorders at the Henry Ford Medical Center (Department of Neurology) in Detroit, Michigan. His academic interests have focused on medical speech-language pathology and neurologic communication disorders. He has been involved in the development of widely used outcome measures in voice and swallowing disorders and communication quality. Johnson is an American Speech-Language-Hearing Association Fellow, has received the Honors of the American Speech-Language-Hearing Association and National Student Speech Language Hearing Association, and is a Distinguished Scholar in the National Academies of Practice.

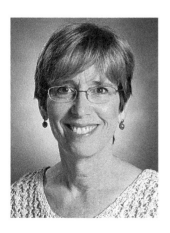

Barbara H. Jacobson, PhD, CCC-SLP, ASHA Fellow, served as Associate Professor at Vanderbilt Bill Wilkerson Center for 9 years working in medical speech-language pathology administration, clinical education, and as a clinician in acute care. Prior to that, she was Associate Professor in the Vanderbilt Voice Center. She was a senior staff speech-language pathologist at Henry Ford Hospital in Detroit, Michigan, from 1988 to 2003 where she established a Voice Production Laboratory. Her clinical and research interests are in functional and patient-reported outcomes, medical speech-language pathology, and neurogenic voice disorders. Jacobson is a co-author of the *Voice Handicap Index* (1997) and *Dysphagia Handicap Index* (2012). She is an American Speech-Language-Hearing Association Fellow.

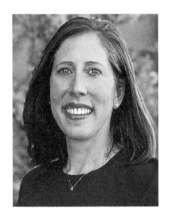

Megan E. Schliep, PhD, CCC-SLP, MPH, is an Assistant Professor in the Department of Communication Sciences and Disorders at MGH Institute of Health Professions in Boston, Massachusetts. She also holds a clinical appointment as a speech-language pathologist at Spaulding Rehabilitation Hospital in Boston, Massachusetts. Her research focuses on poststroke aphasia and explores the implementation of standardized assessment practices across the care continuum and identification of clinical predictors to inform recovery trajectory, with a focus on interdisciplinary research–practice partnerships.

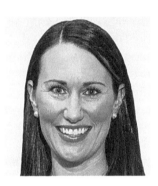

Bridget J. Perry, PhD, CCC-SLP, is an Assistant Professor in the Department of Communication Sciences and Disorders and the Program Director of the Clinical Doctorate in Speech-Language Pathology program at MGH Institute of Health Professions. Her research is focused on improving patient-centered management of swallowing and speech impairments for patients diagnosed with serious illness through the use of novel assessment and intervention methodologies.

CONTRIBUTORS

Abigail T. Burka, PharmD
Associate Professor of Pharmacy and Pharmaceutical Sciences
Lipscomb University College of Pharmacy
Nashville, Tennessee
Chapter 8

Mary L. Casper, MA, CCC-SLP, ASHA Fellow, FNAP
Corporate Rehabilitation Consultant
HCR ManorCare
Toledo, Ohio
Chapter 4

Julia R. W. Haffer, MS, CCC-SLP
MGH Institute of Health Professions and
Spaulding Rehabilitation Network
Boston, Massachusetts
Chapter 3

Barbara H. Jacobson, PhD, CCC-SLP, ASHA Fellow
Retired Faculty
Vanderbilt Bill Wilkerson Center
Vanderbilt University Medical Center
Nashville, Tennessee
Chapter 2

Alex F. Johnson, PhD, CCC-SLP, ASHA Honors, FNAP
Provost Emeritus
MGH Institute of Health Professions
Boston, Massachusetts
Chapters 1 and 6

Jeffrey P. Johnson, PhD, MS, CCC-SLP
Geriatric Research Education and Clinical Center
Audiology and Speech Pathology
VA Pittsburgh Healthcare System
Pittsburgh, Pennsylvania
Chapter 9

Minal Kadam, MA, CCC-SLP, CBIS
Speech-Language Pathology Clinician, Clinical Specialist
Spaulding Rehabilitation Network
Boston, Massachusetts
Chapter 6

Jennifer Loehr, MA, CCC-SLP, COS-C
Executive Director of Acquisitions
Enhabit Home Health and Hospice
Austin, Texas
Chapter 5

Megan L. Malone, MA, CCC-SLP
Speech-Language Pathologist/Associate Lecturer
Kent State University
Kent, Ohio
Chapter 5

Erin L. Meier, MS, PhD, CCC-SLP
Assistant Professor
Communication Sciences and Disorders
Northeastern University
Boston, Massachusetts
Chapter 9

Kaitlyn Johnston Minchin, MS, CCC-SLP
Pediatric Speech-Language Pathologist
Vanderbilt Children's Hospital
Nashville, Tennessee
Kentucky Children's Hospital
Lexington, Kentucky
Chapter 7

Bridget J. Perry, PhD, CCC-SLP
Assistant Professor and Program Director
Clinical Doctorate in Speech-Language Pathology Program
Department of Communication Sciences and Disorders
MGH Institute of Health Professions

Speech-Language Pathologist
Brigham and Women's Hospital
Boston, Massachusetts
Chapter 2

Rachel Pittman, MS-HPEd, MS-CCC-SLP
Assistant Professor and Director
Impact Practice Center
Department of Communication Sciences and Disorders
MGH Institute of Health Professions
Boston, Massachusetts
Chapter 6

Megan E. Schliep, PhD, CCC-SLP, MPH
Assistant Professor
Department of Communication Sciences and Disorders
MGH Institute of Health Professions
Speech-Language Pathologist
Spaulding Rehabilitation Hospital
Boston, Massachusetts
Chapters 3 and 6

Zachary Smith, MS, CCC-SLP
Speech-Language Pathologist
Brigham and Women's Hospital
Boston, Massachusetts
Chapter 10

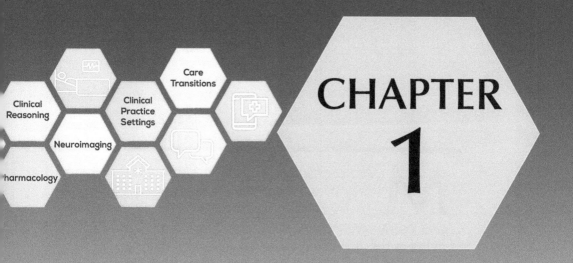

CHAPTER 1

Medical Speech-Language Pathology: Key Concepts

Alex F. Johnson

Chapter Objectives

Upon completion of this chapter, the reader will be able to:

- Introduce and familiarize the reader with the defining characteristics of medical speech-language pathology.
- Provide basic concepts about clinical reasoning in health settings.
- Familiarize the reader with the concept of the continuum of care, as the basis for reading the other chapters in the book.
- Guide the reader toward the use of additional resources to aid practice.

Getting Started

M ost new clinicians find the challenge and opportunity of working in the medical setting to be a wonderful experience. The opportunity to learn and really understand the impact of communication and swallowing disorders in this setting is powerful. Similarly, discovering and appreciating the solutions that the speech-language pathologist (SLP) can add for patients with health issues is impactful. Learning to work together with other disciplines (interprofessional practice) to achieve the best possible outcomes is realized in this setting, as well.

It must also be noted that for the new SLP, the unfamiliar territory of a hospital, skilled nursing facility, or home health setting can challenge clinical reasoning in a way that is not experienced in the safety of the university clinic. This text provides an opportunity for the student or new graduate to learn about these settings and think about the skills and knowledge needed for working in these areas. It also is intended to be helpful for those experienced SLPs transitioning from other settings.

Like every profession, speech-language pathology can be practiced in several contexts. A common approach to understanding the distribution of speech-language pathology services is subdivision into health care and education settings. These two areas encompass most speech-language pathology practices. Additional settings include higher education, research, private practice, industry, and so forth. Interestingly, most of the work in these additional settings is devoted to activities related to either health- or education-focused practice. Because SLPs are generally trained to provide services in many contexts, it is safe to assume that the skills associated with health- and education-based practice can be observed in both types of settings. Consider the clinician in the hospital setting, who spends most of the time dealing with patients with swallowing disabilities and aphasia but receives a referral from a pediatric neurologist for a 6-year-old child with dyslexia and language learning difficulties. Conversely, think about the school-based SLP who spends most of her day with children with language *and reading problems but receives a new student who has swallowing and cognitive problems after a brain injury. In each case, the physical environment is different, the purpose and focus of treatment may be different, yet the client could be seen in either environment.*

This text is designed to serve as a resource for emerging and established clinicians beginning practice in the medical setting, to provide information and support. Thus, the focus here is on features that can help the SLP appreciate the characteristics of the setting (context) and the critical decisions and activities associated with medical speech-language pathology across the continuum of care.

Describing Medical Speech-Language Pathology

Medical speech-language pathology can be considered from two perspectives: (a) the location where services are provided, and (b) the clinical approach to care. The first topic focuses on the various types and approaches of clinical service that occur in and across health settings. In the United States, health care is delivered in many different physical settings: acute care hospitals, rehabilitation settings, specialty hospitals, outpatient settings, and the patient's home. Some patients with chronic conditions are seen by their SLP in skilled nursing or other long-term care facilities. A broad array of specialty hospitals, community health centers, and governmental agencies also provide this type of care.

A second perspective for the discussion of medical speech-language pathology has to do with a clinical practice and decision model, or clinical reasoning. A detailed discussion of clinical reasoning is beyond the scope of this chapter. However, various aspects of clinical reasoning, especially those that are setting specific, are reflected throughout this book. Adapted from medicine, this clinical reasoning model considers the patient's history, any current or chronic health conditions or physical limitations, the setting and functional needs of the patient, any social or societal concerns, the family context, and so forth. In speech-language pathology, as in the other health professions, a cause-and-effect approach for diagnosing a communication or swallowing disorder and generating possible solutions to management of the patient's problem is the overarching concern. In a behavioral science, such as speech-language pathology, this approach involves generating hypotheses about possible explanations for the presenting problem, and then refining tests and observations to confirm or reject these various options. At times, testing allows for observation of a direct physical cause for the problem, but in many cases in speech-language pathology, the cause must be inferred using discipline-specific knowledge. This model has been in use in speech-language pathology for decades, particularly in health-related settings (Nation & Aram, 1977; Tomblin, Morris, & Spriestersbach, 2000). Interestingly, this approach is also applied in many other speech-language pathology settings, including those in community, in schools, in private practice, and in other settings. It is important to note that many individuals with health-related (medical) communication disorders are seen in these community contexts. While their communication impairment may be related to a health condition, they may be participating in social, educational, or vocational activities in their community. The SLP in these settings needs to appreciate the health-related history and concerns of the individual client or patient or student, regardless of the setting. It is, in fact, the interaction among patient health status (causes), resultant difficulties in communication or swallowing function, available treatments, functional outcomes, and the patient's perspectives and goals that define the boundaries of medical speech-language pathology.

It also makes sense to clarify the use of the term *medical*. This term, as a descriptor for health condition–focused speech-language pathology practice, has been in use for many years. In a previous reference text, Johnson and Jacobson (2017) reviewed use of this terminology in some detail. In some cases, the use of the term *medical* can cause confusion. More precise, yet cumbersome, terminology might include condition-focused or health-related speech-language pathology services as an alternative. However, the common understanding of the term *medical* in this case is not intended to imply the practice of medicine, rather it relates to the points previously discussed: settings and an approach to problem-solving. A brief, if incomplete, introduction to some of the exemplary contributors to medical speech-language pathology may be found in Appendix 1–A, at the end of this chapter. It is important to acknowledge that there are dozens of additional contributors that could be mentioned, and the reader is invited to augment the list with those contributors who have influenced their own thinking. Review of the primary work of some of these individuals can provide an interesting glimpse into some of the historical thinking, theoretical perspectives, and clinical tools that are in common use across medical speech-language pathology contexts of practice.

Clinical Reasoning Tools for the Novice Speech-Language Pathologist

It can be helpful for new clinicians to map out the likely continuum for their specific patient. This can serve as an alert to communicate carefully and deliberately both within the current team and with the next team in the continuum. For new clinicians, being both deliberate and anticipatory regarding collaboration across the continuum, can enhance quality and efficiency of care, and can produce the best clinical outcomes for the patient. Deliberation and anticipation can be thought of as two critical clinical reasoning processes that help all clinicians, especially new ones, focus on the needs of the patient within the scope and context in which they are being seen.

Deliberate Practice

Deliberate practice involves a concentrated focus on a skill or activity or on a set of decisions. To develop expertise with a new or complex skill, one needs repeated and focused experience. Dudding et al. (2017) have written about the important role of deliberative practice in clinical teaching. Paired with expert feedback and self-evaluation (reflection), deliberate practice is an effective approach to establishing competence in new skills. Ericson (2008) described deliberate practice as a highly structured training experience that is focused on improvement of performance in a specific domain and leads to expertise. Applied to speech-language pathology, one could imagine that learning to make reliable perceptual judgments about voice or speech samples of varying types requires practice. Typically, these skills are learned through highly specific training exercises in the classroom and laboratory. Initially, learners acquire this skill by focusing on discrete elements (pitch, loudness, quality, intelligibility) separately. Eventually, clinicians improve their skills and advance to being able to reliably make these judgments with real patients in the clinical setting. However, it is important to acknowledge that each step toward integrated decision-making in the "real world" requires focused and repeated practice, sequenced over time, in increasingly challenging situations. Perceptual judgments, psychomotor abilities, diagnostic test administration and interpretation, and clinical decision-making are some of the most salient SLP skills that lend themselves to acquisition through deliberate practice. Tools that can help someone learn these skills include apps, checklists, organizers, and templates. In addition, the importance of external feedback and mentoring cannot be under-estimated. These elements, human ones, are particularly helpful in the earliest stages of learning.

Deliberate practice is not unique to speech-language pathology. Atul Gawande, a surgeon, highlights this concept in his best-selling book, *The Checklist Manifesto* (Gawande, 2010). This author effectively describes the use of simple checklists to get things right in health care. He documents improvements in surgical procedures, intensive care units, and emergency situations using this cueing mechanism. The decision to be deliberate about patient manage-ment keeps a clinician's attention on the patient and the primacy of their needs in the clinical interaction. In a busy clinical setting, the distractions of multiple demands, personal interruptions, or benign forgetfulness can allow for clinicians to omit or overlook key factors. Deliberate practice mitigates these errors.

Anticipatory Practice

Anticipatory practice focuses on the larger system of care and addresses the patient's needs as their condition or the location of care changes. Consideration of what the patient will need in the future, at the next point of care, may change steps or actions that a given clinician takes at a specific point in time. An early description of anticipatory practice was provided by Pridham et al. (1979). In this article, the authors described application of anticipatory practice on two scenarios—maternal /child health and surgical management and follow-up. Expert clinicians, from any discipline, make recommendations and provide interventions that reflect the long-term goals of any patient in the context of their capabilities and the capability of the system needed to sup-port them. For example, a clinician may recognize that a patient has a motor speech disorder (dysarthria) and has trouble being understood by family and friends. Understanding the cause of the dysarthria (chronic versus degenerative) sheds light on the patient's immediate and future needs and likely outcomes. These observations and decisions become automatic as clinicians gain knowledge and experience. However, it is common for clinicians, early in their practice, to err because of their limited anticipatory knowledge.

In deliberate practice, one learns relevant skills and develops expertise in appropriate implementation. In anticipatory practice, one learns to project the patients' needs along the continuum of care. Figures 1–1A and 1–1B summarize these two important foci in the process of clinical reasoning.

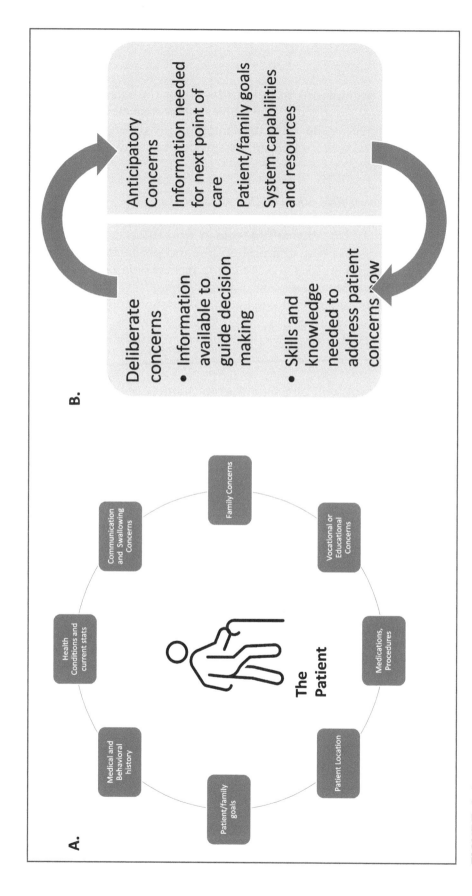

FIGURE 1-1. A. The patient in context. **B.** Deliberate and anticipatory practice in medical speech-language pathology.

An example might help to highlight the interaction between these two perspectives on clinical expertise development. One might consider the ways they might apply differently to a graduate student, a new clinician, or a more experienced clinician.

Case Example: Deliberate and Anticipatory Practice

The patient is a 50-year-old woman who sustained a stroke and is having trouble with comprehension and production of both written and spoken language. She is currently being seen by the SLP in an acute stroke unit in a university medical center. The SLP will want to be sure to evaluate and monitor communication skills and check motor speech and swallowing capabilities.

The deliberative practice decisions for this clinician will be as follows:

- What tools will be useful for repeatable, accurate, and precise measures of change during this acute stage of recovery?
- What information about language, speech, and swallowing will be most useful for those providing care for the patient?
- What information will be of benefit to the patient and her family?
- Are there any short-term compensatory tools that could be useful in the current (acute stroke unit) setting?
- Do I (the SLP) have the competency to gather and prioritize the information needed, to use appropriate assessment tools, to diagnose the communication disorder, and to provide appropriate recommendations, especially for the current point of care?

The anticipatory questions that the clinician might consider:

- When will this patient be discharged?
- What are the various services they will need upon discharge? Who will be providing speech-language pathology services for this patient, if needed? In what setting will speech-language pathology services be provided?
- What information or actions could help with the transition to the next point of care?
- What is the best way to transmit the important information to the next provider?

■ Is there any speech-language pathology–specific information that should be highlighted for case managers, physicians, or other providers who are focused on the patient's future needs?

A second rationale for focusing our discussion in this text around settings of practice (rather than the more typical approach of focusing on specific communication disorders) is that it allows for a patient-centric discussion. Patients who exhibited health-related speech, language, or swallowing disorders rarely present with a single prototypic problem. Rather, it is most common for the patient to exhibit multiple symptoms, numerous health-related concerns, a unique set of environmental and personal issues, and so forth. Considering the needs of the patient at a specific moment in time, while understanding where they have come from and where they will go, seems like an important perspective. Hopefully, this organizational model will help new clinicians appreciate their own role and its variations, depending on where on the continuum of setting that they are seeing the patient. An implicit goal of this book is to assure that SLPs recognize their critical role at both the point of care with their patient, as well as doing everything possible to assure the best outcomes as the patient moves through the system.

The approach proposed so far has been one that focused on clinical reasoning across the continuum of care. Regardless of the type of patient, the location of the patient in the continuum, or the relevant clinical questions, a model that focuses on necessary decision-making, deliberative and anticipatory practice, and reflection increases the likelihood of competent care for the patient and assures the best outcome. New clinicians are sometimes frustrated by this highly specific and deliberate approach to practice development. Individuals who have studied the acquisition of expertise in health providers (Benner, 2001) indicate that as competence is developed, many aspects of clinical reasoning become more flexible and automatic. Thus, it makes sense for new clinicians to focus on the deliberate approach to learning so that they can move toward independent and efficient models of practice.

The Scope of Medical Speech-Language Pathology

The scope of medical speech-language pathology can be described as including specific clinical areas (voice disorders, neurogenic language and communication disorders, motor speech disorders, psychiatric and developmental conditions, and dysphagia). Table 1–1

TABLE 1–1	Speech, Language, and Swallowing Disorders Frequently Encountered in Medical SLP
Condition	**Typical Causation**
Cognitive Disorders: Memory, attention, organization, social communication	Traumatic brain injury, dementing illnesses, other neurodegenerative conditions
Language Disorders: Aphasia, dyslexia, dysgraphia	Stroke, traumatic brain injury, dementing illnesses, brain tumors
Speech Disorders: Apraxia of speech, dysarthria	Stroke, movement disorders, neuromuscular diseases, neurodegenerative conditions, traumatic brain injury
Voice and Upper Airway Disorders: Dysphonia, aphonia, neurogenic voice disorders	Benign and malignant growths, neurologic conditions, tracheotomy, head and neck surgeries, respiratory diseases and conditions
Swallowing Disorders: Dysphagia	Tumors, neurologic conditions, digestive disorders, pulmonary disorders, burns
Psychogenic Disorders: Functional communication and swallowing disorders	Stress, emotional concerns, anxiety

provides a summary of the types of speech, language, and swallowing conditions that are commonly observed across the various health settings.

It is a common, almost universal, observation among new clinicians that despite having excellent graduate coursework in these areas, they rarely feel prepared for the in vivo experience. Seeing patients with communication disorders in the context of their social, family, and health conditions and experiencing the collective impact on quality of life can be breathtaking and humbling. Particularly in the acute setting, when patients are at the height of their own vulnerability and frailty, the experience for the new clinician can be unsettling, even frightening. The best clinicians in these settings learn to approach every patient with deep respect, curiosity, and keen observation skills. Knowing about a communication or swallowing disorder is quite different than knowing a patient who is experiencing that disorder.

Another perspective, which serves as the central organizing feature of this text, is based on setting. Each health care setting can have patients with a variety of health conditions. However, each setting has distinct purposes and activities related to care of the patient. In this text we consider these functions and activities in some detail. It is assumed that students reading this material will have completed (or be completing) the required graduate study in speech-language pathology and will have been exposed to specific content information for the diagnosis and management of various disorders.

The Continuum of Care in Medical Speech-Language Pathology

One concept that helps to explicate this approach for consideration of health settings is the concept of a continuum of care. According to one source (Evashwick, 1989), the continuum of care is a concept involving an integrated system of service delivery that guides and tracks patients over time through a comprehensive array of health services. The concept of a continuum allows for consideration of critical decisions and activities over the course of an illness or condition. As you can imagine, speech-language pathology services can be inserted almost anywhere across the continuum. To illustrate this concept, Figure 1–2 provides a continuum model as a road map, comparing two different patients.

In this example, Patient A (Figure 1–2A) is a 22-year-old singer who notices hoarseness and reduced singing range and checks in with her primary care provider, who refers her to an otolaryngologist. Her road map consists of three providers (primary care, ENT, SLP) and three settings (outpatient medical, outpatient SLP, home). Compare that to Patient B (Figure 1–2B), another 22-year-old, who survived a motor vehicle crash (MVC) and sustained a traumatic brain injury. His road map (continuum) reveals a much more complicated picture consisting of at least eight major setting changes, and a likelihood of several dozen different providers (a conservative estimate) over the course of treatment. One can imagine that the complexity differences for these two patients are immense. Thus, when thinking of continuum of care, the clinician can anticipate several different factors that are likely to affect outcome. These include communication within settings (across the care team, including the family/patient), communication during transitions from one setting to the next, shared decision-making, evidence-based treatment, and so forth. In general, the more complex the patient's medical problems, the more providers, settings, and complicated decisions are involved. Embedded in all this clinical activity are many opportunities for clinical communication exchange, some of which can be quite complex, requiring clinical knowledge

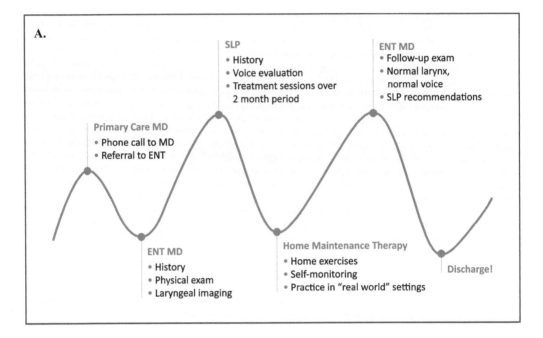

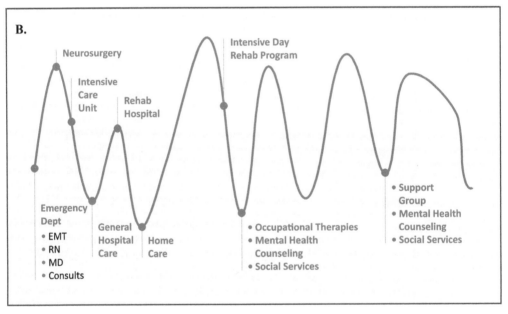

FIGURE 1–2. Continuum of care. **A.** Patient A: 22-year-old singer with vocal nodules, hoarseness, and vocal fatigue. **B.** Patient B: 22-year-old survivor of motor vehicle accident.

and expertise and deep understanding of the patient's and family's needs at each step along the way.

In summary, medical speech-language pathology can be considered to consist of three distinguishing characteristics:

▪ the practice of speech-language pathology in the context of medical care across a variety of health settings;

▪ the use of cause–effect diagnostic and treatment decision-making principles in serving individuals with communication and swallowing disorders; and

▪ the use of efficient communication and collaboration across settings to assure efficiency and quality of care, thereby reducing cost and increasing efficiency and quality.

Snapshot of Medical Speech-Language Pathology

The American Speech-Language-Hearing Association (ASHA) produces a biennial summary of SLP Health Care Trends. At the time of this writing, the most recent survey results (ASHA, 2022) show the following trends: 18% work in general hospitals; 18% in home health care; 32% in outpatient clinics or offices; and 21% in skilled nursing facilities. Other prominent settings include pediatric hospitals and rehabilitation hospitals.

In general, for individuals entering practice in these areas, the development of basic to advanced competency in the areas of aphasia, cognitive communication disorders, voice disorders, dysarthria, and swallowing impairment should be a priority.

Safety and Risk in Medical Speech-Language Pathology

Historically, the field of speech-language pathology has not been overtly focused on issues of safety and efficiency, when compared to other health disciplines. For instance, within the fields of medicine, nursing, and pharmacy, there are subspecialty areas and professional organizations devoted to these topics. In these fields, there is a direct linear relationship between certain practices and patient morbidity or mortality. It is obvious that administering the wrong drug, failing to note certain patient disease indicators, or making errors in surgical or medical treatment can have devastating effects. Thus, there is a large literature on medical safety, infection control, and assurance of quality outcomes in these other disciplines.

In medical settings, as speech-language pathology has moved into areas of greater risk and introduced more invasive clinical procedures, the physical risk to the patient is increased. Other risks associated with speech-language pathology practice may have a less linear relationship to patient outcome but also need to be considered by every clinician. It is important to remember that sometimes errors involve taking an inappropriate action (e.g., making an inappropriate recommendation), failing to take an appropriate action (e.g., failing to communicate recommendations in a timely way), or making a clinical error (e.g., misdiagnosis or misinterpretation of test results). Table 1–2 provides a summary of common errors observed in the medical setting.

As this text goes to publication, the entire world is in the process of recovering and adjusting to the broad effects of the COVID-19 pandemic. In this most recent context, the preeminence of infection control involving repeated vaccination and use of a variety of personal protective equipment is now well known. While the devastation of this epidemic is moving toward resolution, a new aware-

TABLE 1–2 Potential Medical Speech-Language Pathologist Errors in Practice

	Possible Error	Example
1	Failure to communicate significant findings to other providers of care	Not informing patient's physician of an observed worsening of mental status
2	Technical errors in administering or interpreting clinical tests or procedure results	Using a standardized tool inappropriately
3	Providing advice outside the scope of practice	Recommending a specific medication to the patient
4	Failure to use existing information about patient safety or limitations	Encouraging a patient to stand or walk without assistance (if needed)
5	Inappropriate application of general information that should be available to all speech-language pathologists	Misdiagnosis of a communication or swallowing disorder
6	Failure to communicate risks or precautions to stakeholders	Forgetting to document necessary safety precautions for swallowing
7	Failure to comply with patient safety protocols, including infection control	Failure to use personal protective equipment as required
8	Failure to comply with the ASHA Code of Ethics or with state or federal laws	Guaranteeing outcomes of service
9	Failure to follow legal requirements for documentation, coding, or billing	Billing for the wrong dates of service or miscoding, so as to increase revenue
10	Provision of any potentially high-risk procedure without demonstrated competency	Performing endoscopic procedures without training or supervision

ness of how disease is transmitted has left most, if not all medical institutions with new requirements for masking, gloves, and eye protection as a minimum form of personal protective equipment.

Clinicians entering all the settings discussed in this book need to be prepared in the use of personal protective equipment, know vaccination requirements, and become familiar with risk management for disease transmission overall. Those who work in high acuity settings may need additional special training to protect their patients, colleagues, and themselves.

Roles for Speech-Language Pathologists in Health Care Settings

It may be helpful to consider the various roles that SLPs experience in the course of their work in health settings. Clinical practitioner, educator, and leadership functions are interrelated roles taken on by every SLP. Occasionally, these responsibilities are titled positions within an organization and make up most of a particular job. Clinician, supervisor, instructor, manager, and director are all examples of terms that suggest a defined role or scope that make up a specific job. Regardless of job title, though, every SLP has responsibilities from each category. Every speech-language pathology clinician is also a leader and (hopefully) an educator. Care must be taken to develop capabilities in each of these areas to be most effective.

Clinical Practitioner

Most of the work in speech-language pathology is focused on the safe, efficient, and effective delivery of speech and language services to patients. Accordingly, there are documents, journals, websites, and hundreds of other resources to guide practice across the spectrum of human communication disorders. It is safe to say that the bulk of preparation in our graduate programs is focused on this aspect of professional function, as well. Accreditation documents and licensure requirements all specify the content and scope of what SLPs need to learn. This is further defined as new graduates enter the workplace and additional expectations, beyond the very basic entry level, are delineated for the new professional. It is important to note that in speech-language pathology, as well as other health professions, certification requirements are changing to include a deeper focus on interprofessional practice, ethics, and justice and equity for persons served.

Clinical Educator

The role of the clinician as educator is an implicit part of the job. It is rarely delineated clearly in job descriptions, and it is unfortunately not often presented as a set of professional skills to be developed and mastered. There are two primary educational domains that clinicians should explicitly learn: patient-related education and education of learners (students, fellows, new staff members). These are two different skill sets, but they are of equal importance to the discipline, and to those served by SLPs.

Helping patients understand the goals, activities, and outcomes of their treatments is essential to both progress attainment and patient satisfaction. Because communication disorders, especially in patients with multiple problems, can be somewhat invisible, it is important that the nature and extent of the problem be clearly explained to the patient and the family. Verbal explanations should be supplemented with appropriate reading materials, videos, or other resources appropriate to the language level of the recipient. SLPs in health settings should not assume that other providers can adequately explain communication disorders to their patients. Skilled and experienced clinicians learn to titrate the amount and type of information for the patient in a way that is informative, helpful, and promotes the best outcome. Offering too much information or too little will generate confusion and misunderstanding. Similarly, it is essential to understand the linguistic and cognitive readiness of the patient or family in the education process. In this educator role, the SLP must think of what Nation and Aram (1977) referred to as the "client complex." The client complex includes the patient, the family, and caregivers, as well as other professionals involved with the patient. Teaching nurses, other therapists, and physicians about communication and swallowing needs is essential in assuring patient safety and outcome.

The second educational focus is devoted to those entering the profession or the setting: students, fellows, and new staff members. In general, students are very interested in exposure to health settings as part of their education. Similarly, postgraduate clinical fellowships are highly desirable. The various approaches to teaching in these settings are increasingly supported with evidence. Tools of clinical assessment and observation, feedback, and debriefing can be of great benefit to the learner. Recently, the Council of Academic Programs in Communication Sciences and Disorders (CAPCSD) has produced a series of instructional courses on supervision and on the use of simulation. This information should be helpful to those who want to learn to be better prepared to educate learners in the health setting.

The educational paradigm across health professions is almost always developmental, with the learner moving gradually from novice states to one of advanced expertise. This is also true in medical speech-language pathology. Providing guided pathways that move learners from very basic protocols and clinical reasoning to advanced skills in diagnosis and interpretation, as well as integration with information from medicine, nursing, and physical and occupational therapy is helpful to learners. For some learners, exposure and immersion in health settings is the only framework needed. These individuals can quickly assimilate and apply new learning with a high level of performance accuracy and competence. However, most learners benefit from a more deliberate linear experience with clear milestones, expectations, assessments, and feedback. This approach is geared to assure the development of necessary competencies.

Johnson and Jacobson (2017) provide a summary of helpful educational models and goals for preparing medical SLPs. Some goals of their educational model included (a) establishing a clear connection between learned content and the real clinical world; (b) providing internships and fellowships that are both learning-centric and patient-centric; (c) assuring that learners' safe competencies, especially around high-risk issues, are documented; (d) assuring that high-value continuing education experiences are available.

Clinical Leadership

Leadership can be considered from two perspectives. At various points in their career, experienced SLPs frequently become titled leaders (manager, director, supervisor). These titled roles distinguish the leadership focus of a certain job. Usually, these leaders are responsible for program development, hiring and supervising, managing budget, scheduling staff for various responsibilities, and other functions that assure smooth and coordinated delivery of services. A second, less obvious aspect of leadership involves all professionals, regardless of their title. Advocating for patients or for the profession, developing new programs or processes for patient care, participating in committees, initiating improvements, or helping others understand the needs of a specific patient are activities that require leadership skills and knowledge. An important emerging area of leadership content of vital importance involves responsibility for advocating for populations that have been disadvantaged or have had less access to care. Sound clinical capabilities and sophisticated leadership skills combine to form the most gifted clinicians.

Conclusion

This overview provides a glimpse into the issues and topics considered in this book. The rich history, dynamic growth, and critical importance of medical speech-language pathology practice are all important considerations for readers to understand. In the following chapters, provided are specific opportunities to explore the landscape of necessary knowledge and practice competencies that are necessary to succeed in medical speech-language pathology.

Questions for Discussion

1. What are the differences and similarities between medical and educational speech-language pathology practices?
2. In this chapter, we provided a brief listing of several important figures in the development of medical speech-language pathology. From your readings or experience, can you add another example of a "history-maker?" What is your rationale for choosing that individual?
3. Think about deliberative practice and anticipatory practice. Apply these concepts to a client or patient you have seen in your own clinical experience.
4. Consider the opportunities for leadership that apply to all clinicians. Can you identify one or more situations where you have seen these applied by an SLP in a non-titled role?
5. Having read this chapter, identify one or more lingering questions that you have about medical speech-language pathology? What is not clear? Be deliberate (focus on your own knowledge now and what you need to know) and anticipatory (What would you like to learn? What would benefit you as a learner as you move through this text?).

References

American Speech-Language-Hearing Association. (2021). *Highlights and trends: Member and affiliate counts, year-end 2022.*

American Speech-Language-Hearing Association. (2022). *2021 SLP Health Care Survey: Survey Summary Report*, 66.

Benner, P. (2001). Creating a culture of safety and improvement: A key to reducing medical error. *American Journal of Critical Care, 10*(4), 281–284.

Dudding, C. C., McReady, V., Nunez, L. M., & Procaccini, S. J. (2017). Clinical supervision in speech-language pathology in the United States: Development of a specialty. *The Clinical Supervisor, 36*(2).

Ericsson, KA. (2008). Deliberate practice and acquisition of expert performance: A general overview. *Academic Emergency Medicine: A Global Journal of Emergency Care, 15*(11), 988–994.

Evashwick, C. (1989). Creating the continuum of care. *Health Matrix, 7*(1), 30–39.

Gawande, A. (2010). *The checklist manifesto: How to get things right.* Henry Holt and Company.

Johnson, A. F., & Jacobson, B. H. (2017). Educational perspectives for medical speech-language pathology: From concept to competency. In A. F. Johnson & B. H. Jacobson (Eds.), *Medical speech-language pathology: A practitioner's guide* (3rd ed., pp. 9–17). Thieme.

Johnson, A. F., & Jacobson, B. H. (Eds.). (2017). *Medical speech-language pathology: A practitioner's guide* (3rd ed.). Thieme.

Nation, J. E. & Aram, D. (1977). *Diagnosis of speech and language disorders.* Mosby.

Pridham, K. F., Hansen, M. F., & Conrad, H. H. (1979). Anticipatory problem solving: Models for clinical practice and research. *Sociology of Health & Illness, 1*(2), 177–194. https://doi.org/10.1111/1467-9566.ep10478953

Tomblin, J. B., Morris, H. L., & Spriestersbach, D. C. (2000). *Diagnosis in speech-language pathology* (2nd ed.). Singular Thomson Learning.

APPENDIX 1–A
A Short List of Some Key Figures in Medical Speech-Language Pathology

Contributor	Key Areas of Contribution	Exemplary Publications
Hildred Schuell	Aphasia	Schuell, H. (1955). *The Minnesota Test for the Differential Diagnosis of Aphasia.* University of Minnesota.
	Aphasia	Wertz, R. T., Collins, M. J., Weiss, D., Kurtzke, J. F., Friden, T., Brookshire, R. H., . . . Resurreccion, E. (1981). Veterans Administration cooperative study on aphasia: A comparison of individual and group treatment. *Journal of Speech and Hearing Research, 24,* 580–594.
Leonard LaPointe	Aphasia	LaPointe, L., & Stierwalt, J. A. G. (2018). *Aphasia and related neurogenic language disorders.* Thieme Medical Publishers.
Audrey Holland	Aphasia	Holland, A. L., & Elman, R. J. (2001). *Neurogenic disorders, and the life participation approach: The social imperative in supporting individuals and families.* Plural Publishing. Holland, A. L., & Nelson, R. L. (2013). Counseling in communication disorders: A wellness perspective (2nd ed.). Plural Publishing.
Nancy Helm-Estabrooks	Aphasia	Helm-Estabrooks, N., Albert, M. L., & Nicholas, M. (2014). *Manual of aphasia and aphasia therapy* (3rd ed.). Pro-Ed.
Daniel Boone	Voice	Boone, D. R., McFarlane, S. C., Von Berg, S. L., & Zraick, R. I. (2020). *The voice and voice therapy* (10th ed.). Pearson.
Robert Hillman	Voice	Hillman, R. E., Stepp, C. E., Van Stan, J. H., Zañartu, M., & Mehta, D. D. (2020). An updated theoretical framework for vocal hyperfunction. *American Journal of Speech-Language Pathology, 29,* 2254–2260.
Joseph Stemple	Voice	Stemple, J. C., Nelson, R., & Klaben, B. K. (2014). *Clinical voice pathology: Theory and management* (5th ed.). Plural Publishing.

Contributor	Key Areas of Contribution	Exemplary Publications
Frederick Darley Arnold Aronson	Motor Speech Disorders	Darley, F. L., Aronson, A. E., & Brown, J. R. (1969). Differential diagnostic patterns of dysarthria. *Journal of Speech and Hearing Research, 12*, 462–496.
Joseph Duffy	Motor Speech	Duffy, J. R. (2019). *Motor speech disorders: Substrates, differential diagnosis, and management* (4th ed.). Elsevier.
Kathryn Yorkston	Motor Speech	Yorkston, K. M., & Beukelman, D. (1981). Communication efficiency of dysarthric speakers as measured by sentence intelligibility and speaking rate. *Journal of Speech and Hearing Disorders, 46*(4), 374–378.
Mark Ylvisaker	Traumatic Brain Injury	Ylvisaker, M. (1997). *Traumatic brain injury rehabilitation: Children and adolescents* (2nd ed.). Elsevier.
Katherine Bayles	Dementia	Bayles, K., McCullouth, K, & Tomoeda, C. (2020). *Cognitive-communication disorders of MCI and dementia: Definition, assessment, and clinical management* (3rd ed.). Plural Publishing.
James Nation and Dorothy M. Aram	Diagnosis/Treatment	Nation, J. E., & Aram, D.M. (1984). *Diagnosis of speech and language disorders* (2nd ed.). Little Brown, and Co.
Robert West	General Medical Speech-Language Pathology	West, R. (1936). *Disorders of speech*. College Typing Co.
Robert Miller, Michael Crary, Michael Groher	General Medical Speech-Language Pathology	Miller, R., Crary, M., & Groher, M. (1990). *Medical speech-language pathology*. Aspen Publishers.
Lee Ann Golper	General Medical Speech-Language Pathology	Golper, L. A. (1992). *Source book for medical speech pathology. (Clinical Competence Series)*. Cengage Learning.
Joan Arvedson	Pediatric Medical Speech-Language Pathology	Arvedson, J. C., Brodsky, L., & Lefton-Grief, M. A. (2020). *Pediatric feeding and swallowing: Assessment and management* (3rd ed.). Plural Publishing.
Jeri Logemann	Dysphagia	Logemann, J. A. (1983). *Evaluation and treatment of swallowing disorders*. PRO-ED.
Susan Langmore	Dysphagia	Langmore, S. (2001). *Endoscopic evaluation and treatment of swallowing disorders*. Thieme.

continues

Contributor	Key Areas of Contribution	Exemplary Publications
Ann Kummer	Craniofacial	Kummer, A. W. (2020). *Cleft palate and craniofacial conditions: A comprehensive guide to clinical management* (4th ed.). Jones and Bartlett.

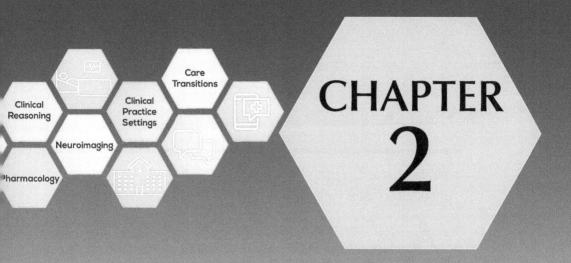

CHAPTER 2

Acute-Care Medical Settings

Bridget J. Perry and Barbara H. Jacobson

Chapter Objectives

Upon completion of this chapter, the reader will be able to:

- Describe the characteristics of an acute care medical setting for speech-language pathology services.
- Discuss common kinds of consultations received by medical speech-language pathologists.
- Explain the primary considerations for assessment and treatment for various types of consultations received by speech-language pathologists in acute-care medical settings.
- Familiarize the reader with the members of the interprofessional team in acute-care medical settings.

Introduction

Role of the Speech-Language Pathologist in Acute Care Settings

*A*cute care is the level of health care where patients seek short-term, active treatment for severe injuries, episodes of illness, urgent medical conditions, or during recovery from surgery. Acute-care settings are complex, fast-paced environments in which patients move in and out of the system quite rapidly. Speech-language pathologists (SLPs) in acute care serve as consultants called upon to diagnose and treat swallowing, cognitive communicative, language, speech, and voice impairments caused by a wide array of medical conditions (Getting Started in Acute Care Hospitals, *n.d.*). SLPs are tasked with providing professional recommendations and short-term treatment plans to physicians and health care provider teams within the hospital as well as to patients and their family and/or caregivers. As such, SLPs working in acute-care hospitals or medical centers are required to have a strong grasp of medical diagnoses, procedures, and terminology as well as a good understanding of the various roles and responsibilities of other health care professionals within the acute-care environment (Getting Started in Acute Care Hospitals, *n.d.*).

About Acute-Care Hospitals

There are several kinds of acute-care hospitals, with the most common being community hospitals. According to the American Hospital Association, in 2020 there were 5,139 community hospitals spread across the United States that range in size from small (6–99 beds) to medium (100–399 beds) to large (more than 400 beds) (AHA Stats, n.d.). In addition to community hospitals, there are approximately 200 federally owned and operated acute-care hospitals across the country as well as a small number of specialty acute-care hospitals, including hospitals whose care is focused in areas including psychiatry, cancer, surgery, cardiology, orthopedics, or otolaryngology, to name a few (AHA Stats, n.d.).

Depending on the size and organization of the hospital, the number and kind of units in each hospital will vary from hospital to hospital. Patients are typically placed on hospital floors/units based on their primary reason for admission and/or their level of complexity or sickness. Generally, acute-care hospitals will include at least one intensive care unit (ICU), where the sickest patients in the hospital are closely monitored and treated. Larger hospitals may have numerous ICUs where patients are grouped by reason for admission to maximize resources and efficiency (Table 2–1). Depending on the kind of provider and the hospital organizations, some providers might see patients only within a specific unit, while other providers might move from unit to unit seeing a wide array of patient populations.

TABLE 2–1	Examples of Specialized Units and Common Diagnoses or Etiologies Treated in Them
Unit	**Diagnosis/Etiology**
Medical	Infection, cancer
Trauma	Car accident, violent accident
Burn	Electrical, gas, fire burn
Thoracic	Lung transplant, lung surgery, lung cancer
Cardiac	Heart attack, heart failure
Cardiac surgery	Heart transplant, heart surgery
Surgical	Gastroesophageal surgery, colorectal surgery
Neurological	Stroke, head trauma
Neurosurgical	Brain surgery

Acute-Care Speech-Language Pathologist Caseload

While SLPs' caseloads can vary widely from hospital to hospital, per the American Speech-Language-Hearing Association (ASHA), older adults (>70 years of age) make up more than 50% of the patients seen in this setting (Getting Started in Acute Care Hospitals, n.d.). The most common primary medical diagnoses seen by SLPs are stroke (35%) followed by respiratory disease (13%) (Getting Started in Acute Care Hospitals, n.d.). In terms of SLP-specific diagnoses, dysphagia is the most common impairment treated and assessed in this setting, distantly followed by impairments in spoken language comprehension, spoken language expression, motor speech, and memory (Getting Started in Acute Care Hospitals, n.d.).

Depending on the hospital size and the speech-language pathology department preferences, SLPs within an acute-care hospital may see patients across populations and units or may specialize within a small number of units within the larger hospital setting. Regardless of where they spend most of their time, SLPs in acute-care hospitals are typically expected to be able to assess, treat, and manage patients across the hospital who present with swallowing, communication, and cognitive–linguistic impairments.

Caseloads for SLPs in acute-care settings can vary widely both between hospitals and from day to day within hospitals. Caseloads may range in size from 6 patients to upward of 20 patients per SLP depending on the size of the department, the complexity of the caseload, and the hospital census. Successful management of a SLP's caseload requires the ability to appropriately prioritize patients according to their care and discharge needs, the ability to be flexible to the ever-evolving needs of both the patient and the hospital, and the ability to work efficiently and effectively within an interdisciplinary team setting. Depending on the hospital size, location, and specialty, members of the interdisciplinary team may vary, but effective collaboration is critical to providing safe, effective, and patient-centered care (Figure 2–1).

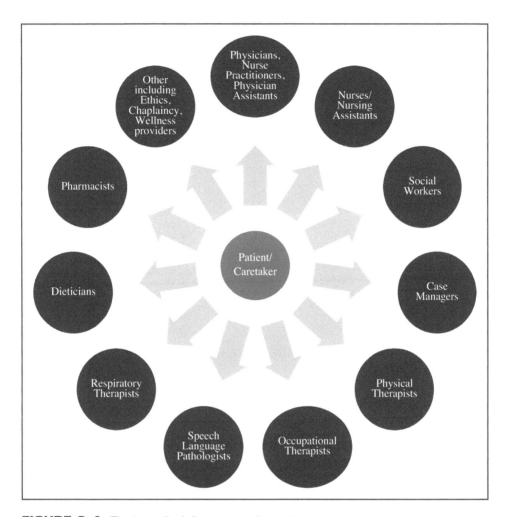

FIGURE 2–1. The interdisciplinary team in acute care.

Speech-Language Pathology Consultations in Acute-Care Settings

A written order or consult is required for an SLP to evaluate and treat an inpatient in the acute-care setting. Referrals for speech-language pathology consultations are requested by a variety of services, most commonly from neurology, medicine, and otolaryngology (Table 2–2). Typically, consults are addressed within 24 to 48 hours of being placed. Due to the nature of acute-care hospital

	Common Speech-Language Pathology Diagnoses and Etiologies Treated by Medical Specialties

TABLE 2–2 Common Speech-Language Pathology Diagnoses and Etiologies Treated by Medical Specialties

Medical Specialty	Common Speech-Language Pathology Diagnoses	Common Etiologies of Diagnoses
Medicine	Swallowing, cognitive communication impairments	Infection, chronic obstructive pulmonary disease (COPD)
Gerontology	Swallowing, cognitive communication impairments	Dementia
Neurology	Swallowing, language, cognitive communication impairments	Stroke, traumatic brain injury, neuromuscular disease, neurodegenerative disease, neuro-oncological disease
Neurosurgery	Swallowing, language, cognitive communication impairments	Stroke, traumatic brain injury, neuro-oncological disease, benign brain lesions, arteriovenous malformations
Otolaryngology	Swallowing, language, cognitive communication impairments	Head and neck cancer
Pulmonology	Swallowing impairments	COPD, cystic fibrosis, pulmonary hypertension, interstitial lung disease, lung cancer
Plastic surgery	Swallowing, communication impairments	Facial surgery, facial reconstruction, burn,
General surgery	Swallowing impairments	Traumatic injury, esophageal surgery, colon surgery, exploratory laparotomy, endocrine surgery, laparoscopic Nissen fundoplication
Gastroenterologists	Swallowing impairments	Esophageal reflux, gastritis, esophageal dysphagia, Barrett's esophagus,
Cardiothoracic surgery	Swallowing, communication impairments	Heart transplant, coronary artery bypass grafting, heart valve repair, aortic aneurysm repair, insertion of ventricular assist device or artificial heart, lung transplant, lobectomy, wedge resection, esophagectomy, gastrectomy
Cardiology	Swallowing impairments	Heart failure, structural heart and valve disease, coronary heart disease
Oncology	Swallowing, language, cognitive communication impairments	Advanced cancers
Palliative Care	Swallowing, language, cognitive communication impairments	Advanced cancers, advanced neurologic disease

settings, at least one SLP is typically present in the hospital 7 days a week during the daytime shift.

The first step to completing a consultation of any kind is a thorough medical chart review. From the medical chart review, it is critical for an acute-care SLP to determine the following:

1. What kind of consultation was placed (swallowing, language, cognitive communicative, etc.)?
2. Why was the consult placed (preemptively, suspected difficulty, observed difficulty, discharge planning purposes)?
3. Why was the patient admitted to the hospital?
4. What is the patient's current mental and respiratory status?
5. How does the patient's current mental and respiratory status compare to the patient's baseline mental and respiratory status?
6. What medical comorbidities (in addition to the reason for hospital) does the patient have?
7. What does the patient's past medical history include?
8. What kinds of evaluations/tests/scans/procedures has the patient had in the past and during the current hospitalization?
9. Does the patient have any allergies?
10. What do the patient's living and social support situations include?
11. Are there are any language, socioeconomic, and/or cultural factors to consider?
12. Are there safety precautions to consider (infection precautions, bed precautions, oral intake status)?

With a thorough understanding of the patient's background, history, and current hospitalization, the SLP should be well-positioned to (a) determine the prioritization of the consult and (b) complete any consultation effectively and efficiently.

Upon completion of a medical chart review and prior to entering a patient's room, SLPs in acute-care settings frequently speak with the nurse charged with managing the patient's care to check in. As things can change quickly in acute-care medical settings, a nurse check-in prior to seeing a patient ensures that the SLP has the most up-to-date information on the patient's status and helps prevent potential safety events and/or errors such as feeding a patient who was recently ordered to have "nothing by mouth" (NPO) for a newly ordered procedure or sitting a patient upright who was recently placed on head-of-bed precautions. With approval from the nursing staff, the SLP will then gather materials needed, take appropriate infection control measures, and see the patient for the appropriate consultation. Initial steps for all SLP consultations can be found in Figure 2–2.

---

1. Identify that you are seeing the correct patient using a minimum of 2 unique identifiers (e.g. Name, Birthday, MRN)

2. Patient-reported history (as able)
    a. History of recent medical events and current hospitalization
    b. History of prior impairment

3. Hemodynamic status
    a. O_2 requirements and O_2 saturation
    b. Respiratory rate
    c. Blood pressure
    d. Stability (need for suctioning, continuous veno-venous hemofiltration (CVVH), hemodialysis (HD), noninvasive ventilation (bilevel positive airway pressure [Bi-PAP], continuous positive airway pressure [CPAP])

4. Cognitive-behavioral assessment
    a. Hearing
    b. Vision
    c. Alertness
    d. Attention
    e. Ability to follow simple commands
    f. Orientation

5. Oral-sensory motor exam
    a. Oral cavity
        i. Oral mucosa appearance
        ii. Dentition
        iii. Secretion management
    b. Face, lip, jaw, and tongue assessment
        i. Symmetry
        ii. Strength
        iii. Range of motion
        iv. Speed
        v. Coordination
        vi. Sensation
        vii. Cranial nerve related findings
    c. Voice/phonation
        i. Volume
        ii. Quality
        iii. Glottal coup
        iv. Cough

FIGURE 2–2. Components of an initial speech-language pathology consultation.

Dysphagia Consultations

Assessment

Dysphagia assessment is the most frequent referral for SLPs in acute-care medical settings. Common reasons for consultation include things such as "nurse observed coughing with/after PO," "difficulty tolerating PO," "concern for aspiration," "difficulty swallowing pills," and "evaluate swallowing safety." The primary goal of a dysphagia assessment is to evaluate the patient's ability to consume oral intake safely and efficiently. Completion of dysphagia assessments is a top priority in acute-care settings, as patients who are suspected of having dysphagia may be restricted from eating, drinking, and/or taking critical medications until seen by an SLP. The initial steps for a dysphagia assessment, including a patient history and oral mechanism examination, can be found in Figure 2–2. Upon completion of an oral mechanism examination, in most cases, a clinical evaluation of swallowing that includes a variety of liquid and solid consistencies is attempted. In some cases, the patient may be deemed unable or unsafe to participate in PO trials during the case history or oral mechanism exam, at which time the assessment is typically deferred to a later date.

Recommendations

Results from the clinical evaluation of swallowing are critical to informing next steps, which may include initiation of an oral diet, performing an instrumental swallowing assessment (videofluoroscopic swallowing study [VFSS] or fiberoptic endoscopic evaluation of swallowing [FEES]) to obtain additional information, or lastly, recommending that the patient be made NPO temporarily. Recommendations made from a swallowing assessment must take several factors into account, including:

- Swallow function: Is there evidence of swallowing impairment?
- Mental status: Can the patient remain awake and alert enough to consume meals?
- Further assessment: Can the patient follow simple commands to participate in further assessment? Does the patient have any restrictions that prevent them from either leaving their room to go to radiology or having an endoscope inserted into their nasal passage? How many exams can the hospital perform on that day?
- Patient/caregiver goals/preferences: What is the patient's/caregiver's goals for their care? Do they understand their

diagnosis? Are they amenable to further testing/modified diet consistencies? Do they understand the risks associated with their impairment and recommendations?

Upon completion of a dysphagia consultation, an initial diet recommendation is made, and a treatment plan is established. For patients who are deemed to be at high risk for aspiration across all liquid and solid consistencies, NPO may be recommended. In this case, the SLP is frequently asked to weigh in on the estimated time they expect the patient to be able to resume some form of PO diet consistently. If the anticipated return to PO is less than 24 to 48 hours and the patient does not have critical medications, the medical team may decide not to place an alternate source for nutrition (i.e., nasogastric tube or percutaneous gastrostomy tube) while they await the patient's return to PO nutrition. If the SLP feels that the patient's return to PO may be more than 48 hours, the medical team may choose to place a nasogastric tube, which would allow the patient to receive nutrition, hydration, and medications while they await improvements in swallowing function. In some cases, the SLP may prognosticate that swallow recovery may not take place during the patient's hospital stay or at all. In those instances, depending on the underlying medical condition causing the dysphagia, the medical team may discuss the surgical placement of a percutaneous gastrostomy (PEG) tube with the patient, family, and/or caregiver. The medical team should incorporate the patient's overall medical prognosis as well as the patient's preferences and goals of care when determining whether a PEG tube is medically appropriate.

Because of the often rapidly changing medical conditions of patients within an acute-care setting, follow-up visits that include reassessments of swallowing function and diet tolerance are frequent. Patients are seen for follow-up and treatment anywhere from two to five times per week depending on their medical condition and need. The SLP is tasked with keeping the medical team informed of initial diet recommendations, changes in diet recommendations, treatment plans, and short-term prognosis as well as with educating patients, family members, and/or caregivers as appropriate.

Treatment

The frequency of dysphagia treatment sessions provided to each patient in acute-care settings can vary widely from 1 to 5 days per week. The frequency of therapy sessions is determined by the SLP as part of the treatment plan and depends on a variety of factors including the patient's level of impairment, ability to participate in therapy sessions, and ability to do therapeutic exercises independently, as well as hospital and speech-language pathology census. Treatment for dysphagia in this setting includes both compensatory strategies (e.g., head turn, chin tuck, etc.) aimed at minimizing or eliminating aspiration and exercises targeting physiologic deficits of the swallowing mechanism (e.g., reduced hyoid elevation and/or excursion, reduced base of tongue to posterior pharyngeal wall contact). Instrumental assessment of swallowing function via VFSS or FEES is needed to identify the primary physiologic deficits contributing to the swallowing impairment so effective compensatory strategies and targeted therapeutic exercises can be prescribed.

Language and Cognitive Communication Consultations

Assessment

For patients admitted with neurologic disease or injury, consultations for language and/or cognitive communication impairments are common. Consultations may be stated as "aphasia," "difficulty with communication," "patient not following commands," and so forth. The primary goals of language and cognitive communication assessments in acute care are to identify cognitive communicative impairments and provide treatment that first targets those impairments that impact patient–provider communication and/or impact a patient's ability to discharge to their home safely. Language and cognitive communication assessments in acute care can vary in form from patient to patient and hospital to hospital depending on the patient's ability to participate, the census of the SLP and the hospital, and the plan for the patient's discharge. In cases where the patient's ability to participate is limited, the SLP caseload is very full, and/or the plan for the patient's discharge is to an acute-care rehabilitation facility where more formal assessment will take place, informal language assessments that provide a general sense of the patient's ability to communicate their care needs with their medical providers may be administered. In other instances, such as when language and/or cognitive communicative impairments may be identified as the primary impairment, more formal assessments may be conducted to ensure the patient is discharged to the appropriate level of care and receives the necessary follow-up. In cases where formal or complete language assessments are warranted, discharge recommendations should call for formal cognitive communicative SLP assessment at the next level of care.

Recommendations

Following either informal or formal assessment, SLP recommendations will typically include a plan for follow-up treatment as well as strategies to help facilitate patient-to-provider communication, including things like "ask simple yes/no questions," "encourage patient to use gestures," "repeat critical messages frequently," and so on. If augmentative and alternative communication (AAC) devices are deemed appropriate, the SLP may provide the patient with no-tech or low-tech solutions such as an eye blink strategy, letter board, or picture board. In some hospitals, more high-tech devices such as iPads may be available for patient use under certain conditions. Some patients have their smartphones with them while in the hospital and can use an app to communicate. Additionally, SLP recommendations will include language indicating what level of care the patient may require upon discharge to best meet their therapeutic needs.

Treatment

The frequency and duration of language and/or cognitive communicative impairments in the acute-care setting vary widely from patient to patient depending on factors such as the patient's ability to participate, the patient's anticipated discharge level of care, the hospital census, and so on. In cases where the patient can participate and the SLP's caseload allows, patients may be seen for therapy as many as five times per week. For patients who have difficulty participating or are expected to discharge to an acute rehabilitation facility where intensive therapy will be provided, treatment may be deferred or limited in the acute setting if the SLP caseload is full. Language and/or cognitive communicative therapeutic activities should be targeted to those deficits that directly impact a patient's ability to communicate their care needs with their medical providers or that limit their ability to discharge home.

Motor Speech Consultations

Assessment

Consultations for motor speech consultations are most frequently placed for patients who are hospitalized for neurologic disease or injury and commonly include phrases such as "garbled speech," "difficulty with speech," and "speech." Assessment of motor speech in acute-care settings is typically subjective. Upon completion of a case history and oral mechanism exam, the SLP should assess the five speech subsystems including respiration, phonation, articulation, resonance, and prosody using syllable-, phrase-, sentence-, and conversational-level tasks and classify the type of motor speech disorder present. The overarching goal of a motor speech assessment in an acute-care setting is to determine the patient's ability to clearly communicate their care needs to their medical providers. In some cases, the motor speech systems can be used to establish or support the medical diagnosis (Duffy, 2018).

Recommendations and Treatment

In this setting, treatment for mild motor speech impairments that do not impact a patient's ability to communicate their care needs is limited. Strategies aimed at minimizing the mild impairment such as using a slow rate of speech, using clear speech, or increasing speech volume may be reviewed with the patient during the initial consultation. The impairment and appropriate strategies are typically noted in the patient's initial consultation note with an indication that the patient needs SLP follow-up at the next level of care or as an outpatient upon discharge depending on the patient's discharge disposition. For those with motor speech impairments that significantly impact a patient's ability to communicate their care needs, the SLP may provide more frequent treatment aimed at improving the patient's communication ability. During treatment, the SLP may review and practice recommended speech strategies and exercises as appropriate or help implement alternative communication techniques including writing or text-to-speech.

Voice Consultations

Assessment

Voice changes are common in patients in acute-care settings and are commonly seen in patients following intubation, cardiothoracic surgery, and neurologic injury. Consults for voice assessments may include statements like "weak voice after intubation/surgery," "wet voice quality," or "scratchy voice." Because impairments in vocal function are a risk factor for aspiration, consults for voice assessments are commonly placed and completed within the context of concern for swallowing impairments. Voice assessments by the SLP in acute care are typically subjective. As first steps of a voice assessment, the SLP typically completes a case history and an oral mechanism examination and asks patients to complete a variety of vocal tasks while listening for impairments in vocal quality, pitch, and loudness. Depending on the hospital, because of noted impairments in swallowing function on clinical assessment and observed changes in vocal function, further evaluation of swallowing function via FEES may be recommended. In addition to providing objective information about swallowing function, FEES allows for the visualization of vocal cord function, and as such, structural changes or impairments of the larynx or vocal cords contributing to voice changes may be identified.

Recommendations

In many cases, changes in voice function during acute-care medical hospitalization are a function of the critical illness and resolve with time. As such, most patients with vocal function changes in this setting do not receive voice therapy or treatment during their hospitalization. In some cases, specifically when vocal fold immobility is suspected and thought to be a major contributor to a patient's inability to swallow safely, the SLP may recommend further laryngeal assessment and/or imaging by the otolaryngology department (ear, nose, and throat [ENT]).

Treatment

Voice therapy in acute-care settings is rare. In some instances, ENT may identify a vocal cord paresis or paralysis that the SLP feels significantly contributes to a patient's dysphagia. In these cases, ENT may recommend a vocal fold injection to help bulk up the immobile vocal fold and reduce the size of the glottal gap through which aspiration may occur. In many cases, however, patients are recommended to pursue voice therapy following discharge from the acute hospitalization should their vocal changes continue to persist.

Hearing Loss Consultations

While common for patients in acute-care medical centers, hearing loss is typically not a result of the hospitalization itself. As such, in acute-care medical settings, the SLP's assessment, recommendations, and treatment of hearing loss are specifically focused on optimizing the patient's ability to hear their medical providers. In some hospitals, SLP consults for hearing loss may be rare, while in others, SLPs may be consulted more frequently. In hospitals where SLP consults for hearing loss are rare, when consulted for other reasons, SLPs may comment on a patient's hearing function and intervene as able/needed. Assessment of hearing in this setting is informal and is typically judged to be "functional" or "subjectively impaired" based on conversational-level tasks. SLPs may provide strategies within their initial consultation and follow-up notes to help medical providers communicate with patients with hearing loss more effectively (i.e., speak loudly, overarticulate, use writing to convey message). Additionally, in some hospital settings, SLPs have access to screening audiometers that can be used to conduct hearing screenings and assistive hearing/listening devices such as voice amplifiers that can be provided to patients for use during their hospitalization. Patients with suspected or identified hearing loss should be referred to audiology upon discharge from the hospital, if they have not been previously seen by an audiologist in the past.

Hospital and Departmental Competency

Within the context of the acute-care setting, competency can be considered to be the ability to carry out a specific clinical task with accuracy (e.g., an SLP is competent to perform an examination of the oral mechanism and its function), or it can refer to the ability to use a comprehensive set of knowledge, skills, and behaviors to perform a range of functions that is consistent with the standards of the profession (e.g., ASHA Certificate of Clinical Competence). The Joint Commission (TJC), the accrediting body for many health care facilities, defines competency as an aggregation of knowledge and skills that are measurable. The clinician must demonstrate competency in specific areas through external review. Competency is integral to providing care to patients that is safe and of high quality.

Competencies should be distinguished from clinical protocols or procedures. Protocols describe the steps for a particular clinical procedure; competencies detail the measurable knowledge and skills required to perform that procedure. Clinical competencies are developed for clinical activities that are fundamental to SLP practice in various settings (e.g., administer an aphasia assessment), have an impact on patient safety (e.g., evaluate swallowing function), or have some inherent risk (e.g., suctioning). TJC does not describe the specific competencies required for health care workers. Instead, they provide the general guidelines that competencies should be developed with consideration of the patient populations, patient disorders and diseases, and equipment and technology used in service delivery to these patients.

Most, if not all, health care settings require that new employees complete a series of "onboarding" trainings that are not specific to any particular health care profession. For example, all new staff will complete training in infection control, including units on standard precautions, bloodborne pathogens, and handing hazardous materials. Many trainings are required by TJC to demonstrate compliance with accreditation standards. These trainings are often required to be completed annually. Some trainings will be online with an assessment component at the end of the presentation. Other trainings may be in person. Cardiopulmonary resuscitation (CPR) training is often completed in person with written and practical components. While these requirements appear routine and unexceptional, they assure that the workforce has the most current information, policies, and procedures to ensure patient safety and good outcomes. See Figure 2–3 for examples of institutional trainings and competencies that may be part of the onboarding process and/or required to maintain compliance.

In contrast, departmental competencies are designed to capture the activities for an SLP that are fundamental to clinical practice, are high risk, and are performed frequently. Newly hired clinicians are assessed on their ability to evaluate and treat patients with a variety of diagnoses and on different hospital units (e.g., a stroke patient in a neurointensive care unit versus one in a general medical unit). Depending on departmental needs, SLPs may initially complete basic competencies and then proceed to competencies that involve more training (e.g., FEES). As noted earlier, a competency is not a protocol. Standardized protocols describe the procedure for completing a particular task. See Appendix 2–A for an example of a clinical protocol for the acute-care setting. Both competencies and protocols ensure that SLPs perform clinical tasks with consistency. This is especially crucial in acute care as a patient may have different SLPs who follow them for assessment (both clinical and instrumental) and treatment.

More often, SLP managers are looking for potential employees to have training in various assessment and treatment modalities. For example, students applying for clinical fellowships may want to complete online training (as a student) in the MBSimP program for the standardized interpretation of modified barium swallow studies. Examples of other training that will be helpful for acute-care practice include the McNeill Dysphagia Therapy Program (MDTP), FEES, and LSVT LOUD or SPEAK OUT!, which are treatment programs for patients with Parkinson's disease. While some employers provide funding for training, clinicians may be responsible for funding their own continuing education activities. Additional training may not result in a higher salary or hourly pay rate; however,

---

Infection Control

       Hand Hygiene

       Standard Precautions

       Contact Precautions

       Isolation Precautions

       Airborne Pathogens

       Bloodborne Pathogens

Radiation Safety

Fire Safety

Hazardous Materials Handling

Workplace Violence

Basic Life Support for Health Care Providers (level above basic CPR)

Alert System

       Rapid Response

       Missing Infant, Child, Adolescent

       Adult Fire

       Active Shooter

       Bomb

       Weather (tornado, severe storm)

FIGURE 2–3. Institutional trainings, competencies, and alerts.

SLPs who pursue advanced training may be able to include this experience in their portfolios as they apply for advancement on a professional career ladder. Figure 2–4 provides a framework for determining the development of selected competencies.

See Appendix 2–B for examples of competencies in the acute-care setting (Videofluoroscopic Swallow Study [VFSS], Flexible Endoscopic Evaluation of Swallowing [FEES], Passy Muir Valve [PMV], Tracheostomy Suctioning, Patient Transfers, Vital Signs Monitoring).

Vital signs are monitored in all patient care units. They are recorded by nursing staff at regular intervals throughout a patient's

Competency Development

Individual Skills		Populations/Settings
Oral mechanism exam		Acute care
History taking		Inpatient rehabilitation
Clinical bedside swallowing exam		Skilled nursing facility
Videoflouroscopic swallow study		Infants
Treatment planning		Elderly adults
FEES		Disease-specific (e.g., ALS)
PMV evaluation		Outpatient clinic

FIGURE 2–4. Framework for achieving competency.

hospital stay. In the ICU, SpO_2 (saturation of peripheral oxygen), respiratory rate (RT), heart rate, heart rhythm, and blood pressure often are monitored continuously. However, patients in certain stepdown units may be periodically monitored depending on their diagnosis and medical status. For the SLP, O_2 saturation, respiratory rate, and heart rate are the most important measures to monitor at bedside. Patients with specific diagnoses (e.g., COPD, heart failure) are at more risk for oxygen desaturation. Vital signs can be indicative of patient distress but should be considered within the context of activities at bedside and patient behavior. For example, SpO_2 measured by pulse oximetry is not necessarily indicative of aspiration during dysphagia assessment at bedside (Colodny, 2004).

The process of attaining competency will vary from facility to facility. One example of a competency verification process (depending on baseline knowledge) for a clinical bedside swallowing evaluation might include a pretest (oral or written), assigned selected readings, observation of 10 procedures, documentation of 20 procedures performed by the certifying clinician, completion of 10 evaluations and documentation (possibly with supervision), determination of inter-rater reliability with other clinicians on standardized sample patients, posttest, and sign-off by the supervising clinician. The criteria for satisfactory completion of any competency will be set by the acute-care division or department. Often, new SLP hires will complete the necessary competencies during the initial probationary period.

Special Populations

Tracheostomies and Mechanical Ventilation

SLPs provide communication and swallowing services to patients who have tracheostomies and are on mechanical ventilation. Ventilator-dependent patients are housed in ICUs. Initially, most patients are intubated with an endotracheal tube (usually orotracheal). Although this interval can vary, patients will receive a tracheostomy tube if it is determined that they require ventilatory support approximately 14 days after intubation. Factors that drive tracheostomy tube placement include diagnosis, progress to weaning from the ventilator, medical status, comorbidities (e.g., premorbid respiratory disease), among others. Approximately 10% of patients are on ventilators with tracheostomies in the United States at any time in an ICU setting (Abril et al., 2021; Mehta et al., 2015; Whitmore et al., 2020). A full description of the protocols and competencies required for working with patients on ventilators is beyond the scope of this chapter; however, SLPs who work in acute-care settings should seek education and training in this area prior to working with this population.

Mechanical ventilation supports breathing function for patients with a wide range of diagnoses. Respiratory failure is central to the reason for intubation; patients may have lung disease, require postoperative respiratory support, have progressive neuromuscular disease (e.g., myasthenia gravis), have spinal cord injury, or be post heart or lung transplant. In an international study of patients with acute respiratory distress syndrome (ARDS), 13% required tracheostomy (Abe et al., 2018). Tracheostomy tube placement (within the context of mechanical ventilation) creates a closed system between the ventilator and the patient so that a prescribed volume of air is delivered efficiently to the lungs at a prescribed rate. Ventilated patients initially will have a cuffed tracheostomy tube that is inflated/deflated using a syringe. Because the tracheostomy tube is placed below the level of the vocal folds, patients are unable to produce voice without some mechanism of diverting exhaled air through the upper airway.

Tracheotomy tubes can be cuffed or uncuffed and are manufactured in various diameters and lengths. The inner and outer diameters of the tubes are marked on the outside flange. Tracheostomy tubes have an inner cannula that is removed for suctioning. After tracheotomy, tube size is selected based on the size of the trachea, airflow needs, and breathing efficiency. A tracheostomy tube size that is larger than 7.0 mm has been associated with laryngeal injury after extubation and worse breathing and voice production outcomes (Shinn et al., 2019). For the evaluation of communication with a one-way valve and/or swallowing, it is ideal for the size of the tracheostomy tube to be smaller than 8.0 mm (outside diameter).

Patients are ready for communication assessment when they can maintain an awake state, follow most commands, and respond to most yes/no questions. Options for speech production for patients with tracheostomy on a ventilator include leak speech, use of a one-way valve (e.g., Passy Muir valve) in-line with the ventilator, and a talking trach. Leak speech is achieved by slowly deflating the cuff of the tracheostomy tube until the patient is able to phonate. The quality of phonation is assessed. For evaluating a one-way valve for communicating, the cuff is deflated, voice production is assessed, and the valve is placed on an adaptor that connects to the tracheostomy tube. The valve is open during the inhalation cycle of the ventilator and then closes on the exhalation phase, shunting airflow through the upper airway and out the nose and mouth. Leak speech and one-way valve in-line use involve modifications of the ventilator settings (discussed later). A talking trach (e.g., Portex Blueline Ultra Suctionaid-BLUSA) is used with an inflated cuff and uses an external air source that provides air for phonation through opening about the level of the cuff. Patients can also be suctioned above the cuff as well.

Patients with tracheostomy and ventilator dependence are at risk for dysphagia. Characteristics of dysphagia include uncoordinated swallow pattern, diminished or absent cough reflex, reduced sensitivity at the level of the larynx, and reduced smell and taste. Secretion management can be particularly challenging (Leder, 2002). Clinical bedside swallowing assessment for patients with tracheostomy tubes on mechanical ventilation is similar to that of any clinical evaluation; patients should be awake and alert and be able to follow directions. While there are some methods for screening for aspiration (e.g., modified Evan's blue dye test), these have low sensitivity and significant rates of false-negative findings (Brodsky et al., 2019). Most patients should be evaluated using instrumental assessment (e.g., FEES or VFSS). For most SLPs, patients are best evaluated at bedside using FEES. The logistics for transporting ventilated patients to a radiology suite are quite difficult, and some suites do not have adequate space for the equipment that accompanies the patient. Instrumental evaluation should be performed with a one-way valve in place.

SLPs will always collaborate with a respiratory therapist (RT) when assessing a tracheostomized and ventilated patient's communication and swallowing. The RT is able to modify the ventilator settings so that appropriate gas exchange is maintained while the cuff is deflated (partially or fully). In general, the following ventilator settings are modified: FiO_2 (percentage of oxygen), PEEP (positive end expiratory pressure), V_t (volume of air delivered by the ventilator), and PIP/PAP (peak airway pressure required to provide the V_t). The RT will also help to monitor for any levels of distress in the patient, including changes in heart rate, SpO_2, respiratory rate, work of breathing, color, and responsiveness. They will modify alarm settings so that the trigger level is increased. The RT will return ventilator settings to pretesting levels after communication and swallowing evaluations are completed. Other members of the team may include nurses, pulmonologists, and otolaryngologists. Increasingly, hospitals are using trach teams composed of an SLP, otolaryngologist, and nurse practitioner or physician's assistant to monitor for opportunities to downsize tracheostomy tubes, encourage evaluations for one-way speaking valves, and provide input into decisions to decannulate (i.e., remove the tracheostomy tube) patients when appropriate.

Intensive Care Unit Delirium

In the acute-care setting, patients may be referred for speech-language pathology evaluation to help determine whether a patient is presenting with dementia or delirium. According to the *Diagnostic and Statistical Manual of Mental Disorders* (*DSM-5*), delirium is considered to be a disturbance in attention that evolves in a short period of time and that cannot be explained by other neurocognitive disorders (American Psychiatric Association, 2013). For the purposes of this discussion, ICU delirium is distinct from similar symptoms that occur due to alcohol withdrawal, abrupt cessation of antipsychotic administration, opioid use, or sleep deprivation. In contrast, dementia develops gradually and is a constellation of symptoms involving memory loss among other cognitive changes as well as psychological findings (e.g., depression, anxiety, agitation). Other terms used instead of delirium include altered mental status, ICU psychosis, acute confusional state, confusion, acute brain syndrome, toxic or metabolic encephalopathy, sundowning, and stupor.

The rates of delirium in the ICU range from 20% to 80%, depending on the study. ICU delirium has been linked to increased morbidity, mortality, longer duration of mechanical ventilation, and increased health care costs. Patients who have a prolonged period of delirium in the ICU are at risk for developing post–intensive care syndrome that includes new or worsening deficits in physical, cognitive, and mental health. Patients who have delirium have five times the rate of self-extubation (Balas et al., 2014).

There are three types of delirium that patients can present with in the ICU. Hypoactive delirium is characterized by lethargy, sedation, and stupor. In contrast, patients with hyperactive delirium demonstrate combativeness, agitation, and restlessness. Patients can also exhibit a mixed form of both hypoactive and hyperactive behaviors. Hypoactive and mixed delirium are the most prevalent types. Agitation and sedation are measured at bedside by the Richmond Agitation–Sedation Scale (RASS) (Sessler et al., 2002) (Figure 2–5). In most health care settings, the RASS is used for

Score	Term	Description
+4	Combative	Overtly combative, violent, immediate danger to staff
+3	Very agitated	Pulls or removes tube(s) or catheter(s); aggressive
+2	Agitated	Frequent nonpurposeful movement, fights ventilator
+1	Restless	Anxious but movements not aggressive or vigorous
0	Alert and calm	
–1	Drowsy	Not fully alert, but has sustained awakening (eye-opening/eye contact) to **voice** (>10 seconds)
–2	Light sedation	Briefly awakens with eye contact to **voice** (<10 seconds)
–3	Moderate sedation	Movement or eye opening to **voice** (but no eye contact)
–4	Deep sedation	No response to voice, but movement or eye opening to **physical** stimulation
–5	Unarousable	No response to voice or **physical** stimulation

Procedure for RASS Assessment

1. Observe patient

   a. Patient is alert, restless, or agitated. (score 0 to +4)

2. If not alert, state patient's name and say to open eyes and look at speaker.

   b. Patient awakens with sustained eye opening and eye contact. (score –1)

   c. Patient awakens with eye opening and eye contact, but not sustained. (score –2)

   d. Patient has any movement in response to voice but no eye contact. (score –3)

3. When no response to verbal stimulation, physically stimulate patient by shaking shoulder and/or rubbing sternum.

   e. Patient has any movement to physical stimulation. (score –4)

   f. Patient has no response to any stimulation. (score –5)

FIGURE 2–5. Richmond Agitation–Sedation Scale (RASS). (Adapted from Sessler et al., 2002; Ely et al., 2003; Virginia Commonwealth University holds the copyright to the Richmond Agitation–Sedation Scale).

most patients; in the ICU, it is particularly useful as a measure of day-to-day changes in behavior. When SLPs are working with patients over time, it is beneficial to review the trend of reported RASS scores and use this data to inform modifications in treatment.

It is recommended that patients with delirium be screened at least once every nursing shift (Devlin et al., 2018). There are several options for delirium screening in the ICU. The Confusion Assessment Method for the ICU (CAM-ICU) is one such tool. When administering the CAM-ICU, the screener reports whether mental status has changed acutely or is fluctuating, notes patient responses to directions requiring attention, records the patient's RASS score, and asks the patient to answer questions (e.g., "will a stone float on water?") and follow commands. If the CAM-ICU indicates delirium is present, then the ABCDEF (A2F) bundle can be activated (Figure 2–6). The A2F bundle is a protocol for early mobilization of a patient and has been shown to improve outcomes in several parameters including mechanical ventilation use, restraint-free care, ICU readmissions, and post-ICU discharge disposition (Pun et al., 2019).

Depending on the health care facility, some SLPs manage the implementation of the A2F bundle. As part of the ICU treatment team, SLPs provide and assist in aspects of the bundle, particularly as they relate to engaging and maintaining patients' attention, encouraging communication, and family education. A systematic review of research on early cognitive intervention in patients with delirium indicated that there may be some demonstrated benefit, especially as it relates to delirium incidence, duration, occurrence, and development (Deemer et al., 2020). Research is ongoing on the

---

Assess, Prevent, and Manage Pain

Both Spontaneous Awakening Trials (SAT) and Spontaneous Breathing Trials (SBT)

Choice of Analgesia and Sedation

Delirium: Assess, Prevent, and Manage

Early Mobility and Exercise

Family Engagement and Empowerment

FIGURE 2–6. ABCDEF bundle. (Adapted from Devlin et al., 2018.)

impact of early intervention in ICU delirium. The Critical Illness, Brain Dysfunction, and Survivorship Center maintains a website that provides resources for providers who work with ICU patients and for patients and their caregivers (https://www.icudelirium.org).

Burns

Due to the complexity of major acute burn injuries, patients who have experienced a major acute burn injury require specialized care. As such, these patients are frequently taken to a major acute-care center following their injury to receive care. SLPs in these kinds of medical centers play an important role in the care of patients with burn injuries because of the nature of the injury itself and the nature of the treatment these kinds of injuries require.

Depending on the severity and location of the burn injury, the SLP's role will vary in scope and frequency. The extent of burn injury is commonly described using the percentage of total body surface area (%TBSA) involved in the burn injury. The burn severity rating takes into account %TBSA, depth of injury, location of burn, age, presence or absence of smoke inhalation injury, extent and severity of other co-occurring injuries/conditions/treatments, and delay in resuscitation (*Burn Triage and Treatment—Thermal Injuries—CHEMM*, n.d.). Many patients with severe burn injuries require prolonged hospital stays lasting numerous months, undergo multiple surgeries, require prolonged ventilator support necessitating tracheostomy tube placement, and require alternate sources of nutrition via either NG tube or PEG.

The role of the SLP in this population includes the assessment and management of dysphagia, communication/voice, and in some cases treatment to aid in the prevention of orofacial contracture formation (Rumbach et al., 2016). Nutritional support is of great importance in the management of patients with severe burns (Clark et al., 2017). Due to this injury, burn patients require substantial increases in caloric intake to support life. As such, dysphagia management is the top priority; however, many of these patients will require supplemental nutrition via NGT or PEG regardless of their ability to swallow. Due to the need for frequent surgery and heavy sedation during burn care, it can be a significant challenge for patients with severe burns to meet their nutritional needs via oral intake alone.

In addition to dysphagia management and treatment, because many patients with severe burn injuries will require ventilation support along with tracheostomy placement, depending on the hospital, assisting these patients with communication is an important role of the SLP. The primary goal of communication management in this setting is allowing the patient to express their care needs. Depending on the presence and severity of coexisting injuries that may impact communication, need for sedation, and the presence/absence of delirium, techniques for managing communication may vary widely. For patients who are awake, alert, and oriented but voiceless because of the tracheostomy, the SLP may provide patients with alternate means of communication including writing and/or text to speak as well as work alone or alongside respiratory therapists to help patients achieve voicing by assisting with speaking valve placement and tolerance.

Last, for patients with facial burns, SLPs may provide targeted rehabilitation (including massage, stretching, and splinting) to help prevent contracture formation of orofacial structures. These techniques may be unfamiliar to many SLPs, so training in these areas frequently takes place on the job or during specialized courses, as needed. Additionally, interdisciplinary colleagues, including occupational and physical therapists, may have specialized training in this area as well and provide orofacial contracture rehabilitation to this population. Frequent communication and teamwork within the interdisciplinary burn care team are critical for optimizing patient outcomes.

Palliative Care and Hospice

In the acute-care setting, it is common for SLPs to work with patients who have previously or recently received a terminal diagnosis. While sometimes used interchangeably, palliative care and hospice are two distinct kinds of medical care: palliative care is focused on the management of symptoms from disease or treatment of disease at any stage of a serious illness, and hospice is focused specifically on symptom management in the last 6 months of a terminal illness (*What Are Palliative Care and Hospice Care?*, n.d.). Typically, palliative care teams work in conjunction with primary medical teams, while hospice teams take over the medical management of patients in the final stages of their disease (*What Are Palliative Care and Hospice Care?*, n.d.).

Dysphagia assessment and management is the most common reason for SLP consultation in this population. Unlike other patient populations, in which the primary objective of dysphagia management is to prevent aspiration, for patients receiving palliative care and particularly hospice care, the primary objective of dysphagia management is focused on maximizing eating-related quality of life and minimizing patient discomfort with oral intake. SLPs should play an integral role in the team decision-making process surrounding alternate nutrition for patients with life-limiting illness who are diagnosed with dysphagia. Even though aspiration prevention is not the primary goal of dysphagia management in this population, instrumental swallowing assessments may still be valuable in improving the patient's, SLP's, and medical team's understanding of the risks of oral intake.

In this setting, it is critical for SLPs to understand where the patient is in their course of illness, what the prognosis is for the patient in the short term from a medical perspective, and what the long-term prognosis for swallowing recovery may be. Patients receiving palliative care may be admitted to an acute-care setting somewhat early in their disease process for an acute medical issue that is expected to resolve. As such, conservative management of dysphagia may be warranted. In contrast, a hospice patient may be admitted to the hospital with an acute infection from which they are unlikely to recover. While SLP diet recommendations should always incorporate patient and caregiver preferences, patient and caregiver preferences should take center stage, particularly in circumstances when a patient is not expected to improve from a medical perspective, despite what the SLP may think is safest from a clinical perspective.

Communication facilitation can also be an important role of the SLP in the care of patients who are nearing the end of life. For patients who lose the ability to communicate at the end of life, SLPs may create and/or recommend low-tech AAC devices that allow patients to communicate simple or complex care needs as they are able. SLPs may train caregivers/family members in the use of AAC devices or provide recommendations for how to maximize the communication ability of their loved one.

Cardiothoracic (Heart/Lung) Transplant

While not all acute-care hospitals perform cardiothoracic transplantation, in the major medical centers that do, SLPs serve as an integral part of the care team. As a result of critical illness myopathy, extended intubation, respiratory compromise, and/or nerve damage that can occur during or after surgery, dysphagia is common in this population (Black et al., 2020). Dysphagia following cardiothoracic transplantation has been found to increase hospital length of stay and negatively impact survival (Atkins et al., 2007, 2010), and as such, the primary role of the SLP in this population is the assessment and management of dysphagia with goals of care centered around preventing aspiration. For those patients who require prolonged ventilation and/or tracheostomy placement, SLPs may also play a role in the management of speaking valves for these patients.

For the most part, patients who undergo cardiothoracic transplantation require instrumental swallowing evaluation via VFSS or FEES to advance to oral diets, as silent aspiration is common in this population. Prior to conducting an instrumental assessment, typically the SLP will evaluate the patient at bedside for their readiness to participate. The SLP should assess the patient's respiratory status, mental status, alertness, ability to manage secretions, and ability to travel off the floor or tolerate an endoscope in the nasal cavity prior to scheduling the instrumental assessment. In some cases, it may be several days or even weeks before a patient is able to safely participate in an instrumental exam, during which time the patient typically remains NPO and receives nutrition through either an NGT or PEG.

Once a patient participates in an instrumental swallowing assessment, recommendations for modified diets, compensatory strategies, and targeted therapeutic exercises can be made. Patients who present with dysphagia on instrumental assessment are typically seen for swallowing therapy several times a week during which time the SLP also monitors for any signs of diet intolerance or swallowing improvement. Diet advancements in this population typically require repeated instrumental assessments to ensure safety.

Planning for Discharge

The length of stay (LOS) in acute-care hospitals serves as an important indicator of hospital management efficiency. In 2016, the Healthcare Cost and Utilization Project estimated the average length of hospital stay in an acute-care hospital to be 4.6 days (*Overview of U.S. Hospital Stays in 2016: Variation by Geographic Region #246*, n.d.). Hospital LOS can vary widely from patient to patient depending on factors including but not limited to the reason for admission, treating physician, age, insurance, and social support. Additionally, average LOS has been found to vary from state to state, hospital to hospital, and physician to physician for a variety of reasons ranging from differences in patient demographics, differences in physician preferences, and differences in diagnoses seen, to differences in hospital management.

Increases in hospital LOS have been found to increase patients' risk of infection, reduce quality of life, and create hospital capacity constraints that have been associated with poor patient outcomes, including increased mortality (Siddique et al., 2021). Conversely, premature discharge has also been associated with adverse outcomes, including increased readmission and increased mortality (Siddique et al., 2021). As such, unlike other settings where SLPs provide care, in acute care, LOS is an important factor driving care for all hospital care providers as they seek to provide optimal care, including safe discharge and avoiding prolonged hospital stays. For this reason, SLPs working in acute-care settings often begin to consider a patient's potential discharge needs and post-hospital follow-up plan often as early as during the initial assessment. Additionally, discharge considerations are often a driving factor in how SLPs prioritize assessment and treatment plans for patients on their caseload.

Like many aspects of patient care in the acute setting, discharge recommendations require an interdisciplinary team effort. Depending on a patient's medical condition, preferences, living situation, and home support, following an acute-care hospital stay, patients may be discharged to an acute rehabilitation hospital, long-term acute care hospital, skilled nursing facility, or their home with or without in-home or outpatient therapy. While the primary medical team is responsible for making official discharge recommendations, their decision is made with input from physical therapy, occupational therapy, speech-language pathology, and case management. Physical therapist, occupational therapist, and SLP services are responsible for providing the medical team with the critical information they need to understand the patients' abilities to ambulate, perform essential activities of daily living, communicate, and safely maintain nutrition. Case managers provide background on any social and financial considerations that may impact discharge destination. Once the appropriate level of care is determined, case managers help facilitate patient discharge to the optimal destination at the necessary level of care.

Patient and Caregiver Education and Training

From the time of the initial consultation through the time of discharge, the SLP is responsible for providing each patient and their caregiver or caregivers with education about the patient's diagnosis, prognosis, treatment, and progress. Patients and caregivers have various levels of background knowledge and experience regarding SLP diagnoses, and as such, when providing education, SLPs should use simple language, provide thorough explanations and visual demonstrations, and continuously assess patient/caregiver understanding over the course of the hospitalization. Effective patient and caregiver education is particularly important for patients who are discharged to their home, as they will have less frequent follow-up and oversight than those discharging to a different medical facility. Patients being discharged to their home should be provided with verbal and written instructions for any recommended treatments as well as for their follow-up plan. For patients being discharged to other medical facilities, the SLP should provide a discharge report including a detailed description of any assessments, recommendations, and treatments that took place over the course of the hospitalization to the primary medical team or case manager. This report should be included with the discharge documentation from the medical team and other supporting providers that is sent from the acute-care hospital to the next level of care.

Workflows and Routines

Documentation

In all speech-language pathology practice, timely and accurate documentation is critical for interprofessional communication, for complying with regulatory requirements, and for reimbursement. In the hospital setting, written evaluations and treatment notes and other documented communications allow for coordinated care, meet CMS and private insurer standards, and subsequently, drive billing and reimbursement. During the accreditation process, one of the critical issues that TJC reviews is the ability of health care systems to accurately relay all aspects of evaluation and treatment during a patient's "episode of care" or hospitalization among members of the care team. Clear and specific documentation reduces the risk of medical and surgical errors and allows each health care provider to understand a particular patient's hospital course.

All hospitals have policies that outline the required components of documentation. For acute care, notes (evaluation and progress notes) are typically required to be entered into the electronic medical record (EMR) within 24 hours. Medical record audits are performed on all documentation, and providers are notified and can be officially reprimanded if documentation is not completed within the prescribed time frame. There is also prescribed content. A typical evaluation note might include the following:

- History of admission: This is a description of the events that led up to the admission to the hospital. Often, emergency department observations and findings and diagnostic tests are reported. This is the beginning of the patient's "story."

■ Reason for referral to speech-language pathology: This is a statement of the medical diagnosis and referral question to be answered by this assessment.

■ Medical and surgical history: Details regarding known medical history and past surgical procedures may be populated automatically into the note.

■ Subjective: The SLP provides observations of the patient's general behavior, descriptions of the caregivers who are present, and environmental considerations. For example, the patient's level of alertness, responsiveness to general questions, and other findings are included in this section.

■ Objective: The SLP documents testing and results, including all cognitive, language, speech, voice, and swallowing domains that are required to answer the referral question (e.g., auditory comprehension, speech production).

■ Assessment: This is a statement of the specific communication and/or swallowing diagnosis and degree of impairment (mild, moderate, severe), the underlying medical diagnosis, and general comments about other important factors that might impact the patient's response to treatment in the hospital as well as discharge recommendations (e.g., social and psychological conditions).

■ Education: It is important to provide a description of oral and written education about the communication/swallowing diagnosis (its severity, expected course), recommendations for treatment while the patient is in the hospital and after discharge, and resources that might help the patient and caregiver understand the impact of the disorder. The SLP provides strategies for enhancing communication and/or swallowing for the caregiver. Clinicians also include a statement about patient/caregiver understanding of this information.

■ Plan/Recommendations: Includes a recommendation for the next level of care after discharge (e.g., home health care, skilled nursing facility, outpatient clinic). In some instances, specific recommendations for a therapy program might be included. In the acute-care setting, treatment sessions may be sporadic and are related to the patient's medical status and ability to participate in active behavioral treatment.

■ Goals: In this section, the clinician inserts an initial long-term goal (e.g., speech/language/cognitive skills to functional limits) and short-term goals (e.g., patient will follow one-step commands in 80% of trials).

▪ Prognosis: This is a statement about the potential response to treatment moving forward (e.g., "Rehabilitation potential is fair for the previously stated goals and expected medical course"). This adds to the information that the team uses to plan discharge.

Most hospitals use EMRs that include documentation templates. This includes all the requirements noted earlier. Frequently used phrases can be selected to populate the various sections of the note. For example, if the Ranchos Los Amigos Scale is administered, part of the objective section might look like this:

Abilities consistent with Rancho 2

▪ Demonstrates generalized reflex response to painful stimuli: Consistently present
Comment: Withdraws left upper extremity to nail bed pressure

▪ Responds to repeated auditory stimuli with increased or decreased activity: Consistently present
Comment: Moves feet and left hand

▪ Responds to external stimuli with generalized physiological changes: Consistently present

▪ Responds to external stimuli with gross body movement and/ or not purposeful vocalization: Consistently present

▪ Responds to all stimuli, may be same regardless of type and location of stimulation: Consistently present

In many documentation systems, the SLP has the option to use customized "smart phrases" that are available in assessment and recommendations sections. The clinician "free texts" additional information that clarifies or expands behavioral observations.

The SLP writes progress notes every time there is a patient encounter and a service (e.g., therapy) is provided. Unlike outpatient settings, in acute care this might be a reevaluation of critical aspects of their communication or swallowing as the patient's condition evolves through their hospital stay. Progress notes follow the standard SOAP (subjective, objective, assessment, plan) format and may be templated like evaluations. As in other settings, progress notes that document treatment summarize therapy activities and progress toward specific goals.

Discharge notes are written as the patient leaves the hospital for the next level of care. Ideally, clinicians who are working with the patient in their next care setting will receive these notes; this can depend on whether there is a relationship between the hospital and that facility. In the current health care environment, it can be difficult to communicate between facilities, and SLPs are often dependent on the discharge planner to bundle documentation for transfer. The components of a discharge note include history of admission, initial communication and medical diagnosis, goals and objectives, course of treatment, diagnosis on discharge, and recommendations for further evaluations and/or treatment.

In an environment where a patient's medical status can fluctuate frequently, speech-language pathology documentation provides a valuable track of communication and swallowing function. Ultimately, the goal of well-written and timely documentation is to add to the patient's medical record pertaining to a particular hospital stay and to provide critical information to the care team. Poor documentation has the potential to result in lack of continuity in care, diminished patient safety, overuse of resources and testing, and reduced patient and caregiver satisfaction (Vermeir et al., 2015). Adhering to best practices in documentation improves team functioning overall and better patient outcomes.

In April 2021, the Office of the National Coordinator for Health Information Technology (ONC) Final Rule went into effect. This is part of the implementation of the 21st Century Cures Act (Cures Act), which was signed into law in 2016. The rule requires health care providers to give patients secure access (free of charge) to their electronic health information through their health patient portal. This health information should also be able to be downloaded onto smartphone applications (Open Notes, n.d.). Specifically, patients have access to the following types of records:

- Consultation notes (SLP evaluation)
- Discharge summary notes (SLP discharge summary)
- History and physical notes
- Imaging narratives
- Laboratory report narratives
- Pathology report narratives
- Procedure notes (SLP FEES, VFSS reports)
- Progress notes (SLP treatment notes)

Final implementation is required by 2023. This regulation was designed, among several reasons, to provide more transparency and increased accuracy in communications between patients and health care providers. Ultimately, this will have the intended effect of improving the quality of care.

As a consequence of this rule, it is incumbent upon SLPs to attend to the content, clarity, and language in their documentation. While SLPs will continue to use abbreviations in their medical record entries, the narrative of any evaluation, treatment session, or procedure note should be written logically and clearly. SLPs should avoid any language that is subjective (e.g., "this pleasant, elderly man was seen today for a swallowing evaluation"). They should describe behavior observed during the session accurately and objectively. Taking the perspective of the patient while documenting encounters that will appear in the EHR facilitates writing notes that provide an accurate record of the session.

Billing and Reimbursement

In acute care, SLPs bill for their services just as they do in any other setting. In an outpatient facility, clinicians bill a procedure code (CPT code) that describes the service. For example, when an SLP performs a clinical swallowing evaluation, the CPT code 92610—"Evaluation of oral and pharyngeal swallowing function"—is billed. Clinicians must also enter diagnostic codes (ICD-10 codes); the first code corresponds to the communication or swallowing diagnosis as determined by the SLP, and the second code relates to the medical diagnosis that is the "cause" of the communication/swallowing condition. In the outpatient example presented earlier, the primary diagnostic ICD-10 code—R13.12 (dysphagia, oropharyngeal phase) and the secondary ICD-10 code—I63.9 (stroke) are entered along with the CPT code. A bill is then sent to the insurer for reimbursement. In hospital settings, SLPs also enter procedure codes and diagnostic codes when they submit charges. However, instead of being sent to the insurer directly, the charges become part of a bundle of charges that corresponds to the patient's hospitalization. Every health care provider that evaluates and treats a patient and submits a charge contributes to the bundled care charge. For hospital billing, Medicare and some health insurance companies classify expected hospitalization costs based on Diagnostic Related Groups (DRGs). Each DRG (e.g., stroke) has a predetermined reimbursement rate with modifications based on diagnostic severity, age, gender, and procedures related to the patient and the hospital stay. If the hospital spends less than the expected DRG payment for a particular diagnosis for a patient, it makes a profit. If it spends more than the DRG payment, then it incurs a loss. The hospital is incentivized to provide quality care that reduces the chance of complications and prepares the patient for discharge as soon as they are ready.

In 2012, the Centers for Medicare and Medicaid Services (CMS) added another program that provides penalties for hospital readmissions within 30 days after discharge for certain diagnoses. If a patient returns to the hospital in that time frame, then payments for DRGs are reduced. One of the targeted diagnoses is pneumonia. This is one of the most common reasons for referral to the speech-language pathology service. SLPs can play a critical role in the prevention of readmission for patients with pneumonia. Assuring appropriate evaluation for dysphagia and clear discharge recommendations for diet, compensatory swallowing maneuvers, and swallowing treatment can help prevent readmission. On many hospital units, a series of metrics (number of falls, infection rates) also includes episodes of pneumonia as a quality-of-care measure.

Speech-language pathology departments within a medical center will not see actual revenue for services provided in the hospital. However, they do receive credit in the form of procedure counts; evaluation and treatment visits are accounted for in their budgets. This can impact the number of SLPs that work in acute care. Since acute-care SLPs do not generate "real" dollars for the hospital, this can require SLPs to advocate for their services as necessary for quality patient care, patient satisfaction, and prevention of readmissions. Overall, speech-language pathology services can reduce the length of stay for patients, which benefits the hospital's financial health.

Safety and Infection Control

As providers in a health-care system, SLPs must adhere to a set of practices that ensure patient as well as clinician safety. While SLPs follow safety and infection control measures in every practice setting, there can be more risk associated with SLP practice in the hospital. Patients can be admitted with infectious disease or develop an infection during their hospital stay. Visitors may carry airborne disease into the hospital. The Centers for Disease Control and Prevention (CDC) have developed guidelines for providers to ensure that they are protected and that patients and caregivers are protected (CDC, n.d.).

Safety

"Safety" refers to principles and practices that minimize physical harm to patients and staff. These include patient transfers, protection from harmful substances (e.g., chemicals), and general work-place safety. Part of the orientation process to a hospital setting includes training modules on how to transfer a patient from a lying to a sitting position, transferring a patient from bed to chair, how to handle chemicals safely (use and disposal), and how to respond to hospital-wide alerts (fire, patient cardiac/respiratory arrests, patient leaving floor without permission).

When clinicians transfer patients, they are at risk of injury if they do not practice appropriate technique. According to the National Institute for Occupational Safety and Health, the rate of musculoskeletal injury for health care workers is roughly double that of all industries combined (68 per 10,000 versus 33 per 10,000 workers) (National Institute for Occupational Safety and Health, n.d.). Providers receive instruction in movement based on principles of "ergonomics" or the practice of designing specific tasks that are adapted to the worker's movement. There are guidelines for the amount of weight to be handled by one person as well as specific processes for provider posture and movement. In the hospital, staff work as a team, and SLPs may be asked to help with patient transfers (e.g., from bed to chair). SLPs will adjust a patient's bed position to assure appropriate posture for clinical and instrumental swallowing assessments. Prior to moving a patient, SLPs must always receive the permission of the patient's nurse, as there may be restrictions on head-of-bed elevation for certain patients.

SLPs can be exposed to hazardous chemicals during endoscope processing. As noted earlier, endoscopes require sterilization or high-level disinfection (HLD) depending on a hospital's infection control policy. There are several chemical products that can be used for HLD. These products are designed to remove bacteria and viruses such as HIV and hepatitis A, B, and C, among others, to prevent infection between patients. Each manufacturer or distributor of these products must provide a Safety Data Sheet (SDS, formerly called a Material Safety Data Sheet [MSDS]) for every hazardous chemical. The SDS is required by the Occupational Safety and Health Administration to be written in a user-friendly format. The SDS contains information including the properties of each chemical; the physical, health, and environmental health hazards; ways to protect the user; and safety precautions for handling, storing, and transporting the particular chemical. The SDS is posted in the area where the chemical is used. In speech-language pathology, clinicians will usually come into contact with chemicals during HLD. One example of such a chemical is Revital-Ox RESERT. This is used for processing endoscopes used for FEES, nasoendoscopy, and laryngovideostroboscopy. This chemical does not require special ventilation for its use, but some chemicals used in HLD do.

Protocols for responses to hospital-wide alerts are mandated by TJC. For most hospitals, employees must undergo annual training after their initial training to remain in compliance. See Alert System in Figure 2–3 for examples of alerts that may be broadcasted over the hospital PA system. Many clinicians carry "badge buddies" that are cards attached to an ID badge for ready reference for alerts, fire safety, and hospital police notifications.

Infection Control

The term *infection control* comprises several components. These include standard precautions (formerly "universal precautions") and transmission-based precautions. Standard precautions include hand hygiene, regular personal protective equipment (PPE) use, disinfection and sterilization of equipment, and needle safety and sharps precautions. SLPs typically do not handle needles; however, they may be required to undergo training for the purposes of annual compliance. Transmission-based precautions refer to measures taken when a patient has an infection that requires additional care to prevent transmission to another person.

On hospital units, clinicians perform hand hygiene by using an alcohol-based foam or solution to cover the hands thoroughly. This must be performed on entering and leaving a patient's room, whether or not gloves are worn. Gloves, as a form of PPE, should be (in most instances) worn in patients' rooms, and hand hygiene is performed before putting on gloves as well as after removing them. For patients with certain infections, handwashing with soap and water is performed before leaving their room in lieu of using foam. Assiduous hand hygiene has been demonstrated to reduce the incidence of hospital-acquired infections. Some hospitals have limitations on fingernail length and artificial fingernails to reduce the risk of infection transmission.

A full discussion of endoscope disinfection/sterilization is beyond the scope of this chapter. SLPs use guidance from their Environment of Care (EOC) team to develop appropriate protocols and procedures for disinfection. Because of safety issues related to solutions used for HLD, SLPs who perform this task must undergo training. At times, equipment (e.g., FEES cart with endoscope and computer) is brought into a patient's room where some level of precautions are in place. In that instance, the cart, computer, and any other nondisposable materials are cleaned consistent with EOC guidelines in addition to the endoscope.

Transmission precautions include contact precautions, droplet precautions, and airborne precautions. Expanded PPE use (beyond gloves) is required to work with patients with certain infections. This includes patients with COVID-19, tuberculosis, methicillin-resistant *Staphylococcus aureus* (MRSA), *Clostridioides difficile* (*C. diff*). The type of PPE to be used with a patient should be posted on the patient's door along with the type of precaution. Health care workers may need to wear a surgical or N95 mask, disposable gown, and eye protection (goggles or face shield). If an N95 mask or respirator is used, then the clinician must have completed a fit test. Fit tests ensure that the respirator is comfortable and provides enough seal to prevent entry of infectious material. During a fit test, the SLP will wear a mask/respirator with a plastic hood over the head. A chemical is sprayed (usually a saccharin solution) under the hood, and several tasks are completed (e.g., breathing, speaking, head turning). If the SLP is unable to detect the substance by smell or taste, then the seal is adequate for protection.

For contact precautions, SLPs typically wear a gown and gloves. Contact precautions are indicated for patients with MRSA and *C. diff*. There is a protocol for donning and removing PPE for contact precautions, and there is a designated receptacle (usually red-bagged) for disposal. For droplet precautions, a surgical mask is added to basic PPE. Droplet precautions are indicated for infectious respiratory diseases such as influenza. Finally, airborne precautions require the use of gloves, gown, N95 (or other) respirator, and potentially, face shield. Infections such as COVID-19 and tuberculosis produce aerosols with coughing, sneezing, and talking and can be transmitted to health care workers without protection. SLPs perform several procedures that have the potential to trigger aerosol production (aerosol-generating procedures or AGPs), such as FEES and clinical swallowing evaluation and treatment. Full PPE is always recommended.

Conclusion

Clinical work in acute-care settings is fast-paced, challenging, and requires SLPs to have a strong grasp of medical diagnoses, procedures, and terminology. SLPs working in these settings assess and treat a wide variety of patient populations and serve as critical members of the interdisciplinary care team who are responsible for providing direct patient care as well as educating patients, caregivers, and interdisciplinary team members on patient diagnoses, prognoses, treatment plans, and discharge needs.

References

Abe, T., Madotto, F., Pham, T., Nagata, I., Uchida, M., Tamiya, N., . . . LUNG-SAFE Investigators and the ESICM Trials Group. (2018). Epidemiology and patterns of tracheostomy practice in patients with acute respiratory distress syndrome in ICUs across 50 countries. *Critical Care* (London, UK), *22*(1), 195. https://doi.org/10.1186/s13054-018-2126-6

Abril, M. K., Berkowitz, D. M., Chen, Y., Waller, L. A., Martin, G. S., & Kempker, J. A. (2021). The epidemiology of adult tracheostomy in the United States 2002–2017: A serial cross-sectional study. *Critical Care Explorations, 3*, e0523. https://doi.org/10.1097/CCE.0000000000000523

AHA Stats. (n.d.). https://guide.prod.iam.aha.org/stats/us-hospitals

American Psychiatric Association. (2013). *Diagnostic and statistical manual of mental disorders* (5th ed.).

Atkins, B. Z., Petersen, R. P., Daneshmand, M. A., Turek, J. W., Lin, S. S., & Davis, R. D. (2010). Impact of oropharyngeal dysphagia on long-term outcomes of lung transplantation. *Annals of Thoracic Surgery, 90*(5), 1622–1628. https://doi.org/10.1016/j.athoracsur.2010.06.089

Atkins, B. Z., Trachtenberg, M. S., Prince-Petersen, R., Vess, G., Bush, E. L., Balsara, K. R., . . . Davis, R. D. (2007). Assessing oropharyngeal dysphagia after lung transplantation: Altered swallowing mechanisms and increased morbidity. *Journal of Heart and Lung Transplantation, 26*(11), 1144–1148. https://doi.org/10.1016/j.healun.2007.07.038

Balas, M. C., Vasilevskis, E. E., Olsen, K. M., Schmid, K. K., Shostrom, V., Cohen, M. Z., . . . Burke, W. J. (2014). Effectiveness and safety of the awakening and breathing coordination, delirium monitoring/management, and early exercise/mobility (ABCDE) bundle. *Critical Care Medicine, 42*, 1024–1036.

Black, R., McCabe, P., Glanville, A., Bogaardt, H., MacDonald, P., & Madill, C. (2020). Oropharyngeal dysphagia and laryngeal dysfunction after lung and heart transplantation: A systematic review. *Disability and Rehabilitation, 42*(15), 2083–2092. https://doi.org/10.1080/09638288.2018.1552326

Brodsky, M. B., Mayfield, E. B., & Gross, R. D. (2019). Clinical decision making in the ICU: Dysphagia screening, assessment, and treatment. *Seminars in Speech and Language, 40*, 170–187. https://doi.org/10.1055/s-0039-1688980

Burn Triage and Treatment—Thermal Injuries—CHEMM. (n.d.). https://chemm.hhs.gov/burns.htm

Centers for Disease Control and Prevention. (n.d.). *Isolation precautions.* https://www.cdc.gov/infectioncontrol/guidelines/isolation/index.html

Clark, A., Imran, J., Madni, T., & Wolf, S. E. (2017). Nutrition and metabolism in burn patients. *Burns & Trauma, 5*(1), 11. https://doi.org/10.1186/s41038-017-0076-x

Colodny, N. (2004). Pulse oximetry as an indicator for aspiration: The state of the art. *Perspectives in Swallowing and Swallowing Disorders, 13*, 9–13. https://doi.org/10.1044/sasd13.4.9

Deemer, K., Zjadewicz, K., Fiest, K., Oviatt, S., Parsons, M., Myhre, B., & Posadas-Calleja, J. (2020). Effect of early cognitive interventions on delirium in critically ill patients: A systematic review. Effet des interventions cognitives précoces sur le delirium chez les patients en état critique : Une revue systématique. *Canadian Journal of Anaesthesia, 67*(8), 1016–1034. https://doi.org/10.1007/s12630-020-01670-z

Devlin, J. W., Skrobik, Y., Gélinas, C., Needham, D. M., Slooter. A. J. C., Pandharipande, P. P., . . . Alhazzani, W. (2018). Clinical practice guidelines for the prevention and management of pain, agitation/sedation, delirium, immobility, and sleep disruption in adult patients in the ICU. *Critical Care Medicine, 46*, e825–e873. https://doi.org/10.1097/CCM.0000000000003299

Duffy, J. R. (2018, December 29). Motor speech disorders and the diagnosis of neurologic disease (world) [Review article]. *The ASHA Leader.* https://doi.org/10.1044/leader.FTR1.13162008.10

Ely, E. W., Truman, B., Shintani, A., Thomason, J. W. W., Wheeler, A. P., Gordon, S., . . . Bernard, G. R. (2003). Monitoring sedation status over time in ICU patients: The reliability and validity of the Richmond Agitation Sedation Scale (RASS). *Journal of the American Medical Association, 289*, 2983–2991. https://doi.org/10.1001/jama.289.22.2983

Getting Started in Acute Care Hospitals. (n.d.). American Speech-Language-Hearing Association. https://www.asha.org/slp/healthcare/start_acute_care/

Leder, S. B. (2002). Incidence and type of aspiration in acute care patients requiring mechanical ventilation via a new tracheotomy. *Chest, 122*, 1721–1726.

Mehta, A. B., Syeda, S. N., Bajpayee, L., Cooke, C. R., Walkey, A. J., & Wiener, R. S. (2015). Trends in tracheostomy for mechanically ventilated patients in the United States, 1993–2012. *American Journal of Respiratory and Critical Care Medicine, 192*, 446–454. https://doi.org/10.1164/rccm.201502-0239OC

National Institute for Occupational Safety and Health. (n.d.). *Safe patient handling and mobility.* https://www.cdc.gov/niosh/topics/safepatient/default.html#Patient%20Handling%20Ergonomics

Open Notes. (n.d.). Federal Rules Mandating Open Notes. https://www.opennotes.org/onc-federal-rule/

Overview of U.S. Hospital Stays in 2016: Variation by Geographic Region #246. (n.d.). https://www.hcup-us.ahrq.gov/reports/statbriefs/sb246-Geographic-Variation-Hospital-Stays.jsp

Pun, B. T., Balas, M. C., Barnes-Daly, M. A., Thompson, J. L., Aldrich, J. M., Barr, J., . . . Ely, E. W. (2019). Caring for critically ill patients with the ABCDEF bundle: Results of the ICU liberation. *Critical Care Medicine, 47*, 3–14. https://doi.org/10.1097/CCM.0000000000003482

Rumbach, A. F., Clayton, N. A., Muller, M. J., & Maitz, P. K. M. (2016). The speech-language pathologist's role in multidisciplinary burn care: An international perspective. *Burns, 42*(4), 863–871. https://doi.org/10.1016/j.burns.2016.01.011

Sessler, C. N., Gosnell, M., Grap, M. J., Brophy, G. T., O'Neal, P. V., Keane, K. A., . . . Elswick, R. K. (2002). The Richmond Agitation Sedation

Scale: Validity and reliability in adult intensive care patients. *American Journal of Respiratory Critical Care Medicine, 166,* 1338–1344. https://doi.org/10.1164/rccm.2107138

Shinn, J. R., Kimura, K. S., Campbell, B. R., Lowery, A. S., Wootten, C. T., Garrett, C. G., . . . Gelbard, A. (2019). Incidence and outcomes of acute laryngeal injury after prolonged mechanical ventilation. *Critical Care Medicine, 47,* 1699–1706. https://doi.org/10.1097/CCM.0000000000004015

Siddique, S. M., Tipton, K., Leas, B., Greysen, S. R., Mull, N. K., Lane-Fall, M., . . . Tsou, A. Y. (2021). Interventions to reduce hospital length of stay in high-risk populations: A systematic review. *JAMA Network Open, 4*(9), e2125846. https://doi.org/10.1001/jamanetworkopen.2021.25846

Vermeir, P., Vandijck, D., Degroote, S., Peleman, R., Verhaeghe, R., Mortier, E., . . . Vogelaers, D. (2015). Communication in healthcare: A narrative review of the literature and practical recommendations. *International Journal of Clinical Practice, 69,* 1257–1267, https://doi.org/10.1111/ijcp.12686

What Are Palliative Care and Hospice Care? (n.d.). National Institute on Aging. https://www.nia.nih.gov/health/what-are-palliative-care-and-hospice-care

Whitmore, K. A., Townsend, S. C., & Laupland, K. B. (2020). Management of tracheostomies in the intensive care unit: A scoping review. *BMJ Open Respiratory Research, 7,* e000651. https://doi.org/10.1136/bmjresp-2020-000651

APPENDIX 2–A
Example of a Clinical Protocol*

Acute Care Division
Department of Hearing & Speech Sciences
Clinical Protocol

Protocol Title: Clinical Swallow Evaluation

Providers: ASHA-Certified and state-licensed speech-language pathologists

I. Policy Statement:

Speech-language pathologists (SLPs) use the clinical swallow evaluation (CSE) to determine overall clinical status, cognition, oral structure function, and oral mastication skills as they relate to swallowing. Results are used to determine the presence or absence of dysphagia and readiness to begin an oral diet and take medication orally. Patients with suspected dysphagia may warrant further instrumental evaluation utilizing flexible endoscopic evaluation of swallowing (FEES) or videofluoroscopic evaluation of swallowing (VFSS).

II. Equipment and Supplies:

May include, but not limited to:

1. food/liquid such as
   a. ice chips
   b. water
   c. applesauce/pudding
   d. fruit cocktail
   e. crackers/Fig Newton
2. thickener packets
3. cups
4. straws
5. spoons
6. tongue blade
7. penlight

---

*Courtesy of Acute Care Division, Vanderbilt University Medical Center.

III. Protocol(s):

1. An order from physician or mid-level provider (NP or PA) is entered in the electronic medical record (EMR).
2. Patients are seen based on priority (NPO status, needed for discharge planning).
3. Patient is seen for CSE. If additional instrumental assessment is warranted, then assessment is described to patient. Primary team is contacted, and order is obtained/entered in the EMR for the instrumental assessment.

IV. Procedures:

1. Prior to food trials:
   a. Complete thorough chart review and discuss current medical status with nurse and care team, including baseline swallowing function and diet
   b. Observe overall physical, social, behavioral, and cognitive/communication status
   c. Observe vocal quality at baseline
   d. Observe and monitor physiological status and vital signs, including heart rate, oxygen saturation, and respiratory rate
   e. Observe secretion management skills
   f. Assess cranial nerve function
   g. Complete oral mechanism evaluation
   h. Ensure proper posture and positioning for feeding
   i. Assess status of oral care, and provide oral care if needed
2. Provide food trials while assessing:
   a. Oral stage including
      i. labial seal
      ii. anterior spillage
      iii. oral control of the bolus
      iv. mastication
      v. manipulation of the bolus
   b. Pharyngeal stage including
      i. presence/absence of hyolaryngeal elevation (Note: unable to judge adequately at bedside)
      ii. time required to complete swallow
      iii. behavioral signs and symptoms of laryngeal penetration and/or aspiration
      iv. changes to physiological status/voice quality.

    c. If the patient tolerates all food trials without overt signs and symptoms of aspiration, a 3-oz water test is administered to rule out silent aspiration in most populations.

3. Special Considerations:

    a. Patient status post–lung transplantation—An evaluation is performed, but only ice chips and water trials are given. Given high risk for silent aspiration and poor tolerance of aspiration, these patients are evaluated for readiness to proceed with FEES.

    b. Patient status post-cardiothoracic surgery—The 3-oz water test is contraindicated because evidence suggests this screening tool is not sensitive enough to detect silent aspiration in this population (Dallal-York, 2021).

V. Required Clinician Education/Supervision to Ensure Competency:

<u>Department Requirements</u>

All new clinicians or clinicians new to a clinical service are required to complete a focused evaluation of clinical practice with an assigned senior clinician. The senior clinician will work with the supervisor to establish competency.

The SLP must have appropriate training and demonstrate competency prior to completing CSEs. If the clinician has had recent experience completing CSEs defined as within the prior 12 months, then they are supervised completing CSEs on patients with a variety of diagnoses (general medical patient, ICU patient, patient s/p burn/inhalation injury, and patient with head and neck cancer). They are required to complete at least one CSE on each patient type (minimum four patients). Competency is established when the supervised clinician demonstrates reasonable decision-making for readiness to implement an oral diet vs. recommendation for instrumental assessment based on evidence-based practices and thorough and accurate documentation. At that point, they are deemed competent to complete independent CSEs that may occur within the duration of the focused evaluation of clinical practice. If the clinician does not demonstrate competency, then they continue with supervision of CSEs until the supervising SLP feels that competency has been met. If this is not achieved within the 6 months of focused evaluation, the supervisor may choose to remove the clinician from this service or continue with supervised training to develop competency.

If a clinician does not have recent experience completing CSEs, then they must first complete prescribed readings and then observe at least one CSE for each patient type (minimum of four) with the supervising SLP. Following completion of readings and observations, they then proceed through steps as outlined earlier with supervised CSEs to establish competency.

Annual competency is maintained through participation in monthly Dysphagia Journal Club, continuing education, chart review, and/or direct observation by supervisor or peer.

VI. Documentation:

Results are interpreted and documented in a written report in the EMR. Documentation includes

1. Medical history

2. Dysphagia history

3. Subjective observations, including patient's tolerance of and response to assessment

4. Objective findings, including
   a. cognitive status and alertness at time of evaluation
   b. results from oral mechanism evaluation
   c. oral phase findings
   d. pharyngeal phase findings

5. Assessment statement including diagnosis and recommendations (including diet [liquid/solid], mode of medication administration, compensatory strategies and feeding positions, and recommendation for further instrumental assessment, as appropriate)

6. If patient is going to be followed for therapy, goals are clearly documented

7. Billing and coding:
   a. CPT: 92610 Evaluation of oral and pharyngeal swallowing function
   b. ICD-10: R13.10—dysphagia, unspecified; R13.11—dysphagia, oral phase; R13.12—dysphagia, oropharyngeal phase; R13.13—dysphagia, pharyngeal phase; R13.19—dysphagia, neurogenic; along with a medical diagnosis which is the presumed cause of dysphagia

References

American Speech-Language-Hearing Association. (n.d.). *Adult dysphagia*. [Practice portal]. https://www.asha.org/Practice-Portal/Clinical-Topics/Adult-Dysphagia/

American Speech-Language-Hearing Association. (n.d.). *Dysphagia Competency Verification Tool (DCVT): User's Guide*. https://www.asha.org/practice-portal/clinical-topics/adult-dysphagia/#collapse_5

Dallal-York, J., Leonard, K., Anderson, A., DiBiase, L., Jeng, E. I., & Plowman, E. K. (2021). Discriminant ability of the 3-ounce water swallow test to detect aspiration in acute postoperative cardiac surgical patients. *Dysphagia,15.* https://doi.org/10.1007/s00455-021-10333-0

Suiter, D. M., & Leder, S. B. (2008). Clinical utility of the 3-ounce water swallow test. *Dysphagia, 23,* 244–250. https://doi.org/10.1007/s00455-007-9127-y

APPENDIX 2–B
Sample Competencies

Videofluoroscopic Swallowing Study (VFSS) Competency

Knowledge/Performance Criteria	DNM	NI	MR	ER	FER
Recognizes anatomic landmarks via videofluoroscopy in lateral and anterior-posterior planes					
Identifies the indications and contraindications for VFSS, including appropriate candidacy					
Understands the fundamentals of VFSS recording (e.g., minimum frames/second) to accurately capture swallowing function					
Identifies and explains the risks, benefits, and precautions related to the VFSS					
Follows a standardized protocol for barium consistency administration					
Understands how to minimize radiation exposure risk for the patient					
Understands how to minimize radiation exposure risk for themselves					
Positions the patient appropriately for optimal visualization of anatomy and function					
Trials appropriate interventions, implements postural changes, and alters the bolus or method of delivery to determine the effect on the swallow during the VFSS					
Directs the patient through appropriate tasks as required for a complete and comprehensive examination					
Demonstrates knowledge of signs of patient distress, and identifies indicators for stopping the VFSS					
Detects and interprets abnormal findings in terms of the underlying anatomy and pathophysiology					

Knowledge/Performance Criteria	DNM	NI	MR	ER	FER
Interprets and documents findings in a written report, including swallowing diagnosis, severity, prognosis, recommendations, and goals					
Formulates treatment and management strategies based on patient performance and integrates patient, family, and caregiver input into treatment plan					
Makes appropriate referrals based on findings					
Educates the patient, caregivers, and staff regarding VFSS findings and the subsequent plan of care					

Ratings:

Does Not Meet (DNM): Requires education and training at the introductory level.

Needs Improvement (NM): Requires input from supervisor or other colleagues for routine cases.

Meets Requirements (MR): Demonstrates competency independently in most cases; seeks resources for additional support when needed.

Exceeds Requirements (ER): Independently demonstrates competency across routine to complex cases.

Far Exceeds Requirements (FER): Demonstrates competency at all levels of complexity and provides mentoring or training to other staff.

Knowledge/Performance Criteria	DNM	NI	MR	ER	FER
Recognizes anatomic landmarks via endoscopy					
Identifies the indications and contraindications for FEES, including appropriate candidacy					
Identifies and explains the risks, benefits, and precautions related to the FEES exam					
Adapts the evaluation for the patient's medical diagnosis					
Operates, maintains, and disinfects FEES equipment					
Applies topical anesthetic when clinically appropriate and when permitted by licensing regulations					
Inserts and maneuvers the endoscope to obtain a view that causes minimal discomfort					
Manipulates the endoscope within the hypopharynx to obtain the desired view					
Directs the patient through appropriate tasks as required for a complete and comprehensive examination					
Demonstrates knowledge of medical contraindications, signs of patient distress, and appropriate actions to take if complications arise					
Detects and interprets abnormal findings in terms of the underlying anatomy and pathophysiology					
Assesses vocal fold mobility and laryngeal closure for breath holding, phonation, and cough					
Assesses secretion management, quantity and location of residue, pharyngeal constriction/contraction symmetry, and swallow initiation					
Presents various dyed bolus consistencies					
Determines presence, quality, and timing of any protective responses					

Knowledge/Performance Criteria	DNM	NI	MR	ER	FER
Trials appropriate treatment interventions, implements postural changes, and alters the bolus or method of delivery to determine the effect on the swallow					
Uses endoscopy as biofeedback and educates patients, caregivers, and staff using FEES images either during or after the examination					
Interprets and documents findings in a written report, including swallowing diagnosis, severity, prognosis, recommendations, and goals					
Formulates treatment and management strategies based on patient performance and integrates patient, family, and caregiver input into treatment plan					
Makes appropriate referrals based on findings					

Ratings:

Does Not Meet (DNM): Requires education and training at the introductory level.

Needs Improvement (NM): Requires input from supervisor or other colleagues for routine cases.

Meets Requirements (MR): Demonstrates competency independently in most cases; seeks resources for additional support when needed.

Exceeds Requirements (ER): Independently demonstrates competency across routine to complex cases.

Far Exceeds Requirements (FER): Demonstrates competency at all levels of complexity and provides mentoring or training to other staff.

Passy Muir Valve (PMV) Competency

Knowledge/Performance Criteria	DNM	NI	MR	ER	FER
Describes mechanism and application of PMV					
Describes patient candidacy for PMV					
Identifies tracheostomy tube type and size					
Selects appropriate PMV					
Deflates/inflates tracheostomy tube cuff appropriately					
Follows suctioning protocol, if necessary					
Trials patient for ability to phonate					
Trials patient for PMV toleration and quality of phonation					
Understands monitoring parameters for vital signs during PMV trial					
Describes signs of poor toleration of PMV					
Educates patient and caregiver regarding use and cleaning of PMV					
Educates nursing staff on use and cleaning and places appropriate signage in patient's room					
Determines follow-up if PMV trial is not successful					
Determines augmentative and alternative communication (AAC) modality for patient if PMV trial is not successful					
Documents procedure and communicates with team re: outcome of assessment					

Ratings:

Does Not Meet (DNM): Requires education and training at the introductory level.

Needs Improvement (NM): Requires input from supervisor or other colleagues for routine cases.

Meets Requirements (MR): Demonstrates competency independently in most cases; seeks resources for additional support when needed.

Exceeds Requirements (ER): Independently demonstrates competency across routine to complex cases.

Far Exceeds Requirements (FER): Demonstrates competency at all levels of complexity and provides mentoring or training to other staff.

Knowledge/Performance Criteria	DNM	NI	MR	ER	FER
Completes initial training with respiratory therapy					
Identifies the signs that indicate the need for suctioning					
Identifies the contraindications for suctioning					
Selects the appropriate personal protective equipment (PPE) and describes standard precautions for suctioning					
Explains the procedure to the patient and caregiver					
Describes appropriate patient positioning					
Understands aseptic technique for catheter and basin use					
Monitors O$_2$ saturation and takes appropriate action when needed					
Understands use and adjustment of the vacuum regulator					
Monitors consistency and color of secretions					
Coordinates care with nursing and respiratory therapy					
Documents procedure within evaluation or treatment note					

Ratings:

Does Not Meet (DNM): Requires education and training at the introductory level.

Needs Improvement (NM): Requires input from supervisor or other colleagues for routine cases.

Meets Requirements (MR): Demonstrates competency independently in most cases; seeks resources for additional support when needed.

Exceeds Requirements (ER): Independently demonstrates competency across routine to complex cases.

Far Exceeds Requirements (FER): Demonstrates competency at all levels of complexity and provides mentoring or training to other staff.

Knowledge/Performance Criteria	DNM	NI	MR	ER	FER
Understands risks to patient and self for patient transfer					
Describes patient conditions that may affect transfers (e.g., hemiplegia, sensory deficits, cognitive deficits)					
Identifies transfer and lifting devices that can assist in transfers					
Performs appropriate assessments of patient status prior to transfers (e.g., alertness, physiologic capacity to transfer, proprioception, sensory status)					
Assesses the number of individuals necessary to transfer the patient safely					
Performs transfer as necessary with vital signs monitoring					
Assesses patient's level of pain and comfort after transfer					
Assures all monitors and IVs are in place after session					

Ratings:

Does Not Meet (DNM): Requires education and training at the introductory level.

Needs Improvement (NM): Requires input from supervisor or other colleagues for routine cases.

Meets Requirements (MR): Demonstrates competency independently in most cases; seeks resources for additional support when needed.

Exceeds Requirements (ER): Independently demonstrates competency across routine to complex cases.

Far Exceeds Requirements (FER): Demonstrates competency at all levels of complexity and provides mentoring or training to other staff.

Vital Signs Monitoring Competency

Knowledge/Performance Criteria	DNM	NI	MR	ER	FER
Understands basic physiologic monitoring for inpatients					
Identifies specific vital signs as displayed on electronic monitor					
Understands variables that can affect monitoring (e.g., skin tone for pulse oximetry/SpO_2 monitoring, sensor positioning on finger)					
Describes the range of normal values for SpO_2, respiratory rate, heart rate					
Identifies the lower range normal values of vital signs for specific patients that will trigger alarms as set on monitor					
Understands how to silence alarms when appropriate					
Identifies what SLP assessment and treatment activities require vital sign monitoring (e.g., suctioning, transfers, PMV placement trials)					

Ratings:

Does Not Meet (DNM): Requires education and training at the introductory level.

Needs Improvement (NM): Requires input from supervisor or other colleagues for routine cases.

Meets Requirements (MR): Demonstrates competency independently in most cases; seeks resources for additional support when needed.

Exceeds Requirements (ER): Independently demonstrates competency across routine to complex cases.

Far Exceeds Requirements (FER): Demonstrates competency at all levels of complexity and provides mentoring or training to other staff.

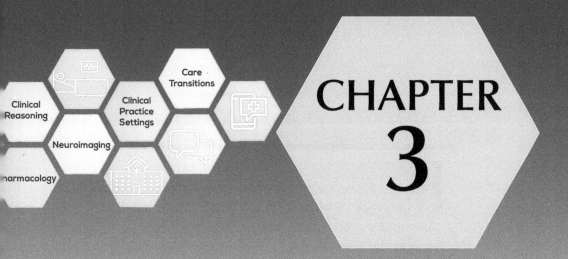

CHAPTER 3

Inpatient Rehabilitation Facilities

Julia R. W. Haffer and Megan E. Schliep

Chapter Objectives

Upon completion of this chapter, the reader will be able to:

- Describe guiding principles for patient care and treatment intensity in inpatient rehabilitation facilities.

- Discuss treatment within the International Classification of Functioning, Disability and Health framework, including restorative and compensatory treatment approaches.

- Provide primary considerations for interdisciplinary care, communication, diagnostic and treatment planning, and documentation.

Introduction

Inpatient rehabilitation facilities (IRFs), also referred to as acute inpatient rehabilitation or "acute rehab," are a common next level of care for many individuals after their acute-care hospitalization. According to the Centers for Medicare and Medicaid Services, IRFs are "freestanding rehabilitation hospitals and rehabilitation units in acute care hospitals. They provide an intensive rehabilitation program, and patients who are admitted must be able to tolerate three hours of intense rehabilitation services per day" (CMS, 2021a). Common medical conditions requiring IRF hospitalization include traumatic brain injuries (TBIs), spinal cord injuries (SCIs), cancer, organ transplants, major burns, complex trauma, strokes, and other neurologic and orthopedic conditions (American Hospital Association IRF Fact Sheet). There are nearly 1,200 IRFs in the United States (CMS, 2022a). The typical length of stay (LOS) in an IRF is dependent on many factors, including the patient's diagnosis and severity, the functional progress made during their IRF hospitalization, and the patient's discharge disposition. The average LOS in inpatient rehabilitation is approximately 13 days, though this may vary considerably based on individual patient needs (CMS, n.d.-a).

Interprofessionalism in the IRF

When an individual no longer requires acute hospital level care but remains at a level of medical need and functional impairment that meets the criteria for inpatient rehabilitation, they may be transferred to an IRF. (More rarely, an individual might be transferred to an IRF directly from home or another care setting if medically and clinically determined by physician referral.)

IRF care includes an intensive and coordinated interdisciplinary team approach (CMS, n.d.-a). Patients in an IRF receive a minimum of 3 hours of therapy per day, at least 5 days per week (typically, Monday through Friday) with some additional therapy hours on the weekend days. Therapy sessions may be provided in a one-on-one format, a group format, or a combination. This includes therapy provided by speech-language pathologists (SLPs), occupational therapists (OTs), and physical therapists (PTs). Typically, patients receive 1 hour per day of individual SLP, OT, and PT intervention. Table 3–1 shows a hypothetical daily schedule for a patient in an IRF.

Although PT, OT, and SLP clinicians work individually with the patient to address goals specific to their area of expertise and rehabilitation service, interprofessional collaboration and communication are key aspects of successful patient care. According to the World Health Organization (WHO, 2010), interprofessional practice is when two or more professionals collaborate without any perceived hierarchy and with full understanding of each other's roles and responsibilities to improve a patient's outcomes and care. Research has shown that there are numerous benefits to interprofessional practice (IPP) including improved patient/family outcomes upon return home, the prevention of communication breakdowns or misinformation, shortened hospital stays, reduction or prevention of readmissions, and reduction of hospital costs. Key aspects that staff members must be able to demonstrate are

TABLE 3–1	Sample Daily Schedule in the Inpatient Rehabilitation Facility Environment
8:00 a.m.	Breakfast
9:00 a.m.	Nursing care/wound care
10:00 a.m.	Physical therapy
11:00 a.m.	Recreational therapy group
12:00 p.m.	Lunch
1:00 p.m.	Speech therapy
2:00 p.m.	Occupational therapy
3:00 p.m.	Meeting with psychologist
4:00 p.m.	(Break)
5:00 p.m.	Dinner

Notes: Blue indicates primary daily therapies; green indicates mealtimes. Therapy may be provided during mealtimes pending patient goals. For example, if the patient has swallowing-specific goals for the use of strategies or maneuvers with oral intake, meals may be an ideal time to provide therapy and promote independence with use of these strategies or maneuvers.

responsibility, accountability, communication, cooperative, assertiveness, autonomy, and mutual trust and respect. Table 3–2 lists many of the essential IPP team members involved in patient care at the IRF level.

Communication among the IPP team members is mandated by CMS and occurs through a weekly "rounds" or "interdisciplinary team conference" meeting. These are led by a rehabilitation physician, and attendance includes a registered nurse, a social worker

TABLE 3–2	Essential Interprofessional Practice Team Members Involved in Inpatient Rehabilitation Facility Patient Care
Speech pathologists	Evaluate and work to improve voice, speech, language, cognitive-communication, and/or swallowing abilities
Physical therapists	Evaluate and work to improve strength, flexibility, endurance, coordination, and balance across a variety of activities such as moving in bed, using a wheelchair, and walking
Occupational therapists	Evaluate and provide re-training in independent living skills, self-care, and upper body/hand functioning, as well as training in the use of assistive technology when needed
Recreational therapists	Create and foster activities to promote the physical, cognitive, emotional, and social functioning of patients
Rehab physicians (physiatrists)	Medical doctors who received specialized training in physical medicine and rehabilitation; serve as the team leader for a patient's rehabilitation, directing medical care and supervising medical residents
Rehabilitation psychologists	Provide counseling to help guide the patient and make recommendations to the care team for best methods of providing support and/or managing behaviors
Neuropsychologists	If on staff, can complete a full battery to extensively evaluate neurocognitive skills
Nursing staff	Oversee daily care, education, and coordination of medical treatments, with various specialists potentially involved including pain management and wound care
Social workers	Provide support to the patients and their caregivers through the rehab process and may assist in establishing needed financial, housing, and logistical support for after discharge
Case managers	Coordinate services during the patient's stay and after they are discharged from the hospital; work with the insurance companies directly
Dieticians	Monitor tolerance for tube feedings and/or oral intake, monitor weights, skin integrity, and bowel regimens, and make recommendations to maximize nutrition and overall healing

or case manager or both, and the PT/OT/SLP to the extent that each of the latter three clinicians is involved in the patient's care. The initial meeting occurs in the first 4 days of a patient's IRF stay in order to establish a plan of care as well as a LOS by identifying an anticipated discharge date (when they will leave the IRF) and disposition (where they will go). This may change through the course of the admission, but best efforts are made upon initial conference to establish such a plan. Meetings are weekly thereafter. The purposes of these meetings are to:

1. "Assess the patient's progress towards the rehabilitation goals,

2. Consider possible resolutions to any problems that could impede progress towards the goals,

3. Reassess the validity of the rehabilitation goals previously established, and

4. Monitor and revise the treatment plan, as needed" (CMS, n.d., pp. 15–16).

Outside of the structured weekly team meetings, it is common for primary care team members to have informal/impromptu conversations to discuss a patient's progress, plan of care, or additional needs. Some facilities may have specific practices in place for more structured ad hoc team discussion, such as to consider fall risk reduction strategies, behavior management approaches, and other individualized patient needs.

Primary Objectives of Inpatient Rehabilitation

During the IRF stay, an individual's plan of care is multifaceted. Care is generally both (a) *restorative*, aimed at improving impairment areas and working toward premorbid levels of functioning, as well as (b) *compensatory*, aimed at identifying and practicing new methods or means of completing activities. To better understand how a care plan is developed, it is important to consider the International Classification of Functioning, Disability, and Health (ICF) framework, which provides a scaffold for examining levels of functioning (Figure 3–1). The ICF was developed by the WHO and was published in 2001 (WHO, n.d.). It is the framework for the field in the professional Scope of Practice for Speech-Language Pathology and provides a useful way to consider the selection of interventions and support patient-centered care (ASHA, n.d.).

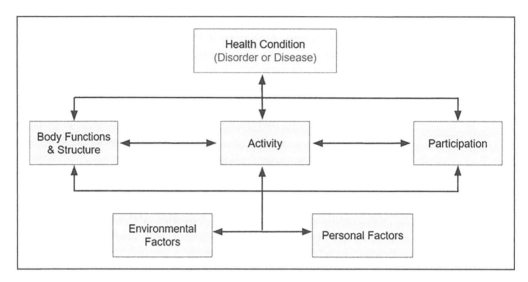

FIGURE 3–1. *Source:* Adaptation of the International Classification of Functioning, Disability, and Health (ICF) Framework. https://www.who.int/standards/classifications/international-classification-of-functioning-disability-and-health

To understand the ICF in practice and how both restorative and compensatory care is provided, it may be helpful to consider an example. If a person were to experience a stroke, for example, that would be the *Health Condition* according to Figure 3–1. The stroke would impact this individual's *Body Functions & Structure*, which may include impairments such as hemiparesis or language (aphasia). Having aphasia would subsequently impact the *Activities* this individual is able to take part in, which would in turn impact their *Participation* or involvement in life situations. Additionally, both *Environmental Factors* and *Personal Factors* have a critical impact on the activities and participation of the individual experiencing the specific health condition and must be considered within the POC to further guide the person-centered care we are providing.

As rehabilitation professionals, the care we provide includes targeting Body Functions & Structure, as we work to restore areas of impairment. In the previous example, this would mean addressing verbal expression and comprehension deficits directly and capitalizing on principles of neuroplasticity to improve linguistic skills. We would also direct our therapy to include compensatory care to support the Activities our clients are able to perform, which has a direct impact on their Participation. In the previous example, this could involve working with the patient to select and use an appropriate alternative and augmentative communication device, which may allow them to return to preferred activities and join in these activities with friends and family. It is important to note that restorative and compensatory care are not an "either–or" option. Rather, it is important to consider both in relation to the individual's areas of impairment, severity, and individual goals to guide the care plan. Further, the focus of therapy may change over time. Initially, intervention may focus on addressing areas of impairment through restorative care, with less of a focus on compensatory strategies. As the patient continues to make gains and progress toward goals becomes more defined, therapy may be shifted to include additional focus on compensatory strategies. These decisions are considered in collaboration with the patient, their families, and the care team.

Assessment and Intervention Considerations

General Assessment Considerations

When a patient transitions to the IRF setting, consultations are placed for each therapy discipline that is indicated to evaluate the patient's current status and determine an appropriate care plan. An important consideration in regard to evaluation is framing the *patient's illness* as the "episode of care" as opposed to treating the *IRF hospitalization* as a separate episode of care. In doing so, we are recognizing that the patient's IRF stay is one step of their recovery course and that we as clinical care team members can and should support continuity of care in their recovery pathway. Further, this framing reminds us, as treating clinicians, to be good stewards of health care resources and to gather any information from previous levels of care to support care planning as opposed to simply repeating testing, potentially unnecessarily. For example, the clinician should obtain results of prior assessments (e.g., prior videofluoroscopic swallow study) and talk to the clinician from the acute-care setting, when able, to establish the best plan of care that reflects the patient's current status and further understand the assessments that have already been completed. It may not be necessary to repeat an exam (e.g., prior example of videofluoroscopic swallow study) upon admission to IRF. Rather, the patient may be best served by waiting until clinical progress is observed for repeat assessment.

Consistent with other levels of care, as part of the assessment plan, the evaluating clinician has a responsibility to speak with both the patient and their care-partners/family members (with patient permission) to learn about the patient and their personal goals. Asking these questions is one aspect of patient-centered care and supports the diversity and inclusion of each of our patients during their hospitalization. Further, this information provides background regarding a patient's baseline status and functioning to better guide therapy activities and goals (e.g., education and literacy levels, vocation, primary language, prior independence with instrumental activities such as financial management).

Standardized Assessment Considerations

During the acute-care hospitalization, the patient may not yet be medically stable, limiting their readiness for intensive therapy, or may be unavailable due to other priority tests and procedures, limiting their time available for therapy services. In the IRF setting, on the other hand, the patient is deemed medically stable and able to tolerate at least 3 hours of therapy per day, with therapy being prioritized. Given that patients participate in each therapy discipline for 1 hour per day, there is often time available to complete more comprehensive assessment procedures, including formal, standardized assessments. For example, in assessing language skills for an individual with aphasia following a stroke, the Western Aphasia Battery–Revised (WAB-R; Kertesz, 2007) may be selected, which provides an Aphasia Quotient (AQ) and Aphasia Classification. To evaluate cognitive skills, the Repeatable Battery for the Assessment of Neuropsychological Status (RBANS; Randolph et al., 1998) or Cognitive–Linguistic Quick Test (CLQT; Helm-Estabrooks, 2001) may be administered, for example, which both provide criterion-based cut scores with descriptive severity ratings. An important benefit of standardized assessment measures is that they can be used to evaluate change. Often, a standardized measure may be administered at admission in order to evaluate patient status, guide the plan of care, and provide initial information to support prognostication. The assessment may be readministered prior to discharge, yielding an updated score from which to measure impairment-based gains.

In addition to diagnosis-specific assessments, there are several other standardized protocols within IRF. A particularly important protocol to the IRF environment includes the *CMS Quality Indicators*, which are part of the IMPACT Act enacted in 2014 (CMS, 2021b). Data collection began in 2018 and includes a "Brief Interview for Mental Status" (referred to as "BIMS") that must be completed for each patient admitted to an IRF setting. The BIMS includes several items, including immediate recall (patients being asked to repeat three words), basic orientation questions (the year, month, and day of week), as well as recall after a short delay (recall of previous words). This information is reported to CMS to standardize the data collected across post-acute settings (e.g., IRF, skilled nursing facilities [SNFs], home health) in order to allow for exchange of information to better understand levels of care and patient severity (CMS, 2021b).

Assessment Interpretation and Intervention Planning Considerations

Following the completion of assessment measures, the SLP will develop an individualized plan of care that becomes a part of the interdisciplinary plan of care. This will consider the SLP diagnosis or diagnoses of the patient (e.g., dysphagia, dysarthria, aphasia, etc.), their individual goals, and their anticipated LOS to allow for time to work toward those goals. Depending on the patient presentation, goals may need to be prioritized to maximize the IRF intervention period. For example, while myriad skill areas may warrant intervention in an individual presenting in a post-traumatic confusional state from an acute brain injury, it may be more important to prioritize basic attention and safe eating and drinking skills before other areas can be of focus. As such, the evaluating clinician must carefully use their assessment to determine the maximally beneficial and individualized plan of care.

An additional element of care planning includes potential referrals to other interprofessional team members based on the identification of need or anticipated need. For example, a referral to the dietician will be imperative for an individual on a modified diet to ensure they are able to meet their needs for nutrition and hydration, or an individual with a severe communication impairment may require timely initiation of the exploration of assistive and augmentative communication (AAC) needs. Some IRFs may have a specialized team or department for AAC technology, while others may have SLP and/or OT clinicians who have skilled experience in that area. Regardless, it is the role of the evaluating and treating clinician to determine the patient's need for support and to initiate or establish AAC options.

Model Systems

Select IRFs have specialized programs of care in SCI, TBI, and burn injury (burn) which are called "Model Systems." Funded by the

National Institute on Disability, Independent Living, and Rehabilitation Research (NIDILRR), "model systems pool information and conduct research intended to improve the long-term functional, vocational, cognitive, and quality-of-life outcomes in individuals with TBI, SCI, or burn injury" (Model Systems Knowledge Translation Center, n.d.). As of 2022, 16 facilities were designated as Model Systems for TBI, 14 facilities were designated as Model Systems for SCI, and 4 facilities were designated as Model Systems for burn injury. In short, a facility that is designated as a Model System is considered "a center of excellence for both treatment and research related to a particular disability" (Moss Rehab, n.d.). Patients at these selected IRFs may be invited to participate in data collection at regular intervals for up to 30 years post injury as part of an ongoing national database. As a result, TBI, SCI, and/or burn programs at these facilities may have discipline-specific (PT/OT/SLP) evaluation protocols that are carried out as part of the Model Systems' research and tracking. Clinicians incorporate these measures into their assessments and may also be involved in ongoing discussions with the research teams to remain up to date with regard to best practice for research methods of assessment collection.

Workflows, Routines, and Requirements of Inpatient Rehabilitation

Patients in an IRF may fall into one of many possible diagnostic categories. For an IRF to maintain a Medicare license (meaning, the facility can be reimbursed by Medicare), 60% of the patients admitted must have a qualifying condition from among 13 possible conditions listed in Table 3–3 (CMS, n.d.-b). Many IRFs, particularly those that are larger, may have a dedicated floor or unit for each specific diagnostic group (e.g., a stroke unit, a brain injury unit, a spinal cord unit, a burn unit). Each unit may provide opportunities for therapy groups and educational sessions for their patients that are specific to the admitting diagnosis.

It is also worth noting that patients from a wide range of diagnostic groups may benefit from SLP intervention at the IRF. While you are likely familiar with the role of the SLP in the rehabilitation of neurologic disorders, our services can be vital in non-neurologic populations as well. For example, patients who have experienced burns may subsequently experience cognitive-communication or voice disturbances or may require orofacial interventions as a result of their injuries. It is important that SLPs recognize the needs of various populations and advocate for the provision of services.

TABLE 3–3	Centers for Medicare and Medicaid Services Compliant Diagnoses for Inpatient Rehabilitation (Inpatient Rehabilitation Facility Classification Requirements)

1. Stroke

2. Spinal cord injury

3. Congenital deformity

4. Amputation

5. Major multiple trauma

6. Fracture of femur

7. Brain injury

8. Neurological disorders

9. Burns

10. Active polyarticular rheumatoid arthritis, psoriatic arthritis, and seronegative arthropathies

11. Systemic vasculidities with joint inflammation

12. Severe or advanced osteoarthritis

13. Joint replacement

Caseload Responsibilities

A caseload is the term used to refer to the number of patients an SLP will be responsible for at a given time. Many SLPs provide care and carry a caseload of patients on a dedicated unit, while others might float throughout a building to care for patients from various diagnostic groups. Some facilities practice rotations, which allow clinicians to provide care on a dedicated unit for a period of time (e.g., a few months) and then rotate to a new unit or area. Even if a clinician's primary practice area is on a dedicated unit or with a primary population, they will need to be able to evaluate and treat patients on other units or with other diagnoses as needs arise. When a clinician has a caseload of patients, they are typically responsible for evaluating their patients, planning for treatment, carrying out interventions, and completing thorough and timely documentation. Additional responsibilities include structured and ad hoc communication with family/caregivers and the rest of the care team, including providing updates at weekly rounds meetings, which you learned about earlier in this chapter. Clinicians may also be responsible for program-specific committees and tasks, such as running a family education group or meeting as part of an inter-professional team to collaborate on improving a hospital process.

Soon you will learn more about the concept of reimbursement, under which it is vital that direct patient care providers (including SLP clinicians) maintain a relatively steady rate of productivity, with billable productivity time measured in direct patient care. This means the majority of a clinician's day (e.g., 80% or more) will be in direct assessment and intervention with patients, with the remaining time (e.g., 20% or less) of the day available for the aforementioned planning, documenting, and communicating responsibilities and other projects. As such, the IRF is a fast-paced, demanding setting that requires strong time management and organizational skills to maintain efficient and effective practice on a daily basis.

Documentation

There are multiple documentation requirements in the inpatient rehabilitation setting. Written documentation is used to communicate information to other care team members and support care plan recommendations, as well as to support reimbursement and justify LOS and discharge recommendations. Further, documented records are often available to the patient and family members, highlighting the importance of accurate, professional, and comprehensive written documentation practices. Specific documentation information is outlined in Table 3–4.

Additional Roles and Responsibilities

Planning for Discharge

The goal of inpatient rehabilitation is not for the patient to stay indefinitely but rather to support patients in developing independence and transitioning to their next level of care. Inpatient rehabilitation is best thought of as "Step 1" of rehabilitative recovery, with patients moving on to a variety of different settings depending on their needs. Some patients may be ready to discharge to their homes following inpatient rehabilitation, while others may still require ongoing inpatient care. For those who discharge to home, many will continue to receive therapy through participation in outpatient treatment or receiving home health care. (Please refer to subsequent chapters on these topics for further information

TABLE 3–4	Inpatient Rehabilitation Facility (IRF) Documentation Requirements
Documentation Type	**Description**
Initial evaluation and plan of care	The initial evaluation report provides a summary of assessment results, including formal standardized assessments and informal/dynamic measures, impressions, diagnosis(-es), and the plan of care.
Daily treatment encounter and therapy minutes log	Daily documentation includes specific therapy activities and performance, daily progress toward established goals, and any other information relevant to the care plan. Daily therapy minutes are documented to ensure IRF requirements are met.
Weekly progress report	Every 7 days, a weekly progress report is required. This report documents notable highlights of the week, progress toward the plan of care, any specific facilitators or barriers, updated therapy goals, and any other information relevant to the care plan.
Discharge report	The discharge report provides a summary of the patient's progress during the IRF hospitalization, results of discharge outcome assessments, whether established goals were met, and discharge information, including whether ongoing therapy services are recommended. This information is particularly helpful to the clinician at the next level of care, should the patient require ongoing services (e.g., outpatient care, home health services).

about the goals of each of these settings.) Other patients may still require additional supportive medical care and may discharge to a SNF, where they may continue to participate in therapy, but generally at a lower intensity than the level provided in the IRF setting.

A critical aspect of discharge planning involves interprofessional communication. As discussed earlier, the SLP communicates closely with the rehabilitation team, including PT, OT, physician, and nursing colleagues, as well as the social worker and/or case manager, to discuss potential plans regarding discharge date and disposition. Decisions regarding discharge plans involve integration of physical, cognitive, and communication needs, as well as more logistical considerations such as the discharge environment and any available caregiver support. Figure 3–2 highlights several example questions that must be considered when making decisions regarding discharge plans. As you can see, these are questions that require the input of the interdisciplinary rehabilitation team and integration of multiple aspects of rehabilitation progress.

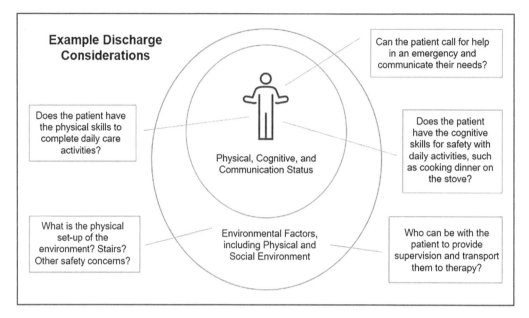

FIGURE 3–2. Example discharge considerations, including Individual Factors and Environmental Factors.

Patient Education and Patient–Family Training

An integral component of a successful inpatient rehabilitation intervention course involves education, training, and preparations for the discharge transition throughout the stay. This includes providing education about the admitting diagnosis and related health topics, reviewing ways to maximize safety and independence at home, and training caregivers in relevant support strategies. While this is an important part of the inpatient rehabilitation course for all patients, it is essential for those who are going home to ensure that they and their caregivers have a complete understanding of the medical, physical, cognitive, and communication needs and supports.

From stroke, to TBI, to SCI, to one of many other possible IRF admitting diagnoses (see further discussion regarding CMS-13 compliant diagnoses for inpatient rehabilitation in the "Caseload" section and Table 3–3), the IRF stay may often be the first time an individual and/or their loved ones have encountered this diagnosis or required such an intensive level of medical care. It is imperative that the interprofessional team provide adequate education about the individual's diagnosis or diagnoses, health risk factors, preventative health information, and available community resources.

The physician and nurse may be primarily responsible for providing medical and medication-related education, but when working with individuals with communication or cognitive impairments, the speech pathologist can play a vital role in assisting to modify and reinforce educational materials to ensure comprehension and retention of important information. The speech pathologist can review information such as medication lists and stroke warning signs in a way that maximizes learning in the context of a patient's individual SLP goals (e.g., reading comprehension, short-term memory). Some facilities may offer education groups within their programs. This provides a cohort of patients with shared diagnoses (SCI, for example) the opportunity to attend a session where medical and rehabilitation information can be provided through presentation, discussion, and handout.

Similarly, an IRF stay may be the first time the individual or their caregivers encounter a speech pathologist and the associated diagnoses (e.g., dysarthria, dysphagia, aphasia, etc.). As such, a successful SLP intervention program will also allow for formal and informal opportunities to educate the patient and their caregivers about the role of the SLP and the goal areas being addressed. In planning for discharge, pre-arranged opportunities for family members and/or caregivers to attend an SLP session can be coordinated by the case manager and are an opportunity for the SLP to provide direct education (handouts, verbal review), demonstration (to highlight the patient's areas of success/impairment and for recommended use of strategies/supports), and training (to allow the caregivers an opportunity to "practice" skills they may need to use at home to support the patient). Specific areas that an SLP might review with caregivers could include how to prepare thickened liquids/modified diet textures; the need for safe swallowing strategies such as chin tuck; support strategies for individuals requiring use of an AAC device; home routine modifications to support memory impairments through the use of calendars, alarms, and other external memory aids; review of behavior management strategies for individuals after a TBI; and so on. While this is beneficial across all cases, it is imperative for those individuals who will be going home. Reflect on Figure 3–2, which you reviewed in the previous section: Answers to many of the questions raised will guide the needed discharge training and education.

An important aspect of patient and family education is the way in which this information is communicated. The definition of health literacy was updated in 2020 in order to capture both (a) personal health literacy and (b) organizational health literacy (CDC, 2022) (see Box 3–1).

Box 3-1

"*Personal health literacy* is the degree to which individuals have the ability to find, understand, and use information and services to inform health-related decisions and actions for themselves and others.

Organizational health literacy is the degree to which organizations equitably enable individuals to find, understand, and use information and services to inform health-related decisions and actions for themselves and others." (CDC, 2022)

Health literacy is important to consider in relation to both the patient and their family members. As clinical providers, we have a responsibility in supporting our patients' personal health literacy skills as well promoting organizational health literacy within our place of work. When providing information and education to patients and family, information should be presented in ways that are easily accessible to all individuals so that they are able to make well-informed decisions regarding their care. Examples of health literacy practices include avoiding jargon and using clear language, using strategies such as verbal and written information to support communication, and providing multiple opportunities for interaction between the clinician and patient/family. Health literacy supports health equity, which is attaining the highest level of health for all people (CDC, 2022). For additional health literacy information and best practices, the CDC Health Literacy website provides a useful starting point and offers many resources to further guide interactions with patients and their family members.

In addition to educating patients and their caregivers, the rehabilitation team should provide specific training and practice for the patient in preparation for and support of the transition to the home environment. First, we recognize the importance of intensive practice and repetition of skills as it is integral to neuroplasticity to support ongoing recovery. While IRF care provides daily (five to seven times per week) therapy, typically within the early weeks of a patient's recovery, subsequent weeks to months will involve therapy at a reduced frequency. It is imperative that patients and caregivers recognize the importance of "homework" and exercise/practice that can be carried out by the individual and/or their caregivers outside of the one-to-one therapy sessions. During the IRF stay, the clinician can begin to introduce programs and tasks aimed at this goal. Second, in preparation for resuming community and home-based tasks, therapeutic activities that target an individual's physical, occupational, and speech therapy goals can be completed within tasks that become increasingly dynamic and provide "real world" application opportunities. See Tables 3–5 and 3–6 for a list of example activities toward both of these goals. Helping a patient identify their strengths, challenges, and use of compensatory strategies in these "real-world" contexts can be a valuable experience in preparation for a discharge back to their home/community, and also provides the therapy team with further insights into the needed supports and precautions at discharge.

Decision-Making Capacity

When an individual is hospitalized, there are many decisions to be made regarding their care and future plans. These decisions are made by either the patient or a representative, such as a health care

TABLE 3–5	Examples of Carryover Exercise Program Tasks
Activity	**Rationale**
Activities or workbooks that can be completed independently by the patient or with support from care-partner/family	Supports carryover of therapy activities and promotes independence in addressing areas of impairment, which may be useful in preparing for discharge home activities.
Assigned work in a therapy app to be completed independently or with support from care-partner/family	Similar to previous, supports carryover of therapy activities and promotes independence in addressing areas of impairment. Therapy apps may be particularly useful for those who were engaged in computer/tablet activities prior to their hospitalization and can be a "natural" next step to promote independence.
Assigned target number of repetitions of prescribed swallowing or voice exercises	Despite the intensive nature of inpatient rehabilitation facility care, some exercises are best completed multiple times per day (e.g., swallowing exercises may be recommended three to five times per day, 10 to 20 repetitions each to address motor weakness/strengthening).
Any task that the clinician asks the patient to complete on their own	Supports patients' independence in building new routines to address specific areas of impairment and participation.

TABLE 3–6	Examples of Dynamic Therapeutic Tasks

Activity	Rationale
Individual community outing (e.g., local pharmacy, coffee shop) with a clinician to guide use of compensatory strategies or practice therapeutic skills in a real-world situation	Provides a functional environment in which to practice new strategies/skills, particularly for premorbid routine activities that may require modifications following the event for which the patient is hospitalized
Group community outing with clinicians and other patients	Provides a highly stimulating and challenging opportunity for the patient to experience being in a community environment, potentially for the first time since their injury, which allows for practice and feedback in all areas of impairment or intervention
Establishing a routine where the patient can signal their nurse call light when medications are due (If the patient does not call by a specified time, the nurse administers the medication per routine protocol.)	Reinforces medication management and training in prospective memory skills for functional activities
Hospital scavenger hunt, which could include finding targets around the building to work on attention, reading a directory to locate specific floors, having an interaction with the front desk to work on verbal expression, for example	Encourages the patient to navigate a new setting, move around in a dynamic environment, and challenge their cognitive and communicative skills

proxy, who can make decisions on behalf of the patient when they are unable to do so. However, those with impaired cognition or a communication impairment (e.g., aphasia) are at risk of losing their autonomy when it comes to ethical issues and decision-making (Brady Wagner, 2003). While SLPs cannot alone determine if an individual has decision-making capacity, they are frequently and appropriately sought to assist in this process. Speech pathologists should be involved in supporting the assessment of decision-making capacity in individuals with communication and cognitive disorders given expertise in assessment of communication strengths and weaknesses and, subsequently, identifying strategies to facilitate communication. Through this involvement, they are able to support the medical team in elucidating a patient's decision-making capacity. For example, an individual with a severe speech or language disorder may be able to indicate their decisions through another modality (e.g., writing, AAC). Conversely, an individual who is a clear verbal communicator but has significant cognitive impairment may be limited in their memory and insight such that they are unable to make safe and thoughtful decisions. The SLP may need to advocate for involvement in the decision-making process by educating other medical team members about their expertise and scope of practice and further demonstrating the benefit of their support (Brady Wagner, 2003).

Safety and Infection Control: Inpatient Rehabilitation Facility–Specific Considerations

An important aspect of patient care in the IRF setting that differs from many other care settings is how aspects of infection control are managed. In the acute care setting, for example, patients spend the majority of their time in their hospital room and typically leave the room only for tests and procedures during their hospitalization. In contrast, a patient in the IRF setting may leave their room several times a day to participate in daily therapies. For example, the patient may go to the rehabilitation gym for physical therapy, to a model "apartment" within the hospital to practice activities of daily living for their occupational therapy session, and to the speech therapy office for their SLP session. Infection control and patient safety continue to be of utmost priority in the IRF setting, while allowing for participation in a variety of activities outside of the patient's hospital room, when appropriate. (For patients on specific isolation precautions, therapy may remain in the patient's hospital room until the patient is cleared to leave the room for activities according to established infection-control protocols.) Given this, proper personal protective equipment is required regardless of the location that therapy is completed. Additionally, infection control includes sanitizing all surfaces according to established protocols to ensure compliance. As learned throughout the COVID-19 pandemic, these protocols and personal protective equipment requirements exist not only to protect the patients we are serving at that specific moment but also to protect care providers in their interactions with other colleagues and other patients, and as they return to their communities at the end of each workday.

Reimbursement

Understanding reimbursement in the IRF setting is important given some of the differences between IRF and other care settings. While this section is not intended to provide detailed information about reimbursement practices, general information regarding IRF reimbursement practices is discussed.

First and foremost, IRF reimbursement operates under a Prospective Payment System (PPS). This is in contrast to a "fee-for-service" or "per-diem" model. Instituted by CMS in 2002, the IRF PPS model reimburses institutions according to a set, predetermined rate for each discharge patient. This rate is determined by multiple factors and utilizes information from patient assessment to classify patients into groups based on clinical characteristics and anticipated resource needs (CMS, 2022b). Even though patients participating in IRF may have different types of insurance, IRF institutions look to CMS as a model, as the institution must submit outcome data for all patients. Importantly, if the institution does not provide the care that they say they will provide, the entire payment for the IRF hospitalization may be denied. This highlights the importance of IRF care being provided according to the required frequency, as well as proper documentation of this care.

These reimbursement requirements link directly to clinician productivity expectations. Only time spent in direct patient contact may be included in billable time calculations. Therefore, expectations for billable productivity (direct patient contact) and nonbillable productivity (supporting activities, such as consulting with colleagues, planning for the therapy session, and completing documentation) are clearly established by the institution (see the section Caseload Responsibilities for more information on clinician caseload).

Conclusion

This chapter has discussed information regarding the structure, considerations, and care provided in the IRF setting, as well as the specific roles and responsibilities of an SLP in this setting. As discussed within this chapter, IRFs serve a wide variety of patient populations, although facilities are required to admit at least 60% of their patients from specific diagnostic groups. SLPs are trained to provide skilled care to a wide variety of patient populations, and treatment most often consists of both restorative and compensatory approaches. Interprofessional practice is integral in providing quality care at the IRF level and supports key domains of care, including discharge planning and education of patients and caregivers. Clinical work in the IRF setting is demanding, fast-paced, and requires strong organizational and time management skills.

References

American Hospital Association. (n.d.). *Fact sheet: Inpatient rehabilitation facilities—A unique and critical service.* https://www.aha.org/fact-sheets/2019-07-09-fact-sheet-inpatient-rehabilitation-facilities-unique-and-critical-service

American Speech-Language-Hearing Association. (n.d.). *International classification of functioning, disability, and health (ICF).* https://www.asha.org/slp/icf/

Brady Wagner, L. C. (2003). Clinical ethics in the context of language and cognitive impairment: Rights and protections. *Seminars in Speech and Language, 24*(4), 275–284. https://doi.org/10.1055/s-2004-815581

Centers for Disease Control and Prevention. (2022). *What is health literacy?* https://www.cdc.gov/healthliteracy/learn/index.html

Centers for Medicare and Medicaid Services. (n.d.-a). *Clarifications for the IRF coverage requirements.* https://www.cms.gov/Medicare/Medicare-Fee-for-Service-Payment/InpatientRehabFacPPS/Downloads/Complete-List-of-IRF-Clarifications-Final-Document.pdf

Centers for Medicare and Medicaid Services. (n.d.-b). *Fact sheet #1: Inpatient rehabilitation facility classification requirements.* https://www.cms.gov/Medicare/Medicare-Fee-for-Service-Payment/InpatientRehabFacPPS/downloads/fs1classreq.pdf

Centers for Medicare and Medicaid Services. (2021a). *Inpatient rehabilitation facilities.* https://www.cms.gov/Medicare/Provider-Enrollment-and-Certification/CertificationandCompllianc/InpatientRehab

Centers for Medicare and Medicaid Services. (2021b). *IMPACT Act of 2014 data standardization & cross setting measures.* https://www.cms.gov/Medicare/Quality-Initiatives-Patient-Assessment-Instruments/Post-Acute-Care-Quality-Initiatives/IMPACT-Act-of-2014/IMPACT-Act-of-2014-Data-Standardization-and-Cross-Setting-Measures

Centers for Medicare and Medicaid Services. (2022a). *Inpatient rehabilitation facilities datasets: General information.* https://data.cms.gov/provider-data/topics/inpatient-rehabilitation-facilities

Centers for Medicare and Medicaid Services. (2022b). *Inpatient rehabilitation facility PPS.* https://www.cms.gov/Medicare/Medicare-Fee-for-Service-Payment/InpatientRehabFacPPS

Helm-Estabrooks, N. (2001). *Cognitive-linguistic quick test.* Pearson Publishing.

Kertesz, A. (2007). *Western aphasia battery—Revised.* Pearson Publishing.

Model Systems Knowledge Translation Center. (n.d.). *About the model systems.* https://msktc.org/about-model-systems#sthash.98qRdUzj.dpuf

Moss Rehab. (n.d.). *The traumatic brain injury model system at Moss Rehab.* https://www.mossrehab.com/traumatic-brain-injury/tbi-model-system-of-care

Randolph, C., Tierney, M. C., Mohr, E., & Chase, T. N. (1998). The repeatable battery for the assessment of neuropsychological status: Preliminary clinical validity. *Journal of Clinical and Experimental Neuropsychology, 20*(3), 310–319.

World Health Organization. (n.d.). *International classification of functioning, disability, and health (ICF).* https://www.who.int/standards/classifications/international-classification-of-functioning-disability-and-health

World Health Organization. (2010). *Framework for action on interprofessional education and collaborative practice.* http://whqlibdoc.who.int/hq/2010/WHO_HRH_HPN_10.3_eng.pdf

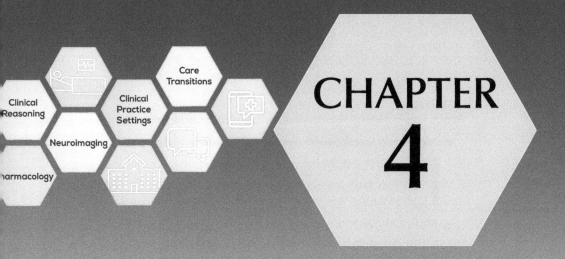

CHAPTER

4

Skilled Nursing Facilities

Mary L. Casper

Chapter Objectives

Upon completion of this chapter, the reader will be able to:

- Describe the characteristics of the skilled nursing facility (SNF) setting for speech-language pathology services.
- Discuss key clinical populations served by the speech-language pathologist in the SNF.
- Explain methods of reimbursement for speech-language pathology services in the SNF.
- Identify the members of the interprofessional team in the SNF.

Introduction

Long-term care in the United States is residential, meaning patients stay at the facility for their care. Different levels of care are provided in long-term care settings, typically after a hospital stay. Assisted living and memory care services are also types of long-term care, but these do not require an initial hospital stay to enter.

This chapter considers the role of the speech-language pathologist (SLP) practicing in long-term care settings, largely known as skilled nursing facilities (SNFs). The range of conditions that lead to communication, cognition, and/or swallowing disorders that are evaluated and treated by the SLP in the SNF setting are examined. Suggestions to meet payer requirements for clinical documentation are reviewed, along with best practices for interprofessional team communication.

Various methodologies for reimbursement, which are an important consideration to understand in regard to long-term care, are discussed, including the Medicare Physician Fee Schedule associated with Medicare Part B and the Prospective Payment System associated with Medicare Part A.

Key Terminology

Centers for Medicare and Medicaid Services (CMS)—The government agency that develops regulations, payment systems, quality measures, and makes agreements with insurance companies to act as administrative contractors.

Medicare Administrative Contractors (MACs)—Insurance companies that are contracted with CMS to process Medicare fee-for-service insurance claims. MACs are based on jurisdictions, for example, Jurisdiction L includes Pennsylvania; Maryland; Delaware; Washington, DC; New Jersey; and two counties in northern Virginia. This means a Medicare beneficiary receiving services in the jurisdiction will have claims sent to that MAC (CMS, 2021).

Skilled Nursing Facility (SNF)—Technically defined by federal regulations, a long-term care facility that meets requirements of participation as a SNF, including 24-hr nursing care, social work, activities, and therapy services. SNFs are licensed by a state to operate a certain number of skilled beds. The SNF may be referred to as "subacute" or "postacute" care.

Long-Term Care—Residential care provided by licensed nurses 24 hr per day.

Omnibus Budget Reconciliation Act 1991 (OBRA)—The sweeping nursing home reform law that requires nursing homes to assure that a person admitted experiences no negative consequences that would not have happened in the community, mandated the use of the Minimum Data Set, and implemented the State Survey process (OBRA, 1987).

Minimum Data Set (MDS)—The federally required comprehensive assessment of each person admitted to a SNF. Sections relevant to SLPs include Section C which includes the Brief Inventory of Mental Status (BIMS; see Chapter 3 for additional discussion), Section K which considers swallowing difficulties and mechanically altered diets, and Section O which collects data about days and minutes of therapy service delivery (CMS, 2019).

State Survey—Annual review of systems and processes in the SNF to assure compliance with safety standards supporting the health and well-being of SNF residents. Conducted by the state health department, referenced against federal guidance. The regulations are often referred to as F-tags. Updates to the regulations are made every 2 to 6 years (CMS, 2022).

Secure Dementia Unit—Care model that provides care to patients with memory loss in a secure environment. Typically, the secure unit has enhanced programming and individualized care planning based on specific cognitive assessments.

Characteristics of Speech-Language Pathology Practice in the Skilled Nursing Facility

Since the 1980s, SNFs have been required to offer speech-language pathology services to their residents. Some SNFs employ SLPs directly, while others offer services via a contract with a provider of physical, occupational, and speech-language therapy. SNFs can range from 30 to more than 300 beds, and SLP staffing is often based on the census. An SLP in the SNF can be the only SLP in the department or may even provide services in more than one SNF. Typically, the SLP works Monday through Friday. Services may be supplemented by SLPs working as needed (PRN) shifts. As in other settings, SLPs working in the SNF are required to have a state license and are usually required to hold the American Speech-Language-Hearing Association Certificate of Clinical Competence or be completing their clinical fellowship (CF).

In recent years, the length of stay for patients in the SNF has been shrinking; a person receives services in the SNF for an average of 28 days (CMS, 2016). Depending on the payer's requirements and the clinical needs of the patient, the SLP may treat the patient 2 to 7 days per week. Patients may be admitted from home or from another SNF; however, most payers require a 3-day hospital stay prior to SNF admission. A wide variety of medical conditions may lead to the need for a SNF stay, including stroke, cardiovascular disease, progressive neurologic disorders, pulmonary disease, orthopedic injury, oncologic conditions, endocrine disorders, dementia, and COVID-19. Patients range in age from 18 to more than 99 years, though the majority are between 65 and 85 years (Health in Aging, 2020). Some SNFs involve the SLP in screening newly admitted patients to make a determination about any communication, cognition, or swallowing needs. Often, this may involve use of a formalized screening instrument such as the Saint Louis University Mental Status exam (Tariq et al,, 2006) or the Yale Swallow Protocol (Suiter et al., 2014) to assess the need for further evaluation. Speech-language pathology services beyond the screening require a physician's order that specifies the approaches, frequency, intensity, and duration of treatment.

Assessment and Intervention Considerations in a Skilled Nursing Facility

Cognitive Loss

Patients in the SNF may have cognitive loss varying from mild cognitive impairment to severe dementia. Downer et al. (2017) studied Medicare beneficiaries in 2013 and 2014 to determine the cognitive status of those discharged to a SNF with a hospital diagnosis of dementia. Their findings indicated:

> [N]early 60% of all beneficiaries were classified as cognitively intact on admission to a SNF, 22% were mildly impaired, 15.4% were mod-

erately impaired, and 3.4% were severely impaired. Among beneficiaries with a hospital diagnosis of dementia, 17.9% were classified
as cognitively intact, 25.8% were mildly impaired, 45% were moderately impaired, and 11.3% were severely impaired. The majority (65.6%) of beneficiaries with no hospital diagnosis of dementia
were classified as cognitively intact, 21.4% were mildly impaired,
10.9% were moderately impaired, and 2.2% were severely impaired.
(Downer et al., 2017)

Some SNFs offer a secure dementia unit that provides specific
interventions designed to address the needs of people with mod-
erate-to-severe impairment. Environmental modifications, activity programming, and clinical assessments (e.g., Brief Cognitive
Assessment Tool [2019]) and interventions (e.g., Montessori-based
approaches [Association Montessori Internationale, n.d.]) or Spaced
Retrieval Training (Benigas, 2015) are common in an SNF with a
secure dementia unit.

Aphasia and Dysarthria

Aphasia and dysarthria, which may occur following stroke or in
conjunction with progressive neurologic conditions like Parkinson's
disease, are common patient populations that an SLP working in a
SNF may encounter. Aphasia treatment focuses on functional communication, while addressing impairment-based deficits in verbal
and written expression and auditory and reading comprehension.

Motor speech production interventions may address respiration, phonation, articulation, and resonance with the target of
functional intelligibility with familiar and unfamiliar listeners. The
SLP administers standardized tests and measures to determine the
areas of focus and the level of deficit. SLPs provide training for
the patient, family, and caregivers on ways to support communication in various situations.

Some patients may benefit from augmentative and alternative
communication (AAC) systems, which may include supports ranging from a "lower-tech" communication board to "higher-tech"–
based digital options. Outside consultants may be enlisted to assess
the patient for the best match for their AAC needs, who would then
work with the primary SLP regarding implementation of the AAC
device. The primary SLP would then work with the patient and
their family to personalize the device for the patient's needs, such
as vocabulary selection.

The SLP in the SNF can deliver care for aphasia and dysarthria
individually or in a group, where two to six patients are engaged

in one activity with the purpose of achieving their individual goals for communication.

Dysphagia

Dysphagia care is primarily provided by SLPs in the SNF, although occupational therapists are sometimes involved in service delivery. As discussed in earlier chapters, dysphagia may be associated with stroke, progressive neurologic conditions, head and neck cancer, endocrine conditions, pulmonary conditions, sarcopenia, dementia, and many other medical conditions.

Clinical assessment of swallowing in the SNF may begin with a screening where the SLP determines whether a comprehensive evaluation is warranted. The clinical swallowing evaluation includes an oral mechanism exam, cranial nerve motor and sensory assessment, and presentation of food and liquid.

In the SNF, access to instrumental assessment of swallowing such as the modified barium swallow study (MBSS) or fiberoptic endoscopic evaluation of swallow (FEES) are typically offered through arrangement with a local hospital or via a contract with a mobile or portable provider of these services. The MBSS and FEES are subject to consolidated billing, meaning that the SNF is responsible for payment and billing. SLPs need to advocate for instrumental assessment of swallowing to accurately assess the structure and function of the swallowing mechanism.

The SLP's treatment of dysphagia in the SNF includes rehabilitation, compensation, and adaptation. Exercises, maneuvers, positioning, strategies, environmental modifications, and diet consistency modifications are commonly included in the patient's plan of treatment. Adjunctive tools such as electromyographic (EMG) biofeedback and neuromuscular electrical stimulation may be available to the SLP.

Diet modification is a common approach to dysphagia care in the SNF. Patients often state that they enjoy eating and wish to continue to eat despite risks for health complications. Patients have the right to make decisions concerning their medical treatment, including those involving consistency-altered foods and drinks. In most cases involving diet restrictions where the consistency or texture of food and drinks is altered, recommendations are preceded by an evaluation by the SLP that identifies swallowing difficulties. When assessing a patient's swallowing capabilities, the patient's health history and overall health status, cognition, preferences, and values are included to formulate the overall professional recommendation. Recommendations are presented to the patient or patient's decision maker, along with options that may be available to choose from. The SLP explains the risks and benefits of each choice, and then the plan of care is formulated. Other members of the interprofessional team such as nurse or social worker may also be involved in the education of the patient about the risks and benefits of any choices and must document any education or support provided in the medical record. The patient's physician is ultimately responsible for ordering diet consistencies as well as educating and having discussions with the patient and patient's decision maker and documenting conversations in the medical record. The physician then issues orders as appropriate. If a patient has a diet order in place that has been agreed upon following this process, and the patient changes from their initial decision, the professional staff should reeducate, document the discussion in the record, and contact the physician to inform them of the patient's status and request for a change.

Long-Term Ventilation Support and Tracheostomy

Patients requiring long-term ventilator support may be cared for in the SNF. SNFs with ventilator units represent a small percentage of SNFs, but when present, the SLP is involved in the care of patients with communication, cognition, and swallowing needs. Patients with a tracheostomy are also commonly cared for in SNFs. The SLP should have familiarity with speaking valves, be knowledgable of different kinds of trach tubes, and participate in any active trach weaning process. Nursing or respiratory therapy manage trach care, while SLPs may be trained to provide suctioning as the state practice act allows.

COVID-19

Beginning in March 2020, the COVID-19 pandemic became prominent in SNFs. Nationwide, the public health emergency led to closure of some SNFs altogether, created COVID-19 isolation units, and required testing and quarantine of newly admitted patients (Ouslander & Grabowski, 2020). Families were not allowed to visit, and patients experienced prolonged social isolation (Simard & Volicer, 2020). As in other medical settings, SLPs and other health care providers had to receive frequent testing and wear personal protective equipment, changing masks, gowns, gloves, and face shields in between patient visits.

Patients admitted to the SNF post-COVID-19 may present with cognitive deficits, along with speech, language, and swallowing difficulties. Long-term ventilation and decreased pulmonary function are associated with "brain fog," voice changes, and dysphagia. Additionally, social isolation required by health precautions affects quality of life with significant impact on SNF patients. Thus, SLPs are called on to facilitate communication and contact.

Interprofessional Collaboration in the Skilled Nursing Facility

The Nutritionist or Registered Dietitian

The nutritionist or registered dietitian is a key collaborator for the SLP in the SNF. While addressing dysphagia, the dietitian addresses that patient's nutritional status, considering factors such as medical history and current conditions, measurements such as weight and height, ability to swallow, food and fluid intake, laboratory values, and medications. The dietitian works closely with the director of food services and the kitchen staff to prepare meals according to menus and specifications for modified food or liquid textures. SLPs and dietitians may discuss the answers to Section K of the Minimum Data Set (MDS), which, as noted in the Key Terminology section, is part of the federally required comprehensive assessment of each person admitted to a SNF. Section K considers swallowing difficulties and mechanically altered diets.

Social Workers

Social workers and SLPs interact to support the patient's effective and appropriate discharge plan. In many settings, the social worker is designated to complete Section C of the MDS (Brief Inventory of Mental Status) and will consult with the SLP on other measures of cognitive status. Social workers are often the primary contact with the patient's family and legal health care decision makers.

Nursing Team

Nurses and nursing assistants provide care and treatment for patients on a 24-hr basis. Nurses deliver medications and serve as a primary contact with physicians and physician extenders. In many states, nurses are the only professionals who can receive orders from the physician. SLPs and nurses collaborate regarding the overall care plan for the patient, communication, cognition, and swallowing needs. Nursing assistants may use care approaches recommended by the SLP including provision of instructions during care, memory strategies, feeding, and mealtime assistance.

Therapy Team

SLPs work closely with physical therapy (PT) and occupational therapy (OT) professionals. The interprofessional rehabilitation team will discuss patients' mobility, self-care, communication, cognition, and swallowing, and using this shared information will make adjustments to a patient's plan of treatment. Meetings to discuss patients' status and discharge plan are usually held weekly. SLPs may deliver co-treatment with PT or OT when coordination between two disciplines will benefit the patient. In the SNF, the rehabilitation department director is often a PT, OT, or SLP.

Regulatory Issues Related to Billing, Reimbursement, and Documentation in the Skilled Nursing Facility

Federal Regulation

The OBRA in 1987 included significant reform in the way that SNFs are required to care for residents and set standards of care for the nursing home setting (OBRA, 1987). The tenets of OBRA suggest that the SNF is responsible to ensure that a resident does not experience a decline in function that they would not have otherwise experienced while residing in the community. Prior to this federal legislation, nursing homes were regulated by each state.

The government maintains quality measurement programs and rating systems based on the results of an annual survey completed by the state health department. The state survey is a federally required annual review of each SNF conducted by the state health department. The results of this survey are based on specific quality measures such as medication rates, falls, and wounds. A national five-star rating program and public reporting of findings helps potential residents and family members compare facilities. In 2016 and 2017, the CMS issued a work plan to promote improvements in care, refine infection control practices, and strengthen the capabilities of the SNF workforce. The work plan sets out requirements of participation allowing the SNF to admit patients and be reimbursed by various insurance companies. The requirements specified expectations for SNFs to demonstrate staff competencies, maintain an inventory of care capabilities, and meet timelines for documentation of the care plan for patients.

State Regulations

As previously mentioned, the state health department completes an annual survey of practices in each SNF based on federal regulations. The SLP may be involved in the state survey process through surveyors' review of documentation, interviews regarding patients, and participation in internal quality assurance and improvement efforts in preparation for the state survey.

All 50 states and the District of Columbia require a license to practice speech-language pathology in a SNF. CFs can be completed in the SNF, and most states have provisional or temporary licensure offering rules around supervision, activities, and documentation of the CF experience that are aligned with the American Speech-Language-Hearing Association CF experience.

Documentation

Admission to the SNF requires a 3-day qualifying hospital stay for Medicare beneficiaries. Traditional Medicare covers up to 100 days in the SNF if the patient is receiving skilled care. Skilled care is defined in the Medicare Benefit Policy Manual as the requirement for 5 days per week of at least 15 min of therapy per day, or daily nursing care for specific conditions such as infection, tube-feeding, wounds, or complex observation and assessment. Numerous other payers reimburse for care in the SNF environment, including Medicare Advantage, commercial insurance, Medicaid, and private payment. Payers may have different documentation requirements, but generally, documentation requirements include medical necessity and skilled care as evidenced in the evaluation, treatment encounter (daily) notes, progress notes every 10 visits or 30 days (whichever is sooner), and discharge summary. Some payers may also require periodic certification by the physician or physician extender. Skilled service is supported in documentation by describing what the SLP did that no other professional was qualified to do. Medical necessity is supported in documentation by describing why the SLP did what they did. Diagnosis selection, administration of standardized tests and measures, measurable and functional short- and long-term goals, and ongoing assessment of barriers to discharge are necessary components of the SLP's documentation.

Reimbursement in the Skilled Nursing Facility

Medicare A

In October 2019, Medicare payment for a skilled stay in the SNF changed to the Patient Driven Payment Model (PDPM). As long as the patient is receiving skilled care (nursing and/or rehabilitation), Medicare will pay for up to 100 days in a SNF after a 3-day qualifying hospital stay. According to Warren (2019), "PDPM reimburses for speech-language pathology services based on any combination of five factors: an acute neurological condition, a cognitive impairment, one or more of 10 comorbidities (for example, apraxia or dysphagia following cerebral infarction), a swallowing disorder, or a mechanically altered diet. SNF reimbursement is higher for a patient with all five factors as compared with only one or two."

Traditional Medicare Part A is an entitlement program where the beneficiary needs to be 65 years old or meet certain other conditions such as disability for 2 years or more, or Black Lung disease. Medicare Part A pays 100% of the cost for the first 21 days in the SNF, then a daily co-pay (established by CMS annually) is charged to the beneficiary. This co-pay may be covered by private coinsurance (CMS, 2022).

Medicare Advantage

Medicare beneficiaries have the option to subscribe to a Medicare Advantage program instead of using traditional Medicare Part A. Medicare Advantage plans are offered through private insurance companies such as United Health Care, Anthem, and Aetna. They may offer additional coverage such as payment for hearing aids or lower co-pays and deductibles for medications. When SNF care is needed, Medicare Advantage plans use a case management approach to make decisions about ongoing skilled care rather than the coverage decision coming from the staff at the SNF as it does with traditional Medicare. Medicare Advantage plans may follow the rules for PDPM payment or may instead pay for an episode of care at the SNF.

A subset of Medicare Advantage, the Bundled Payment Care Initiative (BPCI) combines hospitals, physicians, and SNFs in an effort to reduce the cost of care for certain diagnoses including joint replacement and cardiac care. CMS initiated BPCIs in 2016. BPCIs subcontract with a third-party convener such as NaviHealth or Remedy to apply clinical expertise to decision-making involving case management.

Managed Care and Commercial Insurance

Beneficiaries less than 65 years old or who do not meet Medicare eligibility requirements often have coverage through commercial insurance plans for a SNF stay. These plans usually offer case management for coverage decisions, and as with Medicare Advantage BPCIs, they can use care navigators such as NaviHealth or Remedy to perform this service on their behalf. They can pay for the patient's care in the SNF based on an episode of care, based on fee-for-service payment, or using daily rates that are based on the level of care and services that the patient receives such as the amount of therapy services delivered per day. When paying a daily rate for care and services, these insurance companies may limit the time per day or number of visits that speech-language pathology services are covered.

Medicaid

Medicaid is a federal program, administered in the states, that provides health care benefits to people with limited income and resources. When a patient in a SNF has exhausted their financial resources, they may apply for Medicaid benefits, and when the person qualifies, the stay in the SNF is paid for by Medicaid. If the patient is not eligible for other insurance like Medicare, Medicaid may also pay for therapy services. Each state may have different rules for Medicaid coverage of speech-language pathology services, including prior authorization, fee for services, case-mix methodology, or at the cost to the SNF. Increasingly, states are converting to a managed care approach for Medicaid benefits. Medicaid also pays the 20% co-payment for services furnished under Medicare Part B or Managed Medicare Part B.

Medicare B and Managed Medicare Part B

Medicare beneficiaries can choose to subscribe to Medicare Part B, an optional insurance program that pays for 80% of charges for medically necessary care from physicians and other outpatient services including speech-language pathology services. Medicare Part B requires a physician's certification of the SLP's plan of treatment in order to reimburse for services. Even when the patient resides in the SNF, services furnished under Medicare Part B are considered outpatient. Medicare beneficiaries who have elected to subscribe to a Medicare Advantage plan have the option of subscribing to Managed Medicare Part B. Most Managed Medicare Part B plans require prior authorization for speech-language pathology services, typically granted as a specific number of visits.

Medicare Part B reimburses for speech-language pathology services according to the CMS Medicare Physician Fee Schedule, which sets nationwide payments by Current Procedural Terminology (CPT)/Healthcare Common Procedure Coding System (HCPCS) codes. SLPs are reimbursed for services such as speech-language therapy, swallowing therapy, cognitive skills development, and various evaluation codes described in the Physician Fee Schedule. There are slight variations in the amount that is reimbursed based on geographic location in the United States and based on limits imposed by the particular MAC that processes the claims. Codes can be time-based (either per 15 min or per 1 hr) or service-based (one unit per day regardless of how much time the service is provided).

Spend a Typical Day With Michelle, SNF SLP

Michelle has been a licensed and certified SLP for 10 years. She is employed by a SNF full-time as their only SLP. Michelle has an electronic tablet to complete her documentation and record services as each encounter is taking place. Her SNF has four units on two floors and a census of 112 patients today. There is an SLP office where Michelle can treat patients, or she can see them in their rooms or common areas such as the dining room. She currently has 12 patients on her caseload. In Table 4–1, we see what a typical daily schedule might look like for Michelle.

Michelle delivers care based on her assessment of each patient's clinical needs. She requests orders from the physician for the specific frequency, intensity, and duration of her services. Michelle records services stating the precise minutes as regulations require her to do. Her productivity is measured by dividing the direct patient care time by her time in the facility. On this day, Michelle saw nine patients, completed one evaluation and conducted one group session with four patients.

Time	Activity	Treatment Duration
8:00 a.m.	*Clock in for the day*	
8:02 a.m.	*Prepare for the day* Complete COVID-19 protocol Review daily caseload list and schedule	
8:08 a.m.	*Encounter #1* Mr. C, 82 years old, dysphagia secondary to Parkinson's disease. Orders for 5 times per week for 4 weeks. Dysphagia therapy in Mr. C's room in Unit 1. Include sEMG biofeedback with effortful swallow, assessment of Mr. C's carryover of strategy for alternating solids and liquids.	54 min
9:05 a.m.	*Encounter #2* Mrs. L, 79 years old, mild cognitive impairment and expressive aphasia secondary to Left CVA. Orders for 5 times per week for 3 weeks. Language and cognition therapy in Mrs. L's room in Unit 1. Target problem-solving with functional scenarios as Mrs. L is planning to return home in 6 more days. Review Mrs. L's discharge plan with her and record her progress toward stated goals.	51 min
10:00 a.m.	*Interdisciplinary Consultation* Consult with the dietitian about a newly admitted patient Ms. H on Unit 2 who was reportedly pocketing food. Request physician's orders to evaluate swallowing.	
10:20 a.m.	*Encounter #3* Mr. B, 86 years old, expressive aphasia secondary to Left CVA. Orders for 5 times per week for 4 weeks. Language therapy in the SLP office with Mr. B. Focus on naming, description of function, and making choices. Readminister the Boston Naming Test.	46 min
11:15 a.m.	Attend Rehabilitation Department "stand-up" meeting to review clinical needs of newly admitted patients.	
11:30 a.m.	30-min lunch break	
12:03 p.m.	*Encounter #4* Mrs. S, 75 years old, dysphagia secondary to Multiple Sclerosis. Orders for 3 times per week for 8 weeks. Dysphagia therapy with Mrs. S in the dining room on Unit 3. Training for nursing assistants on positioning and how to cue the patient to take small bites/control volume and complete a lingual sweep after solids.	32 min

TABLE 4–1   *continued*

Time	Activity	Treatment Duration
12:38 p.m.	*Encounter #5*	69 min
	Ms. K, 72 years old, referred for evaluation by nursing when observed to cough after drinking water while taking medications, principal diagnosis of congestive heart failure.	
	Dysphagia evaluation in Ms. K's room on Unit 2. Obtained case history, performed oral mechanism exam, cranial nerve assessment, analysis of performance with food and drinks, discussion of the proposed plan with the patient.	
2:00 p.m.	*Encounter #6*	43 min
	Group therapy with four patients:	
	• Mr. J, 83 years old, Alzheimer's disease	
	• Mrs. P, 78 years old, Lewy Body dementia	
	• Mrs. R, 79 years old, dementia with Parkinson's disease	
	• Mrs. B, 80 years old, Right CVA	
	Cognitive group in the SLP office. Targets include sequencing, thought organization, problem-solving, executive function, and memory for the functional task of medication management.	
2:48 p.m.	*Encounter #7*	32 min
	Mr. J, 83 years old, Alzheimer's disease (also seen in group therapy session just prior). Orders for 5 times per week for 5 weeks. Cognitive linguistic therapy with Mr. J in the SLP office. Using BCAT Working Memory Exercise Book, target problem-solving, sequencing, and categorization.	
3:25 p.m.	*Encounter #8*	39 min
	Mrs. G, 65 years old, dysarthria secondary to traumatic brain injury, status post tracheostomy. Orders for 5 times per week for 6 weeks. Speech therapy with Mrs. G in the SLP office. Focus on pacing, overarticulation, and intelligibility with a familiar listener.	
4:05 p.m.	*Wrap up the day*	
	Complete documentation, review the services recorded, check orders requested earlier, examine the schedule for tomorrow.	
4:23 p.m.	*Clock out for the day*	

Conclusion

The SLP plays a key role in the SNF, delivering skilled and medically necessary services to patients with physician's orders. The long-term care industry is highly regulated in the United States, impacting the SLP's practice in the SNF through documentation requirements, licensure rules, and quality assurance processes. The SLP in the SNF has a diverse caseload, usually over age 65 years, with a variety of etiologies for the patients' communication, cognition, and swallowing capabilities and challenges. The SLP needs to be aware of payer parameters and the employer's instructions for recording services and documenting care. Care for patients in the SNF involves the use of standardized assessment measures, treatment materials, patient and caregiver education, interprofessional collaboration, and thoughtful discharge planning. The SLP may make referrals for instrumental assessment of swallowing and seek support from vendors and specialized SLPs when a patient needs AAC. Speech-language pathology services can be furnished to patients during a short-term stay, a long-term stay, and when the patient resides in a secure dementia unit. Overall, the SLP's work in the SNF involves forming relationships with other health care professionals, patients, and families to support the best possible quality of life and meet the patient's communication, cognition, and swallowing needs.

References

Association Montessori Internationale. (n.d.). *Montessori for Dementia & Ageing.* https://montessori-ami.org/about-montessori/montessori-dementia-ageing

Benigas, J. (2015). Spaced retrieval training: 26 years of growth. *Perspectives on Gerontology, 20*(1), 34–43.

Brief Cognitive Assessment Tool. (2019). *The BCAT test system.* https://www.thebcat.com/bcat-test-system

Centers for Medicare and Medicaid Services. (2016). *Medicare skilled nursing facility transparency data (CY2013).* https://www.cms.gov/newsroom/fact-sheets/medicare-skilled-nursing-facility-snf-transparency-data-cy2013#:~:text=%C3%82%20Nationally%2C%20the%20average%20standardized,of%20stay%20of%2028%20days

Centers for Medicare and Medicaid Services. (2019). *Long-term care facility resident assessment instrument 3.0 user's manual. Version 1.17.1.* https://www.cms.gov/Medicare/Quality-Initiatives-Patient-Assessment-Instruments/NursingHomeQualityInits/Other-Content-Types/

MDS-30-RAI-Manual-v1171-Replacement-Manual-Pages-and-Change-Tables_October-2019.pdf

Centers for Medicare and Medicaid Services. (2021). *Who are the MACs.* https://www.cms.gov/Medicare/Quality-Initiatives-Patient-Assessment-Instruments/NursingHomeQualityInits/Other-Content-Types/MDS-30-RAI-Manual-v1171-Replacement-Manual-Pages-and-Change-Tables_October-2019.pdf

Centers for Medicare and Medicaid Services. (2022, May 4). *Medicare benefit policy manual: Chapter 15—Covered medical and other health services.* https://www.cms.gov/Regulations-and-Guidance/Guidance/Manuals/Downloads/bp102c15.pdf

Centers for Medicare and Medicaid Services. (2022, June 7). *Nursing homes: Medicare and Medicaid programs: Reform of requirements for long-term care facilities.* https://www.cms.gov/Medicare/Provider-Enrollment-and-Certification/GuidanceforLawsAndRegulations/Nursing-Homes

Downer, B., Thomas, K. S., Mor, V., Goodwin, J. S., & Ottenbacher, K. J. (2017). Cognitive status of older adults on admission to a skilled nursing facility according to a hospital discharge diagnosis of dementia. *Journal of the American Medical Directors Association, 18*(8), 726–728.

Health in Aging. (2020). *Nursing homes.* https://www.healthinaging.org/age-friendly-healthcare-you/care-settings/nursing-homes#:~:text=Almost%20half%20of%20all%20people,than%2065%20years%20of%20age

Omnibus Budget Reconciliation Act (OBRA). Pub. L. N. 100–203 § 483.15 (1987). https://www.congress.gov/bill/100th-congress/house-bill/3545

Ouslander, J. G., & Grabowski, D. C. (2020). COVID-19 in nursing homes: Calming the perfect storm. *Journal of the American Geriatrics Society, 68*(10), 2153–2162. https://doi.org/10.1111/jgs.16784

Simard, J., & Volicer, L. (2020). Loneliness and isolation in long-term care and the Covid-19 pandemic. *Journal of the American Medical Directors Association, 21*(7), 966–967. https://doi.org/10.1016/j.jamda.2020.05.006

Suiter, D. M., Sloggy, J. A., & Leder, S. B. (2014). Validation of the Yale Swallow Protocol: A prospective double-blinded videofluoroscopic study. *Dysphagia, 29*, 199–203.

Tariq, S. H., Tumosa, N., Chibnall, J. T., Perry III, H. M., & Morley, J. E. (2006). The Saint Louis University Mental Status (SLUMS) examination for detecting mild cognitive impairment and dementia is more sensitive than the Mini-Mental Status Examination (MMSE)—A pilot study. *American Journal of Geriatric Psychology, 14*, 900–910. https://www.slu.edu/medicine/internal-medicine/geriatric-medicine/aging-successfully/assessment-tools/mental-status-exam.php

Warren, S. (2019). Mechanically altered diets are a factor in new SNF payment system. *ASHA Leader, 24*, 11.

CHAPTER 5

Care Transitions

Clinical Reasoning

Clinical Practice Settings

Neuroimaging

Pharmacology

Speech-Language Pathology Services in Home Health Care Settings

Megan L. Malone and Jennifer Loehr

Chapter Objectives

Upon completion of this chapter, the reader will be able to:

- Describe the history and evolution of home health care.
- Describe the current Medicare reimbursement model for home health care.
- Describe the different services offered by Medicare-certified home health agencies.
- Define the criteria for eligibility of home health services.
- Describe the different roles speech-language pathologists can serve in the home health care setting.
- Describe the process of initiation of care and care planning in home health care.
- Provide examples of how to complete assessment in home health care.

117

- Discuss how to write and develop goals for patients treated in home care.
- List treatment considerations and strategies for the home care setting.
- Describe documentation requirements for home health care.
- Identify several personal safety measures for consideration in home health care.

Introduction

Home health care is a method of providing skilled care to patients in their homes under the direction of a physician. Home health programs include nursing care, therapy, and medical social services. The goal of the home health care program is to help individuals live with greater independence by improving overall functioning in their home. Skilled practitioners including speech-language pathologists (SLPs), nurses, physical therapists (PTs), and occupational therapists (OTs) work to keep patients safely aging in place by promoting an optimal level of well-being and avoiding hospitalization or admission to long-term care institutions. Patients receiving home health services may be living in private residences or residing in a nonskilled facility such as an independent or assisted living facility. Caring for patients in their living environment provides a unique opportunity for the SLP to gain an intimate connection with patients and families that is often not possible in other health care settings. SLPs can offer skilled services with a laser focus on goals and care plans that are meaningful and practical for the patient, family, or caregiver. Home health care can be provided to both pediatric and adult patients. This chapter focuses on working with adults in the home care setting, with many of the areas discussed also having application to home health care with pediatric patients. The reader is encouraged to seek out resources specifically related to pediatric patients if interested in working with that population in the home care setting.

History of Home Health Care

Home health care began at the beginning of the 20th century with visits made to homebound individuals through volunteer groups composed mainly of physicians and nurses. Charitable donations were the main source of funding for in-home services provided to patients who were too sick or infirm to access care outside their homes. As the demand for care of the sick and elderly population grew, additional volunteer services were offered to include physical therapy and social work and proved to be successful in maintaining patient's health and responsible for a significant decrease in mortality rates. In the 1960s, the Medicare and Medicaid programs began to offer reimbursement for these services as an added benefit for beneficiaries. This reimbursement opportunity allowed for home health agencies to expand services to include speech-language pathology, occupational therapy, home health aide services, behavioral health nurses, registered dietician consultation, and so forth, thus creating a broader, holistic approach to care.

How Home Health Agencies Operate

Home health agencies operate as either a public or private entity. A public agency is operated by a state or local government. Examples include state-operated home health agencies (HHAs) and county hospitals. For regulatory purposes, "public" means "governmental." Nonprofit agencies are private (i.e., nongovernmental). These HHAs are often supported, in part, by private contributions or other philanthropic sources, such as foundations. Examples include the nonprofit visiting nurse associations and Easter Seal societies, as well as nonprofit hospitals. A proprietary agency is a private, profit-making agency or profit-making hospital that makes up most home health agencies in the United States.

Today, a large proportion of care that home health agencies deliver is geriatric care. However, home health care plays an important role for patients of all ages with significant acute and chronic illnesses. The U.S. Census projects that by 2030, the proportion of U.S. residents older than age 65 years will have nearly doubled from 2010 (20% vs. 13%) (Ortman et al., 2016). Among the oldest Americans, the census predicts that the population age 85 years and older will double by 2036 and triple by 2049 (MedPAC, 2016), which is why home health care is one of the fastest growing segments in the health care industry. In 2018, there were 11,869 Medicare-certified home health agencies throughout the United States serving 5,125,575 homebound beneficiaries totaling an estimated $103 billion. This number is predicted to reach at least $173 billion by 2026 (CMS, 2018a).

Currently, there is no limit to the volume of services that can be provided to patients if regulations and policies set by governmental oversight agencies are followed (which is addressed later in this chapter). Skilled practitioners develop a plan of care based on discipline-specific evaluations; this plan is then approved by an attending physician. This is similar to most models of care; however, unlike inpatient care, oversight and direct involvement by the physician are limited and require the home health practitioners to manage care through frequent and indirect communication with the attending physician.

The patient care plan is built within an episode of care that is currently a 60-day period. The amount of care and resources are determined at the beginning of care through the Outcome and Assessment Information Set (OASIS), which is a standardized data collection tool that looks at all aspects of patient need regarding level of functioning, physical barriers, community access, diagnosis, and so forth. A patient can be receiving services for multiple episodes of care concurrently or intermittently depending on need. The care and services provided for the patient are calculated at different time periods in the episode (every 30 days) and submitted for reimbursement.

Reimbursement in Home Health Care

The home health care industry has undergone many evolutions over multiple decades regarding reimbursement. As mentioned earlier, these services were initially provided by volunteers, relying on donations from the public. Once social security became a reality, it was not long before home care was included as part of the benefit to Medicare recipients and is the single largest payer for home health services in the United States. Traditionally, reimbursement was offered following the "fee for service" model that allowed for agencies to add on necessary services, as needed, for the patient's plan of care. Currently, this model is evolving toward a "bundled" model of payment that reimburses agencies in lump sums for care given to patients with a focus on quality care and outcomes.

The care, including all resources, provided to a patient is planned and implemented within a 60-day period, or episode of care. A patient can be on service for multiple episodes concurrently or intermittently depending on need. The care and services provided for the patient are calculated at different time periods in the episode (every 30 days) and submitted to the insurance company for reimbursement. Currently, the model for reimbursement is dependent on the patient's diagnosis or clinical characteristics. The Patient Driven Groupings Model (PDGM) adds additional opportunities for payment adjustment including referral source (i.e., is the patient admitting from a hospital or the community?), level of functioning of the patient, comorbidities present, and timing of the episode (whether this is the first or subsequent episode of care).

Patients can receive one or all of these services depending on the complexity of their condition and are reimbursed, in whole or in part, by Medicare, Medicaid, the Veterans Administration, or private insurance. Medicare reimburses 100% for services provided by home health agencies with no out-of-pocket expense to patients. Medicaid, the Veterans Administration, and most private insurance companies also reimburse for these services, some at the same rate as Medicare but most applying limitations to services and reimbursement. All home health agencies must adhere to very strict regulations to ensure that the services provided are appropriate and the patient qualifies to receive these services in order to accept reimbursement.

Regulation

Governmental oversight of health care has become complex over the years, and the home health industry is now highly regulated and closely monitored by state and federal agencies. There are a myriad of rules and regulations that are strictly enforced to ensure that the services provided are effective and safe for the patients. For the SLP to successfully provide home care, it is important to have an understanding about these rules and regulations to ensure that treatment provided complies and is reimbursable. Of course, it is up to the home health agency to ensure that the SLP has the most up-to-date information regarding regulations, and it is up to the SLP to make sure that their practice falls in line with their state practice act.

Home health agencies are highly regulated by local, state, and federal agencies as well as the Centers for Medicare and Medicaid Services (CMS) to ensure patient safety, quality care delivery, and reimbursement parameters are met. CMS maintains oversight for compliance with the Medicare health and safety standards for home health agencies serving Medicare and Medicaid beneficiaries, and makes available to beneficiaries, providers/suppliers, researchers, and state surveyors information about these activities.

CMS developed the Conditions of Participation (CoPs) and Conditions for Coverage (CfCs) that health care organizations must meet in order to begin and continue to receive Medicare and Medicaid reimbursement. These health and safety standards are the foundation for improving quality and protecting the health and safety of beneficiaries (CMS, 2013). The rules apply to all agencies across the United States and are regulated by various local, state, and federal agencies. Some examples of what is included in the CoPs include specific guidelines for documentation, eligibility requirements for patients, care plan development, and care coordination/communication between the SLP and the attending physician.

Eligibility

In addition to ensuring that home health agencies follow regulations and guidelines set for reimbursement, CMS also closely monitors agencies to ensure that patients are eligible to receive these services. Although most private insurance companies provide some reimbursement for home health care, most companies use eligibility requirements established by Medicare. Eligibility criteria are provided at https://www.medicare.gov/coverage/home-health-services and are outlined as follows (CMS, 2019):

1. Patients must be under the care of a physician and receiving services under a plan of care created and reviewed regularly by a physician.
2. Patients must be 18 years or older.
3. Patients may not participate in services that are intermittent or part time.
4. A physician must certify that one or more of the following are applicable:
   a. Intermittent skilled nursing care is needed.
   b. Physical therapy, occupational therapy, or speech-language pathology services are needed.
   c. The amount, frequency, and time period of the services needs to be reasonable, and they need to be complex or determine that only qualified therapists can do them safely and effectively.

d. The patient's condition must be expected to improve in a reasonable and generally predictable period.

e. Patients need a skilled therapist to safely and effectively make a maintenance program for the condition.

f. The home health agency must be Medicare certified.

g. The physician must certify that the patient is homebound. Patients who are homebound are allowed to leave home for short periods of time for medical care and to attend to personal needs, infrequent family events, religious services, or adult day care.

Outcome and Assessment Information Set (OASIS)

The OASIS is a comprehensive assessment designed to collect information related to a patient's health and functional status. The OASIS was developed to provide the data to CMS that are necessary to measure outcomes and patient risk factors. As a result, the OASIS is a key component of outcome measurement and performance improvement and is used to determine reimbursement for care and resources provided by the home health agency.

The OASIS data items address sociodemographic, environmental, support system, health status, functional status, and health service utilization characteristics of the patient. Information is collected at the start of care, 60-day follow-ups, and discharge. The process for administering the OASIS is very lengthy, with over 100 questions related to the patient's past and current functional status. The data collected are detailed and require the SLP to assess systems and functions outside the traditional patient evaluation, such as toileting, bathing, skin integrity, and medication regimen, to name a few. Although the SLP is asked to look at patient aspects that are not normally considered within the SLP scope of practice, the OASIS data collection is supported by the American Speech-Language-Hearing Association (ASHA) as long as the SLP feels competent and confident in the task (Brown, 2017). Although the SLP is recording only objective data through patient/caregiver interview and observation, clinicians should be sure that they are well equipped and educated on the process, as there are specific rules or "conventions" that must be adhered to. It is recommended that clinicians receive OASIS training prior to performing the OASIS assessment to ensure accuracy and efficiency. Most home health agencies offer clinicians specific training on OASIS data collection. Additionally, there are several private continuing education companies that offer specific OASIS training and certification.

Quality Outcome and Patient Satisfaction Ratings

Beginning in July 2015, the Quality of Patient Care Star Ratings were introduced by CMS as a tool to assist people (e.g., family members, caregivers, payers, health care systems, and care organizations) in evaluating home health agencies. This system of reporting is how many patients, physicians, and hospitals choose which agency they wish to partner with by accessing data on the internet (https://www.medicare.gov/homehealthcompare/search .html). The Star Rating summarizes the performance of a home health agency's patient care by displaying information from several different measures in one simple format. The data that comprise the Star ratings come from the OASIS assessments completed at various times during an episode of care. These data help CMS and the public see how agencies are doing in assisting patients with improving function (i.e., ambulating, breathing, transferring) as well as promoting processes to ensure that patients avoid rehospitalization or general decline. There are incentives and penalties for low-performing agencies including an impact on the volume of patients referred to an agency.

In January 2016, the Patient Survey Star Rating (also known as the Home Health CAHPS Star Rating [HHCAHPS]) was added to Home Health Compare. The HHCAHPS uses feedback from surveys of home health patients and caregivers. The Quality of Patient Care Star Ratings can be used together with the HHCAHPS Star Ratings to provide a more comprehensive view of the quality of care provided by a home health agency (CMS, 2016).

Role of Speech-Language Pathologists in Home Health Care

SLPs can play many different roles in the home health care setting. These roles can include clinician/clinical specialist, case manager, educator, collaborator, and advocate, as well as a marketer of services to referral sources and auditor of documentation (Malone & Loehr, 2018). In the role of clinician, SLPs implement the scope of practice dictated by the ASHA, which includes "optimiz[ing] individuals' abilities to communicate and to swallow, thereby improving quality of life" (ASHA, 2016c, p. 5) through the use of evidence-based practice.

SLPs bring a unique skill set to all care settings, but the skilled knowledge of the SLP is particularly impactful to the home care setting. An SLP's strong communication skills, ability to collaborate with others, and ability to translate complex information in a meaningful and understandable manner to patients, caregivers, and other disciplines are of particular importance in home care. This is because the patient and caregivers are acclimating to the home environment following a change in medical status or a hospital or rehabilitation stay, while continuing to cope with either short- or long-term deficits from varying health conditions. In contrast to settings such as inpatient care in hospitals and rehabilitation facilities where patients are monitored continuously by skilled services and provided with assistance with ongoing medical care, patients being seen by home health agency staff are seen less frequently and must implement recommendations more independently. This requires disciplines working in home health, including the SLP, to provide, on an ongoing basis during visits, instruction and education regarding how to maintain or improve overall health and safety, along with recommendations for specific treatment areas. These actions safeguard the patient to remain in the home until they are no longer homebound and can either discontinue skilled services or begin outpatient treatment to continue progress toward identified areas of need.

SLPs in home health can be part of the care team for a patient, serving the role of clinician to assist patients in improving areas of deficit such as difficulties in swallowing, speech, and cognition. In this capacity, if the patient's physician has identified that the patient requires the skilled services of an SLP, an order for evaluation and/or treatment is generated, and the SLP would complete these services in conjunction with the home care agency and the other disciplines from the agency (nursing, physical therapy, occupational therapy, social work, etc.) ordered by the physician to implement care in the home. As a clinician in home care, SLPs perform the skilled services expected in other care settings, such as screening, assessment, and treatment of patients, as well as perform services related to advocacy, prevention and wellness, collaboration, and counseling. Again, the roles of advocate, educator, collaborator, and counselor are particularly pivotal to the home care setting due to the patient's care occurring outside of an established medical facility. Often the disciplines treating the patient in the home may be the only individuals interacting with the patient on a regular basis, making it vital that the roles beyond that of a treating clinician are implemented so the patient remains healthy and safe in the home.

The SLP may also play the role of manager of patient care. Care management includes ongoing monitoring of the patient's health status, identification of changes in the patient's medical conditions, ensuring the patient is maintaining homebound status, and communication of any changes to these areas to the home care agency and the patient's physician. It also includes ongoing education and instruction to the patient and caregivers and documentation of all changes observed and recommendations provided. One scenario when the SLP may play the role of case manager is if the patient is only being seen by the SLP from the home health agency, and other disciplines are not involved in the case. For example, if the patient's physician has identified that the patient only requires skilled treatment related to swallowing deficits, the physician may generate orders to a home care agency for speech pathology services only. In this situation, the SLP would then complete the OASIS assessment for the patient, complete the necessary evaluation measures related to swallowing deficits and/or other aspects in the SLP scope of practice, and manage the patient's care for the care episode. If during completion of the OASIS assessment or at any other point during the patient's episode of care, the SLP identifies additional areas of need that should be evaluated or treated by another discipline (e.g., identifies a wound that would require nursing to become involved or a balance issue that would require physical therapy services), then the SLP would document these needs and communicate to the physician that additional skilled services are required. The SLP would then continue to manage the patient's care with these additional services involved.

An additional role a SLP may fulfill in the home health setting may include marketing of the home care agencies' services to referral sources such as physicians, assisted living facilities, or hospitals. In this capacity, the SLP may meet with these referral sources to provide greater insight and detail regarding the services the agency may provide, including specific information regarding speech-language pathology services. Again, due to the unique skill set of SLPs which includes the ability to clearly communicate information to a variety of individuals, SLPs are well suited to serve in the role as a marketer for an agency. Participating in this role can provide even greater support to the pivotal aspects SLPs can offer to an agency, beyond that of being a treating clinician only.

Documentation of services provided, education given, and collaborative efforts that occur is important in all care settings, as is regular review of the quality of services provided. Often, home care agencies participate in ongoing reviews of documentation from all disciplines within the agency to ensure it meets regulatory standards and provides a detailed description and justification for services provided. Agencies must also participate in regular review of Quality Assurance and Performance Improvement (QAPI) as part of the CoPs by Medicare. SLPs can and should participate in the roles of auditor of documentation as well as collaborator on the agency's QAPI committee. The skills required for both roles are those that SLPs are also likely to perform well due to rigorous training in areas such as attention to detail, how to clearly communicate information, problem-solving, and the ability to critically evaluate information to ensure it supports a given idea, goal, or recommendation. Like that of the role of marketer, SLPs who assist in the review and auditing of documentation and participate in performance improvement within a home care agency provide greater support to the vital role SLPs play in not only patient care but also assisting the agency in other aspects that keep an agency's doors open, which can lead to better outcomes, reimbursement, and improved Star ratings.

Initiation of Care and Care Planning in Home Health

Home health care involves some unique aspects to beginning care with a patient and care planning. Once eligibility has been established (see Eligibility section for more information), the patient may be seen by the disciplines ordered by the physician in the certified home health agency, which includes the services of an SLP. All patient care and services provided through home care must always be coordinated and approved by the patient's physician. Skilled services provided by a home care agency are provided in 60-day increments known as certification periods or episodes of care. As stated earlier in this chapter, home care services provided for the patient are calculated at different time periods in the 60-day certification period or episode (i.e. every 30 days) and submitted for reimbursement. The case manager of the patient's care (either a nurse, PT, or SLP) must complete the OASIS assessment prior to the other disciplines ordered to see the patient complete their evaluations. This is to collect the data required by Medicare to establish patient level of ability and need in a variety of areas to track outcomes of the care provided. Once the OASIS assessment is complete, the additional disciplines ordered to provide care may evaluate the patient.

The number of visits needed by each discipline to treat the patient is determined following each discipline's evaluation of the patient and is communicated to the patient's physician for approval of the amount and frequency of visits requested. This is known as a visit pattern. Each discipline seeing a patient has a separate visit pattern listing the frequency and duration of services the discipline will provide during the certification period. For example, if a patient requires services from a nurse, a PT, and an SLP, the physician will need to approve three different visit patterns provided by each discipline. Visit patterns are typically written with numbers to represent the number of visits per week and for how many weeks the patient will be seen by a discipline, using the abbreviation of "w" to represent "week." For example, a visit pattern listed as 1w2, 2w4, 1w3 would represent a frequency and duration of one visit a week for 2 weeks, two visits a week for 4 weeks, and one visit a week for 3 weeks during the 60-day certification period.

Determination of the number of visits needed to treat a patient depends on a variety of factors. These include severity level of the patient's impairment(s), patient's risk for rehospitalization related to the areas of treatment focus (i.e., "how safe is the patient related to treatment area?"), the number of disciplines involved in care and amount of visits ordered by those disciplines, patient and family schedule (e.g., patient is scheduled for several medical visits outside of home, such as dialysis), and level of caregiver burnout (Malone & Loehr, 2018).

Coordination of care and communication among disciplines are pivotal to determining visit patterns when the patient is first certified for care, when care is resumed due to an inpatient stay (hospital, skilled nursing, etc.) of greater than 24 hr, or when the patient is recertified at the end of a 60-day period in order to provide the best and most needed care to the patient while not overwhelming the patient or family. Provided in Figure 5–1 are some suggestions for strategies to determine visit patterns in home health care.

A final important aspect to care planning in home health care is the scheduling of visits to treat the patient. This is often a difficult task, particularly when several disciplines are involved, the patient is medically fragile and fatigues easily, or the patient requires the presence of a caregiver in order to provide instruction and education regarding patient care and implementation of recommendations. Patients often cite overscheduling of visits and lack of knowledge of the care schedule as top complaints when receiving home care services (Home Care Pulse, 2013). Scheduling of visits requires clear communication and coordination among all disciplines involved in treating a patient, keeping the needs of the patient and their benefit from services as the highest priorities. Using the strategies suggested in Figure 5–1 regarding establishing visit patterns should be assistive in proper scheduling of the patient. Additional strategies that may assist with this process include using an electronic scheduling tool/calendar as part of the patient's electronic medical record so that disciplines can see when other visits are scheduled and plan their visits accordingly, as well as having a paper version of the calendar in the patient's home so that the patient, caregivers, and other disciplines can easily access it to know when visits are scheduled. Disciplines should

---

Strategies for Determining Visit Patterns

- Stagger introduction of disciplines
  - ○ Evaluating discipline should determine at Start of Care the patient's level of severity, examine disciplines ordered by physician, and make recommendations to physician if all disciplines ordered are required to see patient at beginning of certification period or if staggering disciplines would be more beneficial.
  - ○ Evaluating discipline may identify need for other disciplines to be involved in plan of care but should discuss when orders for additional disciplines should be sought and/or request start dates from physician for those evaluations to be further into certification period.
  - ○ Each discipline can complete evaluation visit and determine level of severity and discuss which disciplines are priorities to begin services.
  - ○ If patient is overwhelmed at time of Start of Care with number of visits, physician can be notified, and orders to reschedule evaluations to a later date or to initiate other disciplines later in the certification period can be requested.

- Discuss with team number of visits projected and if that number is feasible for the patient factoring in patient schedule, patient fatigue, and level of caregiver support or burnout.

Communication Among Disciplines Is Key When Determining Visit Patterns!

FIGURE 5–1. Strategies for determining visit patterns.

regularly update both the electronic and paper calendars as schedule changes occur to ensure it is up to date for all who need the information. Each discipline should also call the patient the night before a visit or a few hours prior to the visit to make sure the patient is available and feeling well enough for a visit. A suggestion for SLPs is to possibly schedule visits during meals, as these can be ideal times to address a variety of goals related to swallowing, speech, language, and cognition. Mealtimes are often when other disciplines such as physical therapy, are unlikely to work with a patient, which opens up this time for the SLP to treat the patient effectively, without interrupting the schedule of the other disciplines involved in care (Malone & Loehr, 2018).

International Classification of Functioning, Disability, and Health

A useful tool in developing a patient care plan is the International Classification of Functioning, Disability, and Health (ICF). The ICF, developed by the World Health Organization (WHO) in 2001, is a holistic care-planning model for children and adults. The ICF framework (Figure 5–2) can be used in interprofessional collaborative practice and person-centered care in the scope of practice for speech-language pathology (ASHA, 2019g).

In the practice of home health care, the use of the ICF in care plan development encourages clinicians to consider factors that would influence progress of the patient toward meaningful and practical goals that are very patient specific. Influencing factors (both positive and negative) can be built into the care plan to help justify services and the decisions made to alter the care plan, if necessary. Examples of influencing factors are barriers within the patient's living environment (physical or financial), religious beliefs, education level, and caregiver or patient attitude.

Case Study: Utilization of the International Classification of Functioning, Disability, and Health in Care Plan Development

The following is an example of a case study to help illustrate the use of the ICF in developing a multidisciplinary care plan.

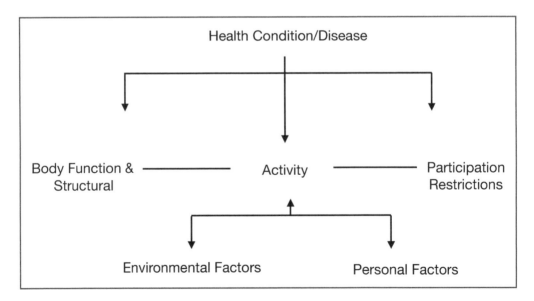

FIGURE 5–2. *Source:* Adaptation of the International Classification of Functioning, Disability, and Health (ICF) Framework. https://www.who.int/standards/classifications/international-classification-of-functioning-disability-and-health

Patient "Mr. WA" is a 78-year-old male who suffered a right-hemisphere cerebral vascular accident (CVA) and was admitted to a home health agency following 2 weeks in an inpatient skilled nursing facility. Patient suffers left hemiplegia, currently uses a wheelchair, and has left visual neglect, mild oral-pharyngeal dysphagia, mild cognitive deficits with short-term memory loss, and motor speech deficits. Mr. WA has no significant comorbidities, however, is now taking multiple medications since the onset of his CVA, including blood thinners. Mr. WA has additional diagnoses of chronic obstructive pulmonary disease (COPD), diabetes, and arthritis. He lives with his wife in a rural area of town, and only his wife is available for assistance. He relies on public transportation to get to medical appointments and do his shopping. Prior to his stroke, he was very active in his church, attending services weekly. Mr. WA has a third-grade education with limited literacy. He is on a very limited income and cannot afford an additional caregiver and reports he cannot afford home repairs or healthy food. The bus stop is 500 ft from his front door on an uneven gravel road. His home is one level; however, he has eight steps up to his front door without handrails. There is minimal lighting throughout the house with no working lights in the kitchen. The home is very cluttered with excessive stacks of magazines and newspapers throughout, creating barriers into the kitchen, bathroom, and bedroom. During the comprehensive assessment (OASIS), Mr. WA was asked what his goal is for discharge. He stated, "I want to get back to living independently and go to church again."

Keeping the patient's overall goal in mind, the SLP must take all of the information from the ICF (Figure 5–3) and together with the rest of the care team, decide what are the priorities and how best to provide care. Safety in the home and reducing the risk for harm, decline, and rehospitalization would be the priority for this patient. While the PTs and OTs may be focused on improving ambulation, the SLP can develop cognitive strategies to ensure that Mr. WA is able to follow the strategies for safe ambulation in the home. In addition, the SLP would focus on goals that would allow him to safely access and take medications as well as prepare food properly for safe oral intake. Additionally, the SLP may be involved in assisting Mr. WA with cognitive strategies that will allow him to access the bus so that he can once again return to the community and what is most meaningful to him.

Case Study: SLP Care Planning in Home Health

Building off of the prior case study, the following will provide examples of decision-making points of the SLP when care planning for this patient, Mr. WA.

Case Study: Patient Summary:

1. **Health Condition:** CVA

2. **Activity Limitations:** Ambulation, Cognition, Swallowing, Vision, Speech

3. **Participation Restrictions:**
   - Following medication regimen
   - Preparing food following safe swallow guidelines
   - Ambulating safely into and throughout home
   - Access to community for food, social needs, medications, medical care

4. **Environmental Barriers:**
   - Stairs into home
   - Safe access within home due to clutter and poor lighting
   - Limited finances

5. **Personal Factors:**
   - Patient's faith and reliance on church
   - Third grade education
   - Wife is overwhelmed by care responsibilities

FIGURE 5–3. Case study: patient summary.

Patient Summary: Mr. WA continues to present with difficulties post rehabilitation stay related to safety, medication management, management of diabetes, ambulation, balance, transfers, swallowing, expressive/receptive language deficits, cognitive deficits, and motor speech difficulties. Primary physician initially orders home health care for the patient for skilled nursing, physical therapy, and speech-language pathology.

Establishment of Eligibility: Home health agency receives physician orders and schedules skilled nursing to complete initial evaluation and OASIS assessment. Nursing determines the patient meets eligibility requirements for home care services, including homebound status and need for skilled services. Nursing sets a visit pattern for skilled nursing visits for 3w3, 2w4, 1w2 (three visits a week for 3 weeks, two visits a week for 4 weeks, and one visit a week for 2 weeks) for the initial certification period. Nursing also orders a home health aide for 3 days a week for 4 weeks to assist with personal care. Physical therapy completes an evaluation the following day and determines a needed visit pattern of 2w7 (two visits per week for 7 weeks) to address ambulation, transfers, and balance. Nursing determines that skilled care from a nurse is pivotal to ensure control and management of diabetes, management of new medications, and education and support to the caregiver regarding many aspects of care, as the patient's wife is very overwhelmed with the role of primary caregiver. Physical therapy agrees to wait to establish treatment orders with the physician until after speech pathology has evaluated the patient.

Speech-Language Pathology Evaluation/Decision Points: The SLP evaluates the patient on Day 3 of episode. Evaluation results determine Mr. WA has moderate impairments in speech and language expression, difficulty processing and following directions, memory deficits, and mild oral-pharyngeal dysphagia. The SLP also notes the high level of stress on Mr. WA's wife and her reported frustration in having difficulty understanding the patient. Mr. WA's wife also reports difficulty in her husband following recommended swallowing/diet recommendations established by the SLP upon discharge from the inpatient rehabilitation facility, resulting in frequent choking and coughing.

Decision Point One: Determination of speech-language pathology visit pattern needed to help patient/caregiver meet goals. The SLP must examine Mr. WA's level of severity, possible impact on safety, and risk for rehospitalization due to identified areas of deficit. The SLP must also account for reported and observed levels of caregiver stress related to these areas. Upon completion of evaluation and examination of those areas, the SLP determines Mr. WA's goals and the number of visits best needed for him to meet these goals, establishing a possible visit pattern of 2w5, 1w3 (two visits a week for 5 weeks and one visit a week for 3 weeks). The SLP meets with the home health agency, nurse, and PT and communicates evaluation findings and recommendations.

Decision Point Two: Interdisciplinary team evaluation and treatment planning. Nursing needs are identified as a priority, maintaining the visit pattern established by the nurse at the start of care. Mr. WA is currently in a wheelchair, and urinary and bowel functions are being addressed by his wife and home health aide with a bedside commode and incontinence products. It is determined that speech pathology services are also a priority at the beginning of the treatment period due to swallowing deficits, particularly due to Mr. WA's established respiratory issues. Physical therapy agrees to adjust the visit pattern to one visit per week for the first 3 weeks of treatment period to allow focus on nursing, personal care, and speech pathology goals. Care planning discussion is documented and both SLP and PT request orders from physician for determined visit patterns.

Decision Point 3: Determination of need for occupational therapy evaluation and when in episode the evaluation should occur.

Following approval of the visit pattern, SLP begins treatment of established goals following the established visit pattern. Upon initiation of treatment, SLP observes Mr. WA having difficulties with fine motor skills and personal care/completion of activities of daily living (ADLs) and discusses deficits noted with Mr. WA's wife and home health aide. SLP communicates with the home care agency and nurse that an evaluation for occupational therapy is needed. It is agreed that occupational therapy should evaluate the patient early in the episode to determine if services are needed immediately or if they can be held until later in the episode. The SLP documents discussion and requests an order for occupational therapy evaluation from the physician to occur during the following week once nursing and speech pathology visits are established.

Decision Point 4: Nurses, PTs, and SLPs determine how and when to schedule visits. The disciplines decide to schedule visits on different days, with the PT scheduling one visit for the first 3 weeks on a day when the nurse visits to allow for patient recovery and to reduce caregiver stress. Established visit times are written on a calendar in the patient's home and in a calendar in the patient's electronic medical record. Occupational therapy evaluation is scheduled for the second week of the episode and is scheduled for a day when nursing visits, but not on the same day as physical therapy, to again allow for patient recovery and to reduce caregiver burden. It is determined that occupational therapy services are needed but can be initiated later in the episode, as the OT has provided some recommendations and strategies for the patient and caregiver to use until services are initiated.

Decision Point 5: Determination of discharge of SLP services. The patient demonstrates rapid progress in priority areas for speech-language pathology services, meeting established goals by Week 5 of the certification period. Upon discussion with the care team, it is determined the SLP will discharge services to allow for an increase in physical therapy visits and initiation of occupational therapy. The SLP provides recommendations for Mr. WA and his wife to continue maintenance of progress. Additional disciplines will monitor the patient to determine if speech therapy services should be resumed in the future.

Common Patients and Conditions in Home Health

SLPs often enjoy a wide variety of different diagnoses and conditions to work with in the home health care setting. Patients receiving home health services frequently have multiple diagnoses and comorbidities that can add an additional challenge for the home health agency when developing a plan of care that will ensure that all of the patient's needs are addressed. With recent changes in the Medicare reimbursement system, it is very important that the patient diagnosis be identified early in the episode (prior to submitting the OASIS to CMS), as reimbursement is primarily determined by category of diagnosis (i.e., neurologic, musculoskeletal, respiratory, etc.). It is important that *all* possible diagnoses (primary and comorbid) are included in the documentation. Each home health agency has a system in place to manage optimal coding for accurate billing.

The National Outcomes Measurement System (NOMS) is a voluntary data collection registry that shows the value of SLP services. According to the NOMS data collected from ASHA members in 2019, the top five primary medical diagnoses of home care clients are as follows:

1. Cerebral vascular accident: 63%
2. Central nervous system diseases: 8%
3. Respiratory diseases: 5%
4. Hemorrhage/injury: 3%
5. Other neoplasm: 2% (ASHA, 2019d)

Furthermore, the top five functional communication measures scored by SLPs working in home care (i.e., functional areas treated in home care) according to the NOMS data collected from ASHA members in 2019 are as follows:

1. Swallowing: 54%
2. Spoken language expression: 37%
3. Motor speech: 29%
4. Spoken language: 26%
5. Memory: 15% (ASHA, 2019d)

SLPs may be working on multiple goal areas simultaneously with their patients. As an example, a patient with a diagnosis of Parkinson's disease may need speech-language pathology services for swallowing as the primary issue and may need additional help to improve motor speech functions.

Assessment in Home Health

Assessing patients in the home care setting offers some unique opportunities for the SLP to evaluate, in the most functional context of all, the patient's home. Here, the SLP can evaluate how the patient is functioning in their daily life within the context of the activities performed throughout the day. Insight can be obtained as to how the patient can manage their own care and deal with situations that arise in the home and with the people they interact with regularly. Assessment areas should most strongly relate to the reason for referral for speech services, but additional areas of need may become apparent during evaluation, which should be further assessed and considered for treatment. For example, a patient may initially be referred for a speech evaluation due to difficulties with swallowing or motor speech deficits, which should be priority areas for evaluation, but the SLP should also assess for additional areas that may also require skilled intervention, such as cognitive skills, receptive and expressive language abilities, and vocal function. As in any setting, assessment of the patient should be an ongoing process and occur on each visit to determine patient progress as well as to identify any new issues that may require intervention (Malone & Loehr, 2018).

The home care SLP has a great deal to accomplish during patient evaluation. Often discussion as to why SLP services are needed and the many areas SLP's can provide intervention for is required because many patients and their families are unaware of this information. "I can speak just fine. I don't think I need a speech therapist" is often the response when the SLP calls to schedule the initial evaluation. It is important to be prepared for this response and provide the patient and family with the reason for the referral as well as how speech services may be beneficial. Even if this explanation occurs over the telephone when scheduling the evaluation, it will likely need to occur again upon arrival at the patient's home. Time to explain the purpose of the evaluation as well as prepare the patient and family for what will occur during evaluation should be factored into the visit. Consent forms and other paperwork required by the home health agency will also need to be reviewed and signed by the patient or their power of attorney. These "housekeeping tasks" must be completed but can also provide opportunities for assessment of the patient. Evaluation of the patient, their environment, and the level of support and understanding of the patient's caregiver (if one is present) should begin as soon as the SLP enters the person's home.

As discussed earlier in this chapter, the SLP may be part of the patient's care team along with other disciplines or may be the sole discipline treating the patient. If the SLP is completing the OASIS assessment (at either Start of Care, Recertification, Resumption of Care, and/or Discharge), the length of the visit and the number of areas to evaluate and document are significant. It should be noted that while the OASIS assessment covers many aspects that may connect with areas an SLP may evaluate, a separate speech therapy evaluation must occur in addition to the data collected when administering the OASIS. This separate evaluation should be done during the same visit, if possible, using both formal and informal measures to evaluate the patient's overall ability to communicate effectively and swallow safely. Because the OASIS is a comprehensive data collection tool that covers many areas, the SLP administering the OASIS can gain great insight into the patient's abilities related to speech, language, and cognition while collecting the OASIS data. This may include the patient's ability to follow directions, recall information, and clearly communicate ideas. As in other settings, the SLP can evaluate patient responses during administration of both formal and informal measures to assess areas not formally targeted in a standardized test or task. For example, the SLP may be administering the "Montreal Cognitive Assessment" (MoCA) (Nasreddine et al., 2005) to the patient, which assesses cognitive functioning, but the SLP can also be evaluating the patient's speech production, receptive language skills, and vocal quality during the assessment. Strengths or deficits noted can be documented and/or further assessed, if needed. During OASIS data collection, the patient is asked about their ability to manage oral medications. When collecting this data, the SLP should be assessing not only the patient's response to the question but also the patient's ability to read their medication bottles as well as their memory and problem-solving skills, all of which are areas that may require intervention from the SLP.

ASHA (2019a) recommends that patients undergo a comprehensive speech and language assessment that includes evaluation of language, communication, and swallowing. ASHA also recommends that comprehensive assessment follow the guidelines set forth by WHO's ICF framework (see "International Classification of Functioning, Disability, and Health" section) (ASHA, 2016c; WHO, 2001), encompassing impairments in body structure or function, comorbid deficits or health conditions, limitations in activity or participation, a patient's personal and environmental factors, and impact of deficits on the patient's quality of life (ASHA, 2019g). Comprehensive assessment can be accomplished through the use of formal and informal measures, as well as through clinical observation and patient/caregiver interview.

When assessing patients in the home care setting, completion of a comprehensive assessment using a balance of formal measures with informal and functional tasks is recommended to gain the clearest picture of the patient's level of functioning. The SLP should use measures that they feel comfortable administering and that will provide the best insight into the patient's abilities.

When choosing formal measures, the SLP should factor in test administration time as well as aspects such as the validity and reliability of the measure. In some cases, administering specific subtests of a formal measure may provide the diagnostic information needed. It is recommended that the SLP examine possible measures to see if individual subtests of a test can be administered and scored to compare with the normative data of the test. If individual subtests of a measure are administered, scoring and reporting of the results may be limited. Figure 5–4 provides a list of possible assessment measures the SLP may consider for use in the home care setting. The list is not exhaustive, nor does any measure listed imply specific endorsement by the authors, but it can serve as a starting point in choosing possible assessments for the home care setting.

Informal assessment tasks can provide additional information regarding a patient's strengths and weaknesses. These tasks should be offered with consideration of the diagnostic question and to further assess the patient's functional needs. For example, informal measures that may be performed during evaluation include tasks such as sustained reading or speaking (2–4 min) to evaluate fatigue,

---

Examples of Assessment Measures that May Be Used in Home Care

✓ St. Louis Mental Status Examination (SLUMS) (Tariq et al., 2006)
✓ Montreal Cognitive Assessment (MoCA) (Nasreddine, 2005)
✓ Arizona Battery for Communication Disorders of Dementia, Second Edition (2019)
✓ The Cognitive Linguistic Quick Test-Plus (CLQT+) (Helm-Estabrooks, 2017)
✓ Allen Cognitive Levels (Allen & Blue, 1998)
✓ Ross Information Processing Assessment: Geriatric (2) (RIPA-G) (Ross-Swain & Fogle, 2012)
✓ Repeatable Battery for the Assessment of Neuropsychological Status (RBANS) (Randolph, 2012)
✓ Spaced Retrieval Screen (Brush & Camp, 1998)
✓ Vision or Reading Screening (Rapid Estimate of Adult Literacy in Medicine, REALM) (Arozullah et al., 2007)
✓ Boston Naming Test (Kaplan et al., 2001)
✓ 3-oz Water Swallow Test (DePippo et al., 1992)
✓ Consensus Auditory-Perceptual Evaluation of Voice (CAPE-V) (ASHA, 2009)
✓ Voice Handicap Index (Jacobson, 1997)
✓ Clinical Swallowing Exam (ASHA, 2016a)
✓ Oral Mechanism Exam
✓ Cranial Nerve Examination

FIGURE 5–4. List of possible assessment measures.

respiration, stress, intelligibility, prosody, pitch, reading comprehension tasks, and sentence-level production tasks to evaluate the
areas previously listed along with the ability to recall and repeat
given information to assess working memory. Other tasks may
include vowel prolongation, percentage correct on structured tasks
(e.g., naming items in categories, recalling lists of given words,
etc.), performance of alternating and sequential motion rates or
diadochokinetic rates to examine jaw, lip, and tongue movement
as well as articulation, and patient response to visual cues and supports to determine ability to respond to compensatory strategies
(Malone & Loehr, 2018). Obviously, the list of informal observations
and tasks that the SLP might include is extensive. However, it is
usually necessary for the SLP to include assessment activities that
exceed those offered by any standardized test. Interview of the
patient and their caregiver to determine personal goals for treatment is also important to complete. Incorporating these goals will
increase functional outcomes as well as patient and caregiver buy-
in into the therapeutic process, supporting practice of skills outside
of treatment, and increased generalization (Malone & Loehr, 2018).

Assessing the patient within their own home provides insight
into the patient's level of functioning on many tasks that may
require skilled intervention by an SLP. Using materials familiar to
the patient and readily available within the home during evaluation is recommended to provide a clear picture of how the patient
is functioning. Some of these familiar objects could include newspapers, books, medication or grocery lists, dining materials, and
so forth.

The following list offers some suggestions for using materials
within a patient's home during evaluation and the skills that may
be assessed using these items (Malone & Loehr, 2018):

1. Use medication bottles or medication list to assess the
   patient's reading ability

2. Use newspaper, mail, and magazines in the home to find
   interesting content to read, discuss, assess recall, etc.

3. Assess barriers to success in the environment and work
   with patient and family toward reasonable solutions (e.g.,
   distance between chair and table, the amount of clutter
   on dining table where patient eats, lighting, ability to read
   written/visual cues from the patient's vantage point, etc.)

4. Evaluate typical meal setup to allow the patient the greatest
   amount of independence to feed self and take recommended
   bite or sip size. Assess patient or caregiver's ability to properly thicken liquids, etc.

5. Use items from the patient's home to assess skills such as confrontation naming, description, sorting, and categorization

Additional factors that should be considered when evaluating a patient in home care include monitoring the patient's level of fatigue and stress, addressing sensory limitations, and preparing materials needed prior to the visit. Patients being seen by a home care agency are typically facing a change in their medical status, have just been sent home from a medical facility, or both. They are tired and adjusting to normal routines at home. Although many tasks need to be accomplished during an evaluation session, the patient should be monitored throughout assessment for signs of fatigue or stress. Bear in mind that if the patient completes the assessment tasks but does so when not feeling their best, the results may not be accurate. Taking frequent breaks throughout the assessment is recommended to allow the patient to rest (these "breaks'" can also be good times for the SLP to complete some documentation, which is discussed later in this chapter). Eliminating distractions when possible (e.g., reduce volume on television) to ensure that the patient can hear questions, commands, and so forth, is also advised. If the patient requires use of glasses, hearing aids, or dentures, it is important that those are used during the evaluation. Schedule evaluations, if possible, for a time during the day when the patient is alert and more likely to be attentive. If some areas are not assessed, document why, and assess in the next session. Because the home care SLP works mainly out of their car rather than an office, materials needed for assessment need to be prepared in advance, organized, and easy to carry into a patient's home. Be sure to have all test forms and other materials prepared and easily accessible to maximize time and efficiency. This is another good reason to use the materials found within the patient's home, when possible. Consideration of these factors will allow for a more successful and productive evaluation visit with the patient.

Goal Development and Writing

Writing goals for intervention areas in home care follows similar procedures as in other care settings. Goals should follow the ICF framework (ASHA, 2019g) and be written to be specific, measurable, achievable, realistic/relevant, and timed (SMART) (Bovend'Eerdt, et. al., 2009). Goals should include the areas identified during evaluation as the greatest need for patient improvement to keep the patient safe and healthy within their home, along with the goals the patient and/or caregivers have identified as priorities. The number of visits requested from the physician to work with the patient is directly influenced by the number/types of goals identified to target during treatment. SLPs should analyze information gathered during assessment, determine goals that will be targeted, and then request the number of visits estimated to successfully target those goals. Sometimes a patient progresses more quickly or slowly than anticipated on goals. If this occurs, the SLP can revise the visit pattern through the physician to reflect these changes. These decisions should always be discussed first with the patient's care team to determine the feasibility of a change in number of visits (i.e., either increasing or decreasing them) to ensure the best outcomes for the patient. There may also be instances where a patient has many treatment areas that require skilled intervention by a SLP, but not all goals can be targeted initially due to the number of other disciplines working with the patient and other patient and caregiver factors. As in other care settings, it is recommended that the SLP prioritize the treatment areas that require intervention initially and set goals for those areas. Because there is no limit to the amount of home care visits a patient can receive if the patient still meets eligibility requirements, the SLP may postpone targeting other identified goals until later in the certification period or in a subsequent certification period.

ASHA provides some excellent resources regarding using the ICF model to develop goals for many different diagnoses, including swallowing, dementia, and dysarthria (ASHA, 2019g). It is recommended that readers access these resources to increase understanding of goal development and writing using the ICF model.

Case Study: Evaluation Decisions and Goal Development

Returning to the case study discussed earlier in this chapter, we now examine the evaluation decisions and development of goals for the patient, Mr. WA. Evaluation results at the start of care determined that Mr. WA demonstrated moderate impairments in speech and language expression, difficulty processing and following directions, memory deficits, and mild oral-pharyngeal dysphagia. Evaluation measures administered to the patient included the St. Louis Mental Status Examination (SLUMS) (Tariq et al., 2006) to evaluate cognitive functioning, a bedside swallowing evaluation conducted during a meal to evaluate swallowing functioning, safety of current diet level recommended at discharge from rehabilitation facility (The International Dysphagia Diet Standardization Initiative [IDDSI] Level 6 "Soft and Bite Sized" for foods and Level 0

"Thin" for liquids [2016]) and use of recommended compensatory strategies (alternating bites of food with liquids, use of slower rate of eating and drinking, and regular checking and clearing of pocketing of foods). Mr. WA was administered the Spaced Retrieval Screen (Brush & Camp, 1998) to evaluate if the technique would be useful to improve recall of important information and was also administered some informal measures to evaluate expressive skills, including intelligibility of speech at the sentence and conversation levels. Evaluation occurred 30 min prior to lunch, during which Mr. WA and caregiver completed home health agency paperwork, interviews, and the administration of both the SLUMS examination and the Spaced Retrieval Screen. Evaluation continued during Mr. WA's lunch to evaluate preparation and setup of current diet as well as safety of swallowing during the meal and use of recommended swallowing compensatory strategies. Speech and language expression was evaluated during both portions of the evaluation through answering of given questions and in conversation. Diagnostic measures chosen and timing of the visit (i.e., planned near patient's mealtime to evaluate swallowing function and safety) were determined based on the deficits noted on Mr. WA's physician referral and information shared with the SLP by the home health agency nurse who completed the initial start of care evaluation and OASIS assessment. Results of assessment included SLUMS score: 20/30, indicating "Mild Neurocognitive Disorder" (as measured by scores for test for "less than a high school education"), with deficits noted in memory/recall, visual spatial skills, and executive functioning/extrapolation. Mr. WA passed the Spaced Retrieval Screen, indicating that the use of the spaced retrieval technique helped the patient recall information. Mr. WA's intelligibility of speech was determined to be approximately 75% at conversation level in known contexts and 50% at the same level in unknown contexts. Mr. WA's intelligibility was improved at word and sentence level using a reduced rate of speech and overarticulation strategies. Mr. WA's caregiver required direct instruction on choice and preparation of food for the meal to be in alignment with diet level. Mr. WA demonstrated a rapid rate of eating/drinking during the meal (greater than 50% of trials) and required cues for 75% of trials to alternate bites/sips as well as to clear pocketed food. Mr. WA required use of short commands and statements (between four and six words on average) and demonstration of tasks/skills to follow instructions and to process information. Mr. WA has a third-grade level of education and limited literacy skills but was responsive to some written and picture cueing to recall instructions, recommendations, and swallowing/eating strategies. The home was observed to be cluttered with limited lighting, particularly in the kitchen area. Instruction and recommendations were provided to Mr. WA and his wife to reduce clutter to reduce fall risk and to increase attention/reduce distraction during meals. Opening of blinds and curtains in the kitchen area to increase natural light during meal preparation and eating was recommended, along with the use of a flashlight, if needed, to increase visibility during meal preparation later in the day. Mr. WA does have lighting available in the living room, so eating of meals in that room was also recommended. Instruction on organizing and preparing Mr. WA's medications in a room with lighting (bedroom, living room, or bathroom) was provided. Possible referral to a medical social worker was documented to help increase the patient and the wife's access to community resources.

Based on evaluation results, the following initial goals were established by the SLP to address areas of need and address patient and caregiver goals. Note that the goals include SMART elements (specific, measurable, attainable, realistic/relevant, and timed) and follow the ICF framework, including the patient's health conditions, effects on body functions/structures, effects on patient's activities and participation, and environmental and personal factors. Clinical reasoning questions were also considered, such as which impairments most affected function, what activities were or are the most important to the patient, and what environmental/personal factors affect participation in activities or situations (ASHA, 2019a):

1. The patient will self-monitor his rate of drinking and eating and use compensatory strategies (alternating bites/sips) to eliminate coughing during meals in 80% of trials with minimal verbal and visual cueing.

2. The patient will check and clear pocketed material in oral cavity in 90% of trials during 30-min meals with moderate verbal cues to reduce risk of coughing/choking.

3. The caregiver will independently demonstrate proper choice and preparation of foods on IDDSI Level 6 diet and recommended meal setup for four out of five meals.

4. The patient will demonstrate recall of intelligibility strategies to improve expression of wants/needs and communication with caregivers at the initial trial of three consecutive sessions using the spaced retrieval technique.

5. The patient will increase intelligibility of speech using provided strategies in 90% of trials at the sentence level with minimal verbal cues to improve self-expression.

6. The caregiver will demonstrate the use of reduced sentence, question, or command length (four to six words) to improve the patient's ability to process and respond to verbal information in 75% of trials over three sessions.

7. The patient will demonstrate responsiveness to written or picture cues to recall how to follow safety strategies to complete activities of daily living in 75% of trials with moderate support.

As stated earlier in this chapter, based on the goals developed, the SLP determined a visit pattern of two visits per week for 5 weeks and one visit a week for 3 weeks (2w5, 1w3) and discussed the plan with the care team. Both Mr. WA and his caregiver met initial goals at the fifth week of treatment, and skilled speech therapy services were discharged to allow for initiation of occupational therapy and increased visits from physical therapy. At the end of the first certification period, it was determined that Mr. WA required continued skilled services from physical and occupational therapy. Nursing services were discontinued, and physical therapy assumed case management responsibilities, including completion of recertification OASIS. A new evaluation was requested from the physician by physical therapy for speech therapy to evaluate and treat the Mr. WA's ongoing cognitive deficits, particularly related to recall of strategies for safe transfers, ambulation, and completion of activities of daily living, including understanding/use of bus schedule, along with addressing Mr. WA's intelligibility at conversation level. The SLP would then complete a new evaluation, develop new goals based on patient performance, and request a new visit pattern from the patient's physician for the second certification period.

Treatment Considerations in Home Health

Treatment in the home care setting follows the same decision-making and methodology an SLP would employ in other treatment settings. Decisions regarding intervention methods should include evaluation of the evidence available to support the use of a particular method or technique. ASHA's Practice Portals are recommended for review for consideration of evidence-based treatment options for a variety of disorders (ASHA, 2019c). The Practice Portal also contains valuable resources related to specific clinical topics, professional issues, patient handouts, and tools and templates that can assist in guiding clinical practice. The Practice Portal can be accessed at https://www.asha.org/practice-portal/

Treatment/intervention in home care should focus on function. SLPs should provide treatment that will increase functional outcomes for the patient and allow them to demonstrate improvement in skills to allow for the greatest level of independence. Treatment may also include instruction to the patient's caregivers and demonstration of recommendations by the caregiver. As in any evaluation, SLPs working in home care should utilize meaningful treatment materials, such as those found in the patient's home, when possible, as well as work within situations that occur or may occur in the patient's home or other settings that the patient may encounter (at church, doctor's office, etc.) to keep treatment as functional as possible. Examples of such situations may include use of strategies in care situations (dressing, bathing, etc.) or practice of strategies in contexts such as conversation with caregivers in person and/or on the telephone, and completion of daily life tasks such as reading mail, managing finances, or managing medications. Treatment methods utilized are dependent upon the diagnosis being treated and the patient's level of severity and should be supported using evidence-based practice. Goals that are written using the ICF framework focus on improving not only the patient's health condition but also the patient's ability to improve in participation in activities, including the patient's personal goals and environmental and personal factors. Therefore, targeting of goals written in this manner during intervention allows for the patient's treatment to be as functional as possible. Diagnoses treated in home care can span from swallowing to language comprehension and expression to cognition. ASHA's Evidence Maps are useful resources for clinicians in finding the latest research related to a variety of diagnoses and disorders (ASHA, 2019b) (the Evidence Maps can be accessed at https://www.asha.org/Evidence-Maps/). Examples of possible treatment methods that may be used in home care, specifically related to cognition or dementia include:

1. Spaced Retrieval Technique to target recall of important information (Benigas et al., 2016; Brush & Camp, 1998)

2. Reminiscence Therapy (Harris, 1997)

3. Use of visual/graphic cues and memory books (Bourgeois, 1992, 2013)

4. Validation therapy (Feil, 1982; Neil & Wright, 2003)

5. Montessori-based methods for dementia (Elliot, 2015)

6. Practice of targeted skills at meals, during daily activities in the home, or during facility activities, if the patient is living in an assisted living facility (Bourgeois & Hickey, 2009; Bayles et al., 2006)

7. Creation of grocery lists, sequencing and recall of use of technology (phone, television, computer, medical alert system, correct use of adaptive equipment, etc.) (Hickey & Bourgeois, 2018)

8. Caregiver interventions for improving communication (Zientz et al., 2007)

Some additional Tools of the Trade that the SLP working in home care may use in treatment are listed in **Figure 5–5**. These tools may be useful to help create written/visual cues to help patient's recall strategies, create checklists/reminders, list what occurred in treatment to aid in patient recall, or assist in communication with caregivers, particularly when the caregiver is not present for a session.

Documentation Considerations in Home Health

Documentation is critical in any care setting. Documentation entails the sharing of information about a patient's diagnoses, assessment

"Tools of the Trade" for Treatment in Home Care:
(Malone & Loehr, 2018)

✓ Index cards (lined or unlined)
✓ Permanent and dry erase markers
✓ Highlighter marker
✓ Adhesive notes
✓ Blank notepaper
✓ Scissors and tape
✓ Dry erase board
✓ Additional lighting
✓ Prepared handouts on different disorders, recommendations, cues, etc.
✓ Colored tape
✓ Velcro or magnets
✓ Clear picture frames
✓ Clear packing tape, laminating pouches or plastic storage bags
✓ Stopwatch
✓ Smartphone or iPad to access websites for education or for use of timer or recording application

---

FIGURE 5–5. "Tools of the Trade" for treatment in home care. Copyright SpeechPathology.com, used with permission.

and treatment of those diagnoses, progress toward goals, recommendations, and communication among a patient's care team and caregivers. ASHA (2019b) states that documentation in health care answer the following questions:

1. Is the service medically necessary?
2. Does the service require the skilled services of an SLP to complete?
3. Are the goals and treatment functionally relevant?
4. How does the service add value to the patient's overall care and health?

Documentation can be used for submission to payer sources for reimbursement of services. In the case of home health care, documentation is typically submitted to Medicare and/or a third-party payer. Payer sources can vary in terms of the documentation they require from clinicians. Most home care agencies have specific paperwork requirements and templates for clinicians to use for documentation. These templates should align with Medicare's requirements for reimbursement of home health services, which include documentation of an evaluation, a plan of care (including diagnoses, treatment goals, amount, duration, and frequency of services), treatment notes, progress reports, and discharge notes (ASHA, 2019e). SLPs in home health care may also complete the OASIS assessment, so completion of this tool would also fall under possible documentation requirements of the clinician. SLPs in home care also participate in choosing the applicable billing codes for patients for reimbursement. Coding should be done with as much specificity as possible regarding the patient's diagnoses being treated or those that contribute to the need for skilled speech pathology services. Often agencies have specific personnel who focus solely on coding and billing, so questions and training from those individuals is useful to ensure the correct codes are used. Additional documentation requirements may include consent forms, case communication forms to document needed communication among care team members, physician communication forms, and missed visit forms. Because the members of a patient's care team are mobile and not physically together often, completion of documentation must occur regularly and be specific regarding a variety of information. This could include "housekeeping-type" information such as the best phone number to reach the patient's caregiver to schedule visits or when the patient has a physician appointment to critical information regarding a change in a patient's medication or vital sign parameters. Medicare requires that agencies with more than 10 full-time employees submit documentation electronically (ASHA, 2019e). Therefore, most SLPs working in home health will be completing documentation using some type of practice management software on an electronic medical record system.

Regular documentation of medical necessity for services provided as well as showing the ongoing need for the skilled services of a SLP are important elements to documentation in health care. The importance of being specific and clear in all documentation cannot be underestimated. Often, the persons or agencies reviewing documentation for coverage and reimbursement are unfamiliar with the services provided by skilled disciplines, including SLPs. Clinicians are encouraged to bear in mind the perspective of an unfamiliar reader when completing documentation to ensure it is as evident as possible as to why a SLP's services are needed, what instruction occurs during visits, and how the patient is progressing. "Unclear, vague, or absent documentation can result in denials by payers and make it difficult for the reader to follow the clinical judgment underlying the diagnosis and treatment" (ASHA, 2019e).

SLPs should employ the same clinical documentation strategies in home care as are needed in other health care settings. This includes justification of medical necessity, skilled service, demonstration of the functionality of services provided, and the value the SLP adds to the patient's care (ASHA 2019e). Using the ICF model is again recommended as a guideline to complete clinical documentation to incorporate these necessary elements (ASHA, 2019g; WHO, 2001).

Some unique aspects to documentation in home care include documentation of a patient's vital signs (see section entitled Vital Signs later in this chapter) or other health information, evidence the patient is homebound, and any changes in a patient's medication (either type, dosage, or frequency) at each visit. Documentation of this information at each visit is critical in order to assess and document any changes in the patient's health that may endanger their safety or require increased medical care by the patient's physician or at a medical facility, such as a hospital. CMS (2017) requires frequent documentation of care coordination (i.e., all discussions between care providers regarding the patient and/or patient's plan of care that occur in person or via telephone or email). Additionally, documentation serves as evidence that each discipline from the home care agency is working to reduce potentially avoidable adverse events such as medication management issues, falls, skin breakdown, and decline due to depression. Typically, clinicians document the prompts they use to probe these areas, the patient/

caregiver responses given, and any clinical observations related to these areas in the documentation templates provided by the home health agency. Other documentation elements that are unique to home care include documentation of visit time, session start and end time, mileage to and from the visit, and signature of the patient, the patient's power of attorney, or another authorized person to prove that the services occurred.

Documentation requirements and the time needed to complete documentation are cited as a top complaint of SLPs working in home health care. According to ASHA's 2017 Health Care Survey (ASHA, 2017), 47% of the SLPs' respondents working in home health agencies or clients' homes reported daily completion of "off the clock" work, which includes completion of documentation. When possible, documentation should occur at the point of service (i.e., during patient visits) to ensure it is thorough and to assist in timely completion. This can be difficult to do when the priority is to provide effective and efficient patient care. Figure 5–6 provides some suggestions/strategies for SLPs working in home care to assist in the completion of documentation.

Health Insurance Portability and Accountability Act of 1996

The Health Insurance Portability and Accountability Act of 1996 (HIPAA) was created to ensure the safety and protection of a patient's personal health information (PHI). Under the Privacy Rule, PHI is "any information that may reasonably allow someone to identify [an] individual . . . such as name, address, insurance information, and information regarding health conditions, treatments, and prognosis and applies to oral, paper, and electronic communication of this information" (ASHA, 2019f). SLPs in home health care must comply with HIPAA regulations to ensure the protection of a patient's PHI. The Privacy Rule does permit instances when this information can be shared, including information regarding treatment, payment, and health care operations, as well as in instances of suspected neglect or abuse of the patient (ASHA, 2019f). The Security Rule is another important part of protecting a patient's PHI. "The Security Rule applies only to electronic protected health information (ePHI). This is in contrast to the Privacy Rule which applies to all forms of protected health information, including oral, paper, and electronic" (ASHA, 2019h). Sharing of PHI should be limited to only those who "need to know," which would include discussion of treatment with other members of the

---

Documentation Strategies for Home Care

✓ Stay organized
- o Know what forms/documents require completion for each patient at each visit. Keep a list if necessary.

✓ Document during sessions as much as possible
- o Provide breaks during treatment for the patient to rest. Use these breaks to complete necessary documentation.
- o Upon completion of each treatment task or any instruction/education provided, take a few moments to document data or information provided.
- o Notify the patient at the start of sessions that documentation will be taking place throughout the session to increase patient knowledge of the process and requirements.

✓ Create "cheat sheets" to help complete forms more quickly
- o Create simple checklists for what should be documented on each required form, along with reminders to include key areas such as medical necessity, description of skilled service provided, and elements of the ICF framework.

✓ Take advantage of "down time" between patients to document
- o Often there may be time between patient visits. Use this time to complete documentation for patients seen earlier in the day.

✓ Use time in car to make care coordination calls (e.g., orders to doctor, discussions with other disciplines, office, etc.)
- o Driving between patient visits provides an excellent opportunity to make any needed phone calls.

✓ Schedule your day to include documentation time
- o Schedule dedicated time either early in the day or at the end of the day to stay on top of documentation demands.

FIGURE 5–6. Documentation strategies for home care.

patient's care team. Discussion of this information should be conducted in a secure manner and only occur when necessary. Home health agencies have specific guidelines for clinicians to follow regarding the protection of patients' PHI. Training regarding HIPAA and protection of PHI is a necessary part of being a clinician in home health care to protect the patient's confidential information. Violations of HIPAA can result in strict penalties, so it is recommended that SLPs have training and education in this area on an ongoing basis.

Unique Aspects of Home Health

The home health environment is diverse and somewhat complex for the SLP. There are several additional aspects of care and job requirements that are unique to this field and important for the SLP to understand to ensure future success with their home health patients.

Employment Options

Depending on the home health agency, SLPs often have many options regarding the status of their employment (i.e., full time, part time, etc.). These options depend on the needs of each agency and availability of SLPs in the service area. Many agencies employ SLPs on a full-time salaried status. This status often comes with additional benefits such as health insurance and paid time off. Working full time for an agency usually means a commitment to the employer regarding hours, productivity, and coverage area. There are other options for most agencies including part-time and as-needed (often referred to as PRN) positions that generally do not include added benefits and would not have productivity requirements.

Transportation

Most home health agencies offer reimbursement for mileage accrued by the SLP with amounts varying from agency to agency. CMS factors mileage rates and distances (urban or rural agencies) into the rates for reimbursement for agencies. Some agencies offer company cars to their employees to offset the burden of accruing mileage on personal vehicles. This is a way for an agency to capitalize on advertising, as well.

Equipment Care and Handwashing

Home health clinicians are mobile and rely on portable equipment. Most clinicians use tote bags with multiple pockets to store and carry necessary equipment and tools from patient to patient. The equipment, known as car stock, is most often provided and replenished as needed by the home health agency. As part of regulation and oversight into patient safety, home health agencies must ensure that their field staff are transporting and handling equipment properly. There are specific procedures for washing hands, sanitizing equipment, storing and removing equipment from the clinician bag (clean bag technique), and keeping clean areas in the clinician's vehicle. Although each agency follows procedures similarly, regulations may vary from state to state, so it is important for the field clinician to receive training and education regarding agency-specific policies.

Vital Signs

Since patients are mainly homebound, home health clinicians are sometimes the only connection to the world outside of the home. Routine monitoring of vital signs is important as it is often the first indicator of patient decline. There are many instances where the monitoring of vital signs at the onset of a patient visit has led to the detection of a serious health issue that could have resulted in illness or even death. Most home health agencies require all field staff, regardless of license or discipline, to take vital signs with each visit. This includes, at minimum, blood pressure, pulse, temperature, and respiration rate. Additional required vital signs may include patient weight, oxygen saturation, heart and lung auscultation, and a measurement of patient's pain level using a standardized pain scale. Most SLPs do not receive formalized training in school with regard to monitoring vital signs. If the SLP does not feel competent in monitoring vital signs, it is important to inform the agency supervisor. Agencies should ensure that all clinicians are given sufficient training to ensure safe and accurate recording of vital signs. Agencies typically provide the necessary equipment and training for accurate and efficient vital sign monitoring.

Elder Abuse

Due to the intimate nature of the services provided in home health care, the field clinician may uncover situations in the patient's own living environment that pose a threat to the patient. It is very important for the clinician to understand the definitions of elder abuse, the different types of abuse, and the responsibility of the field clinician and/or home health agency that is caring for the patient. Furthermore, it is important that the field staff take time to educate their patients and caregivers regarding elder abuse as part of their patient rights. Each state may have different laws pertaining to elder abuse, and each agency may have different policies in place to ensure that patients are instructed in their rights (as part of the

Conditions of Participation). When abuse or neglect are suspected, all members of a patient's care team are designated as mandated reporters of this information and are required to document any concerns and observe and report them to the home care agency, law enforcement, and/or the local Adult Protective Services (APS) agency (National Center on Elder Abuse, 2019). Home care agencies have specific protocols regarding reporting of suspected abuse or neglect, as does each state in the United States. The National Center on Elder Abuse is an excellent resource regarding this topic. Please see their website (https://ncea.acl.gov/) for more information. The definition and types of elder abuse as stated by the Centers for Disease Control and Prevention (CDC, 2019) are as follows:

1. Elder abuse is an intentional act, or failure to act, by a caregiver or another person in a relationship involving an expectation of trust that causes or creates a risk of harm to an older adult. (An older adult is defined as someone age 60 years or older.)

2. Physical Abuse: the intentional use of physical force that results in acute or chronic illness, bodily injury, physical pain, functional impairment, distress, or death. Physical abuse may include, but is not limited to, violent acts such as striking (with or without an object or weapon), hitting, beating, scratching, biting, choking, suffocation, pushing, shoving, shaking, slapping, kicking, stomping, pinching, and burning.

3. Sexual Abuse or Abusive Sexual Contact: forced or unwanted sexual interaction (touching and nontouching acts) of any kind with an older adult. This may include forced or unwanted:
   a. Completed or attempted contact between the penis and the vulva or the penis and the anus involving penetration
   b. Contact between the mouth and the penis, vulva, or anus
   c. Penetration of the anal or genital opening of another person by a hand, finger, or other object
   d. Intentional touching, either directly or through the clothing, of the genitalia, anus, groin, breast, inner thigh, or buttocks

4. These acts also qualify as sexual abuse if they are committed against a person who is not competent to give informed approval.

5. Emotional or Psychological Abuse: verbal or nonverbal behavior that results in the infliction of anguish, mental

pain, fear, or distress. Examples include behaviors intended to humiliate (e.g., calling names or insults), threaten (e.g., expressing an intent to initiate nursing home placement), isolate (e.g., seclusion from family or friends), or control (e.g., prohibiting or limiting access to transportation, telephone, money, or other resources).

6. Neglect: failure by a caregiver or other responsible person to protect an elder from harm, or the failure to meet needs for essential medical care, nutrition, hydration, hygiene, clothing, basic activities of daily living or shelter, which results in a serious risk of compromised health and safety. Examples include not providing adequate nutrition, hygiene, clothing, shelter, or access to necessary health care; or failure to prevent exposure to unsafe activities and environments.

7. Financial Abuse or Exploitation: the illegal, unauthorized, or improper use of an older individual's resources by a caregiver or other person in a trusting relationship, for the benefit of someone other than the older individual. This includes depriving an older person of rightful access to, information about, or use of, personal benefits, resources, belongings, or assets. Examples include forgery, misuse or theft of money or possessions; use of coercion or deception to surrender finances or property; or improper use of guardianship or power of attorney.

Safety

Home health care workers, while contributing greatly to the well-being of others, face unique risks on the job to their own personal safety and health. During 2007 alone, 27,400 recorded injuries occurred among more than 896,800 home health care workers. Home health care workers are frequently exposed to a variety of potentially serious or even life-threatening hazards. Some of the dangers include overexertion; stress; exposure to weapons or illegal drugs; verbal abuse; exposure to bloodborne pathogens; temperature extremes; unhygienic conditions, including lack of water, unclean or hostile animals, and animal waste; as well as other forms of violence in the home or community. Long commutes from worksite to worksite also expose the home health care worker to transportation-related risks (CDC, 2008). The following are a few safety tips for the home health clinician:

1. Familiarize yourself with your destination. If venturing into unknown territory for the first time, it is a good idea to

study and plan the route in advance. Planning in advance will improve efficiency and eliminate frustration if there are unexpected deterrents such as road closures and heavy traffic patterns.

2. Always have situational awareness. Although infrequent, there are times when the clinician encounters situations that may cause feelings of unease. This can include strangely behaving people and homes with weapons and aggressive animals, to name a few. The clinician should be mindful of the situation and leave the home immediately if there is a threat to personal safety. If there are weapons or animals (aggressive or not) in the home, the clinician can request in advance that these items are put out of sight for the duration of the visit.

3. Conceal car stock. When parking the vehicle at the patient's home, it is a good idea to conceal any items left in the car. If the car has a trunk, it is a good idea to put items in the trunk. If there is no trunk, use a dark colored cloth to camouflage items and reduce risk of theft.

4. Parking the car. When parking, make sure to do so in a well-lit area, and if possible, park with the front of the vehicle facing the street to make the exit easy and straightforward.

5. Keep in touch. Always let your home health agency know where you are as you are traveling from patient to patient. This ensures that someone is aware of your whereabouts in the event that you are in need of assistance on the road.

6. Personal safety equipment. Each home health agency has a policy regarding field staff carrying weapons for personal safety (i.e., handguns, mace, knives). Many agencies prohibit carrying weapons into patient homes and even having them in their vehicles. Clinicians should check with their agency for specific policies regarding personal safety equipment.

7. Protect yourself from insects. Occasionally, clinicians are required to visit patients in unclean environments. Even homes that appear to be clean can be infested with bed bugs or other insects or rodents. Following clean bag technique will greatly reduce the risk for any of these creatures to end up in your bag. Additionally, wearing shoe covers and an additional outer layer of clothing can be helpful. Be sure to remove protective clothing and place in a plastic bag before getting into your personal vehicle or entering another place of residence. In working in homes that may have an infestation, consider only bringing into the home what is needed to care for the patient during that visit.

8. **Take breaks during the day.** Many home health clinicians are tasked with spending a great amount of time in the car. Driving for long periods in between visits can become exhausting. It is important to take breaks during the day where you can stretch and walk around so as to remain alert when behind the wheel.

9. **Keep your eye on the weather.** Some areas of the country experience extremes in weather that can change dramatically in a short period of time. It is important to always be mindful of changing weather conditions and always make sure that your car is well equipped should you become stranded. This pertains to cold weather as well as warm weather conditions. Part of being weather conscious is ensuring that your car stock is protected from extreme temperatures, as some products can melt or crack during extended exposure to these temperatures.

Ethical Considerations

All medical personnel are required to follow the same ethical standards and rules that are set for all health providers, regardless of the discipline or chosen health care industry. Health care ethics pertains to a set of moral principles and values that guide professionals in making decisions toward patient care. There are some unique ethical challenges that may arise for the home health care clinician. These challenges may be particularly challenging due to the isolated nature of the work environment and not having immediate feedback or resolution by management or colleagues. The following are some ethical questions or considerations specific to the home health care environment:

1. Is the patient "homebound" if the patient has dementia and leaves the home regularly, despite questionable safety?

2. The patient and/or caregiver is unable or unwilling to follow through with recommendations from the SLP and can only maintain their level of functioning with involvement from a skilled professional. Should home health services continue?

3. The patient has reached their highest level of functioning necessitating discharge to outpatient services yet cannot safely get to an outpatient facility. Does the home health agency discharge from service?

These scenarios and many more present themselves every day in the home health profession. If there is ever a question regarding ethics, the home health professional should bring it to the attention of the agency director and/or care team for discussion and resolution.

Summary

Home health care is a dynamic and unique care setting for SLPs. It allows for patient care to occur in the environment of a patient's home, which provides the opportunity for functional treatment of goals within the context of a skilled care team. SLPs working in home health care can engage in a variety of roles within this setting, providing interesting and challenging experiences for the SLP. As in any care setting, home health care has a variety of specific requirements and procedures that are important to know when considering working in this setting. However, the SLP who works in home health often recognizes the many rewarding aspects of their work (namely, working with patients and their families in their homes to reach functional goals and working closely with other disciplines) and that these aspects far outweigh any of the challenges that may exist.

Glossary

Adult Protective Services (APS): Adult Protective Services (APS) is a social services program provided by state and/or local governments nationwide serving older adults and adults with disabilities who are in need of assistance. APS workers investigate cases of abuse, neglect, or exploitation, working closely with a wide variety of allied professionals such as physicians, nurses, paramedics, firefighters, and law enforcement officers.

Centers for Medicare and Medicaid Services (CMS): The Centers for Medicare and Medicaid Services is a federal agency that administers the nation's major health care programs, including Medicare, Medicaid, and CHIP.

Certification Period (also known as "Episode of Care"): A home health certification period is an episode of care that begins with a start of care visit and continues for 60 days. If at the end of the initial episode of care the patient continues to require home health services, a recertification of services is required.

Conditions of Participation (CoPs): These are federal regulations that participating health care facilities must comply with in order to receive funding from the Medicare and Medicaid programs.

The Health Insurance Portability and Accountability Act of 1996 (PL 104–191) (HIPAA): Federal law designed to improve the efficiency and effectiveness of the nation's health care system.

Outcomes Assessment and Information Set (OASIS): The OASIS is a standardized data collection tool that looks at all aspects of patient need with regard to level of functioning, physical barriers, community access, diagnosis, etc.

Protected Health Information (PHI): This is information about an individual, including demographic information, that relates to the individual's past, present, or future health or condition, the care provided, or the payment history of the individual.

Privacy Rule: The Privacy Rule is part of HIPAA and is intended to prevent covered health care providers from using or disclosing health information without patients' authorization or other legal authority.

Quality Assurance and Performance Improvement (QAPI): This is a systematic, comprehensive, and data-driven approach to maintaining and improving safety and quality in health care while involving all home health care disciplines in practical and creative problem-solving. Mandated to occur through the Conditions of Participation by the Centers for Medicare and Medicaid Services (CMS).

Security Rule: Part of HIPAA that establishes national standards to protect individuals' electronic personal health information that is created, received, used, or maintained by a covered entity. The Security Rule requires appropriate administrative, physical, and technical safeguards to ensure the confidentiality, integrity, and security of electronic protected health information.

SMART Goals: This is a method of developing and writing goals that states that goals should be written to be specific, measurable, achievable, realistic/relevant, and timed.

Visit Pattern: Frequency and duration of visits by a skilled service. Includes number of visits per week and for how many weeks a patient will be seen by a discipline during a certification period. Each discipline treating a patient has a separate visit pattern that must be approved by the patient's physician.

References

Allen, C. & Blue, T. (1998). *Allen Scale/cognitive levels*. https://allencognitive.com/allen-scale/

American Speech-Language-Hearing Association Special Interest Division 3, Voice and Voice Disorders. (2009). *Consensus Auditory-Perceptual Evaluation of Voice (CAPE-V)*. https://www.asha.org/siteassets/uploadedFiles/ASHA/SIG/03/CAPE-V-Procedures-and-Form.pdf

American Speech-Language-Hearing Association. (2016a). *Clinical swallowing exam template*. https://www.asha.org/uploadedFiles/AAT ClinicalSwallowing.pdf

American Speech-Language-Hearing Association. (2016b). *Code of ethics* [Ethics]. https://www.asha.org

American Speech-Language-Hearing Association. (2016c). *Scope of practice in speech-language pathology* [Scope of practice]. https://www.asha.org/uploadedFiles/SP2016-00343.pdf

American Speech-Language-Hearing Association. (2017). *ASHA 2017 SLP health care survey: Practice issues*. https://www.asha.org

American Speech-Language-Hearing Association. (2019a). *Dementia: comprehensive assessment*. https://www.asha.org/PRPSpecificTopic.aspx?folderid=8589935289&section=Assessment#Comprehensive_Assessment

American Speech-Language-Hearing Association. (2019b). *Documentation in health*. https://www.asha.org/practice-portal/professional-issues/documentation-in-health-care/

American Speech-Language-Hearing Association. (2019c). *Evidence maps*. https://www.asha.org/Evidence-Maps/

American Speech-Language-Hearing Association. (2019d). *Getting started in home health*. https://www.asha.org/slp/healthcare/start_home.htm

American Speech-Language-Hearing Association. (2019e). *Health information privacy: Frequently asked questions*. https://www.asha.org/practice/reimbursement/hipaa/privacy/#Ferpa

American Speech-Language-Hearing Association. (2019f). *HIPAA security rule: Frequently asked questions*. https://www.asha.org/practice/reimbursement/hipaa/securityrule/

American Speech-Language-Hearing Association. (2019g). *International classification of functioning, disability, and health*. https://www.asha.org/slp/icf/

American Speech-Language-Hearing Association (2019h). *Person-centered focus on function: Swallowing*. https://www.asha.org/uploadedFiles/ICF-Swallowing.pdf

American Speech-Language-Hearing Association. (2019i). *Practice portal*. https://www.asha.org/practice-portal/

Arozullah, A. M., Yarnold, P. R., Bennett, C. L., Soltysik, R. C., Wolf, M. S., Ferreira, R. M., . . . Davis, T. (2007). Development and validation of a short-form, rapid estimate of adult literacy in medicine. *Medical Care, 45*(11), 1026–1033.

Bayles, K. A., & Tomoeda, C. K. (2019). *Arizona Battery for Communication Disorders of Dementia* (2nd ed.). Pro-Ed.

Bayles, K. A., Kim, E., Chapman, S. B., Zientz, J., Rackley, A., Mahendra, N., . . . Cleary, S. J. (2006). Evidence-based practice recommendations for working with individuals with dementia: Simulated presence therapy. *Journal of Medical Speech-Language Pathology, 14,* xiii–xxi.

Benigas, J. E., Brush, J. A., & Elliot, G. M. (2016). *Spaced retrieval step by step: An evidence-based memory intervention.* Health Professions Press.

Bourgeois, M. S. (1992). *Conversing with memory impaired individuals using memory aids: A memory aid workbook.* Northern Speech Services.

Bourgeois, M. S. (2013). *Memory books and other graphic cueing systems: Practical communication and memory aids for adults with dementia.* Health Professions Press.

Bourgeois, M. S., & Hickey, E. M. (2009). *Dementia: From diagnosis to management—A functional approach.* Psychological Press.

Bovend'Eerdt, T. J., Botell, R. E., & Wade, D. T. (2009). Writing SMART rehabilitation goals and achieving goal attainment scaling: A practical guide. *Clinical Rehabilitation, 23*(4), 352–361. https://doi.org/10.1177/0269215508101741

Brown, J. (2017, August 1). What's my scope? *ASHA Leader, 22*(8). https://leader.pubs.asha.org/doi/full/10.1044/leader.OTP.22082017.40

Brush, J., & Camp, C. (1998). *A therapy technique for improving memory: Spaced retrieval.* Menorah Park Center for Senior Living.

Centers for Disease Control and Prevention. (2008). *Home health hazards.* https://www.cdc.gov/niosh/docs/2010-125/pdfs/2010-125.pdf

Centers for Disease Control and Prevention. (2019). *Elder abuse definitions.* https://www.cdc.gov/violenceprevention/elderabuse/definitions.html

Centers for Medicare and Medicaid Services. (2013). *Conditions of Participation.* https://www.cms.gov/Regulations-and-Guidance/Legislation/CFCsAndCoPs/index

Centers for Medicare and Medicaid Services. (2016). *Quality of care fact sheet.* https://www.cms.gov/Medicare/Quality-Initiatives-Patient-Assessment-Instruments/HomeHealthQualityInits/Downloads/QoPC-Fact-Sheet-For-HHAs_UPDATES-7-24-16-2.pdf

Centers for Medicare and Medicaid Services. (2017). *Medicare and Medicaid program: Conditions of Participation for home health agencies.* https://www.federalregister.gov/documents/2017/01/13/2017-00283/medicare-and-medicaid-program-conditions-of-participation-for-home-health-agencies

Centers for Medicare and Medicaid Services. (2018a). *Home health quality reporting.* https://www.cms.gov/Medicare/Quality-Initiatives-Patient-Assessment-Instruments/HomeHealthQualityInits/index

Centers for Medicare and Medicaid Services. (2018b). *Medicare and home health care.* https://www.medicare.gov/sites/default/files/2018-07/10969-medicare-and-home-health-c are.pdf

Centers for Medicare and Medicaid Services. (2019). *Home health services.* https://www.medicare.gov/coverage/home-health-services

DePippo, K. L., Holas, M. A., & Reding, M. J. (1992). Validation of the 3-oz water swallow test for aspiration following stroke. *Archives of Neurology, 49,* 1259–1261.

Feil, N. (1982). *Validation: The Feil method: How to help the disoriented old-old.* Feil Productions.

Harris, J. L. (1997). Reminiscence: A culturally and developmentally appropriate language intervention for older adults. *American Journal of Speech-Language Pathology, 6,* 19–26.

Harris-Kojetin, L. D., Sengupta, M., Lendon, J. P., Rome, V., Valverde, R., & Caffrey, C. (2019). Long-term care providers and services users in the United States, 2015–2016. *National Center for Health Statistics. Vital Health Stat, 3*(43).

Helm-Estabrooks, N. (2017). *Cognitive linguistic quick test-plus (CLQT+).* Pearson.

Hickey, E. M., & Bourgeois, M. S. (2018). Cognitive and communicative interventions. In E. M. Hickey & M. S. Bourgeois (Eds.), *Dementia: Person-centered assessment and intervention* (pp. 168–213). Routledge.

Home Care Pulse. (2013). *Top 10 complaints from home care clients.* https://www.homecarepulse.com/articles/top-10-complaints-from-home-care-clients/

The International Dysphagia Diet Standardization Initiative. (2016). https://www.iddsi.org/framework/

Jacobson, B., Johnson, A., Grywalski, C., Silbergleit, A., Jacobson, G., Benniger, M. S., & Newman, C. W. (1997). The Voice Handicap Index (VHI): Development and validation. *American Journal of Speech-Language Pathology, 6*(3), 66–70. https://doi.org/10.1044/1058-0360.0603.66

Kaplan, E., Goodglass, H., & Weintraub, S. (2001). *Boston naming test.* Pro-Ed.

Malone, M. & Loehr, J. (2018). *Home health for speech language pathologists.* https://www.speechpathology.com/slp-ceus/course/home-health-for-speech-language-8666

Medicare Payment Advisory Commission, (2016), *June 2016 Report to the Congress: Medicare and Health Care Delivery System. Executive Summary.* MedPAC. https://www.medpac.gov/document/http-www-medpac-gov-docs-default-source-reports-june-2016-report-to-the-congress-medicare-and-the-health-care-delivery-system-pdf/

Medicare Payment Advisory Commission. *July 2021 data book: Health care spending and the medicare program.* MedPAC.

Nasreddine, Z. S., Phillips, N. A., Bédirian, V., Charbonneau, S., Whitehead, V., Collin, I., . . . Chertkow, H. (2005). The Montreal cognitive assessment, MoCA: A brief screening tool for mild cognitive impairment. *Journal of the American Geriatrics Society, 53*(4), 695–699. https://doi.org/10.1111/j.1532-5415.2005.53221.x

National Center on Elder Abuse. (2019). *Frequently asked questions.* https://ncea.acl.gov/FAQ.aspx

Neal, M., & Wright, M. (2003). Validation therapy for dementia. *Cochrane Database of Systematic Reviews*, 2003(3). https://doi.org/10.1002/14651858.CD001394

Ortman, J. M., Velkoff, V. A., & Hogan, H. (2014). *An aging nation: The older population in the United States, current population reports* (P25–1140). U.S. Census Bureau. https://www.census.gov/prod/2014pubs/p25-1140.pdf

Randolph, C. (2012). *Repeatable Battery for the Assessment of Neuropsychological Status*. Pearson.

Ross-Swain, D., & Fogle, P. (2012). *RIPAG:2 Ross Information Processing Assessment—Geriatric* (2nd ed.). Pro-Ed.

Tariq, S. H., Tumosa, N., Chibnall, J. T., Perry, M. H., 3rd, & Morley, J. E. (2006). Comparison of the Saint Louis University mental status examination and the Mini-Mental State Examination for detecting dementia and mild neurocognitive disorder—A pilot study. *American Journal of Geriatric Psychiatry*, *14*(11), 900–910. https://doi.org/10.1097/01.JGP.0000221510.33817.86

World Health Organization. (2001). *International classification of functioning, disability and health*.

Zientz, J., Rackley, A., Chapman, S. B., Hopper, T., & Mahendra, N. K. E. (2007). Evidence-based practice recommendations for dementia: Educating caregivers about Alzheimer's disease and training communication strategies. *Journal of Medical Speech-Language Pathology*, *15*, 53–64.

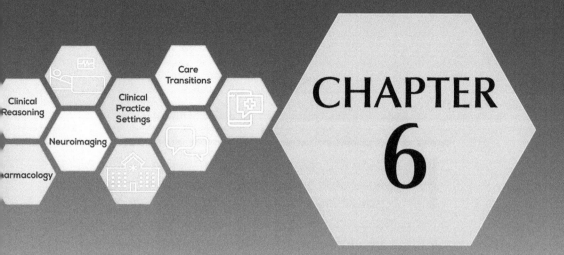

Outpatient Care and Ongoing Therapy Services in Health Settings

Minal Kadam, Megan E. Schliep, and Alex F. Johnson

Chapter Objectives

Upon completion of this chapter, the reader will be able to:

- Explain guiding principles and considerations in outpatient treatment.
- Provide key insights for clinical planning and decision-making.
- Consider various treatment models and modes of delivery.

Introduction

Previous chapters in this text focused on speech-language pathology services in inpatient settings, including acute care, inpatient rehabilitation, and long-term care. In this chapter, we provide considerations regarding outpatient speech-language pathology services. The outpatient setting consists of a diverse array of locations including hospital outpatient departments, general rehabilitation centers, speech and language clinics and centers, physician offices, and speech-language pathologist (SLP) private practices. It is beyond the scope of this chapter to provide detailed discussions of these different contexts for service delivery. Rather, in this chapter, we discuss common considerations that occur across outpatient speech-language pathology service settings.

Almost every SLP has experienced service delivery in an outpatient setting as part of their clinical training. Most graduate students in the United States have their very first clinical education experiences in the closely supervised setting of the university clinic. Over the course of their graduate practicum, this early experience is complemented by experiences in other outpatient settings, where the student experiences increasing levels of responsibility and independence. Students frequently comment that the real-world setting is substantially different from the experience of the university clinic. It is important to note that the earliest experiences in the university clinic are designed to provide the time, space, and supervision necessary for earliest learning of foundational skills for the developing SLP, while the real-world setting is focused on client care, meeting the demands of a busy clinical setting, and providing access to services to meet the needs of as many clients as possible.

Referrals for outpatient therapy may come from many different sources. Examples of referral pathways may include:

1. Clients who have recently discharged from an inpatient setting who receive recommendations for ongoing therapy. Future therapy services are typically coordinated by the inpatient case manager, who

makes arrangements for outpatient speech-language pathology, physical therapy, and/or occupational therapy evaluations and ongoing treatment.

2. *Clients who are referred by a primary care provider or specialist who has documented a change in the client's speech-language, cognitive-communication, or swallowing status.*

3. *Clients who request a referral from their physician due to changes that they or their families have observed.*

For purposes of discussion, this chapter is organized around topics common to the delivery of outpatient services. It is intended to serve as a basic guide for the new clinician starting practice in this setting.

Guiding Considerations in Outpatient Care

Continuity of Services

For clients who have received services in an acute, rehabilitation, or long-term setting, the transition becomes critically important. From a client-centered perspective, understanding the services previously received, the progress demonstrated by the client, and any other medical interventions that are ongoing is essential. As part of building the therapeutic relationship with the client, it is vital that the clinician work to understand the client's—and their care partners'—perspective of their communication and swallowing status and goals. It is also beneficial for clinicians to understand the perspective of the clients and their families on prior treatment, such as if they found it beneficial, if it matched their goals, and if it matched their expectations. Approaching the client with an attitude of genuine concern, respect, and information about the services previously provided are all components of quality speech-language pathology services.

The tools and methods for accomplishing this transition include review of documentation from the previous point of care, conversation with the referring SLP, and interviews with the client and the family. Often, the most frequently overlooked source of information is communication with the previous SLP who provided care for the client in an earlier level of care. (Of note, it is important to seek permission from the client prior to reaching out to their prior care providers.) One brief conversation can eliminate unnecessary duplications of tests and procedures, insights about the client that may not be obvious from the other sources, and discovery of particular tasks or tools that have facilitated improvement.

The Outpatient Evaluation

For clients who have not been hospitalized prior to their outpatient encounter (e.g., following stroke or other acute medical event), the outpatient setting may be their first contact with an SLP. Other clients, who have been seen in acute or rehabilitation settings, may come with more referral information and may have experience with speech services in one of these settings. In any case, the outpatient clinician initiates the building of the therapeutic relationship, establishing initial goals, and attending to the client's social or vocational concerns and the educational needs of the client.

During the evaluation, the SLP will typically verify previously gathered information or may collect new information about the client's history. Most experienced clinicians will note that by simultaneously attending to the information being presented and speech and language production, along with the client's organization of information being shared, they can gain significant (and efficient) insight into the client's perspectives and assumptions about their own communication and/or swallowing problems. A conversational format for collecting this information can reveal what the client understands and believes (e.g., "my doctor told me I will never improve that much"), affording the clinician an opportunity to understand the client's perspective. Here, *motivational interviewing* provides a strong framework for collaborative communication that can help the client and clinician understand the client's perspectives and priorities, which will in turn inform the direction of their care. Motivational interviewing is a client-centered approach to addressing feelings associated with changes from their illness or injury (Miller & Rollnick, 2013). Originally intended for psychotherapy in substance abuse, motivational interviewing uses a line of questioning intended to strengthen and support a client's motivations for change through exploring their personal values and perspectives (Rollnick & Miller, 1995). Motivational interviewing guides the conversation with emphasis on bolstering the client's ability to identify their own capacity for change. In this style of interviewing, the client and clinician are equal partners within a discussion.

Over the course of the evaluation, the clinician makes structured and informal observations, completes standardized and dynamic assessments, and establishes the diagnosis. Selection of appropriate assessments is based on the chart review, reason for referral, and the aforementioned interview. There are a great number of standardized assessments available, each of which can provide valuable diagnostic information. Tierney-Hendricks and colleagues (2022) explored outcome measurement practices in aphasia, for example, and surveyed clinicians across the continuum of care about their assessment and treatment practices. Assessments that clinicians in the outpatient setting reported frequently using include the Western Aphasia Battery–Revised (WAB-R; Kertesz, 2007); Boston Diagnostic Assessment of Aphasia, Third Edition (BDAE-3; Goodglass et al., 2000); Boston Naming Test–2 (BNT-2; Kaplan et al., 2001), Cognitive-Linguistic Quick Test-Plus (CLQT+; Helm-Estabrooks, 2017), and the Repeatable Battery for the Assessment of Neuropsychological Status (RBANS; Randolph et al., 1998). These assessments provide a simple, predetermined protocol for gathering initial data. It is not always possible to collect the required information within the initial evaluation. In these cases, the clinician must prioritize the collection of data needed to establish a plan of care and further set a plan to engage the client in diagnostic therapy in future sessions. At the end of any evaluation, providing feedback to the client and establishing realistic goals together is a critical part of developing the client's trust and buy-in for treatment.

Focus of Care

As clients present for services in the outpatient setting, they may be seeking diagnostic evaluation or determination of potential for successful treatment. They may also be referred as part of a comprehensive multidisciplinary program. Additionally, it is common for clients to be seeking the professional services of a clinical specialist in voice, neurogenic communication disorders, cognitive-communication disorders, augmentative communication disorders, or dysphagia.

The focus of care for persons with communication disorders varies by the client's condition, the referral question, and the client's point in the recovery process. Once a speech-language diagnosis is established and the client's initial concerns are addressed, a determination is made about the ensuing treatment. The question as to whether the client can benefit from treatment that is focused on impairment or activity levels or is more focused on return to activities of their daily life is a critical and ongoing consideration for the clinician and client to explore together.

As opposed to a dichotomy of functional versus impairment focus, it is helpful to think of all rehabilitative care as a continuum, with the clinician identifying the most appropriate starting point in the continuum. For some clients, usually early in their treatment, a focus on physical systems that support speech or swallowing can be most appropriate. As treatment progresses, the decision to move to treatment that focuses on the activities of communicating, talking, reading and writing, speaking, or swallowing provides a critical transition toward more functional skills. As the ability to use some of these skills emerges, the clinician advances the focus of treatment to consideration of participation in life activities that require speech, language, or swallowing.

Not all clients will follow this continuum directly. One does not need to perfect individual skills in order to participate in daily or vocational activities. Clients often achieve return to activity through a combination of restoration and compensation. This dual approach allows a return to school, work, or prior functions without requiring the complete recovery from or resolution of impairments. This approach is particularly important for clients with severe neurologic and physical conditions in which full recovery from impairment may not be expected.

Goal Setting

Outpatient services may be a "last stop" for a client before resuming particular life activities or may be provided as the client simultaneously resumes activities. These activities may include returning to work, returning to school, and resuming household responsibilities. Once the evaluation has been completed, the clinician will have identified impairments and their severities and will collaborate with the client to establish a plan of care. In prioritizing goals, it is crucial to focus on the client's priorities and areas they identify as the most challenging or most impactful in their lives and daily activities. A client-centered approach to treatment ensures that the client's values, choices, and preferences are considered when selecting targets of intervention. The client-centered care philosophy is based in Carl Roger's person-centered therapy (Rogers, 1950). This approach is rooted in the belief that all clients have the ability to direct their own care and, therefore, should drive the direction of intervention and participate in goal writing.

When establishing the plan of care, clinicians must plan for both long-term goals and short-term goals. Long-term goals should be set based on the client's functional goals and consider the client's prognosis. What activities does the client want to resume? What level of independence is the client expected to achieve in the chosen activities? The clinician then helps to determine what target is attainable within the expected time frame of care and the support that will be needed to achieve the goal. The short-term goals are the tactical goals that work toward achieving the long-term goal. In these, there may be an initial focus on impairments as described earlier. For example, in order to achieve the goal of participating in book club discussions (long-term goal), an initial short-term goal may target improving confrontational or responsive naming. As in all settings, goals should always be written within the SMART framework, in which goals must be specific, measurable, attainable, realistic, and time-bound (Bovend'Eerdt et al., 2009). It is not within the scope of this text to instruct on development of SMART goals, however, this is an important area of development for clinicians that requires ongoing practice.

Once goals have been identified, the next decision a clinician has to make is selecting treatment approaches that are appropriate and effective for the client. Selection of treatment approaches should be tailored specifically to each individual client. There are evidence-based treatment protocols that clinicians can employ such as the Verb Network Strengthening Treatment (VNeST) protocol (Edmonds et al., 2009), the Sentence Production Program for Aphasia (SPPA) program (Helm-Estabrooks & Nicholas, 2000), or the Attention Process Training Program (Sohlberg & Mateer, 1987), to name a few. Some treatment protocols may require purchasing materials. More often than not, treatment plans combine multiple evidence-based approaches that best fit the individual's needs.

As the client progresses toward their long-term goals, the therapy activities that are selected should increasingly simulate real-life conditions. This can be achieved by taking the client out of the more-structured therapy room and into different settings to promote generalization of skills outside, while maintaining necessary cueing and support from the clinician. Clients may also bring in family or friends with whom to practice or who may be trained in cueing strategies to help the client apply what is learned in therapy in the natural setting. "Homework" or home practice and application is crucial to generalizing trained skills for functional use and greater independence. As opposed to the home-care setting, where therapy is happening in the client's everyday environment, outpatient clinicians typically have fewer opportunities to facilitate carryover into the natural setting. Much relies on the client's willingness to comply with home practice and recommendations. Family support again becomes a key strength in assisting with this carryover.

The time frame in which goals are set in the outpatient setting is considerably longer than in earlier points in the client's care. Long-term goals can be set for up to 12 weeks, in comparison to the typical few days in acute care or 2 to 3 weeks in inpatient rehabilitation facilities. As a result, short-term goals can be for as short as 1 week and up to 4 weeks at a time before a progress note is required to update goals. Due to the complex nature of clients' lives and participation, clients may be seen in speech services for long episodes of care. Even as one functional goal is achieved (i.e., resuming responsibility as financial manager in the home), there may be additional activities that are important to the client, such as returning to work or being the primary caregiver for their children/parents. In these longer episodes of care, clients may be encouraged to take breaks from therapy to fully engage in life participation at their current level of functioning and participate in an established home program for practice and carryover. They can then return for additional services to target specific participation goals that they find are still limited after engaging in daily activities. The relationship between an outpatient therapist and their clients may often be ongoing.

Billing, Coding, and Documentation of Services

Clinicians in the outpatient setting are directly involved with billing of services. Billing involves knowledge of Current Procedural Terminology codes (referred to as CPT codes; American Medical Association, 1999), which are the designations for the type of treatment that is provided, as well as knowledge of *International Classification of Diseases, Tenth Revision, Clinical Modification* codes (referred to as ICD-10 codes; World Health Organization [WHO], 2016), which are the designations for the diagnoses being treated. Insurance companies generate policies that dictate which treatments are applicable and reimbursable for specific diagnoses. Clinicians must be aware of these general policies and use the appropriate diagnosis that matches the treatment provided while also aligning with the policy requirements. For example, one insurance may cover the cost of *"Treatment of speech, language, voice, communication, and/or auditory processing disorder; individual"* (CPT code 92507) when coded with the diagnosis of "aphasia" (ICD-10 code R47.01), while another insurance may only cover this service when coded with the diagnosis of "aphasia due to acute stroke" (ICD-10 code I63.9). If the insurance does not cover the treatment code for a diagnosis that applies to the client's current status, it may mean that the client will not be able to receive services through their insurance. Private payment is accepted by many clinics; however, most individuals either cannot or choose not to pursue this route. It is a part of the role of the SLP in this setting to understand these limitations and provide clients with the education they need to continue their recovery wherever they may be along the continuum.

In addition to treatment codes and diagnoses, the outpatient clinician must be aware of a component of billing codes called "modifiers," which must be applied to treatment codes in various situations. For example, all outpatient services require special modifiers (e.g., the modifier "GN") to be attached to the billing. Other modifiers include those for teletherapy and designating medical necessity.

Billing claims would be incomplete without proper documentation of services. Documenting services is important for reimbursement, as well as for tracking a client's progress and keeping a record of provided treatments, client responses, and outcomes for later review. By maintaining clear documentation, the clinician affords themselves, as well as future treating clinicians, a clear picture of the client's treatment history. This helps the current clinician identify effective interventions and assist with planning ongoing treatment or determining readiness for discharge. Documentation should be clear and specific enough for a second clinician to easily understand and pick up services where the first clinician left off if assuming care of a client. Clear data on progress toward goals are an important part of good documentation practices. Since goals are written to be "measurable," measurement of outcomes should be included within the documentation. Data may be tracked in the form of numerical percentages, number of occurrences of a behavior, or completion of functional goals or activities.

As with most medical documentation, speech-language pathology notes also typically use the SOAP note format. SOAP notes include four main sections: subjective, objective, assessment, and plan. Within these four areas, the clinician can document the client's perspective and current status in *subjective*, the data associated with the treatments provided within the *objective*, the clinician's observations and *assessments* as a result of these data, and the *plan* for upcoming sessions and continuing care.

Documentation may also be used for future clinicians and medical providers during chart reviews in future treatments, by payor sources to determine eligibility for reimbursement, and in some cases, this documentation can be subpoenaed for court proceedings. With this in mind, the SLP must be sure that the notes are specific but generally understandable to an outside reader.

Family and Client Education

In all settings and at all points of care, family and client education is crucial to the rehabilitation process. During outpatient services, family and client understanding are key to compliance with exercises and carryover of trained strategies. In order to promote client engagement and buy-in for therapy, the client benefits from an understanding of their condition and the selected interventions. In the case of clients with cognitive impairments, family and caregivers may take on the responsibility of carryover and implementing home practice. For this reason, they must be educated in not only the conditions and interventions but also in effective cueing and scaffolding for their loved ones at home. Families and clients can receive education by way of verbal descriptions, demonstrations, written handouts, and video examples.

Along the same vein, involving family and social support in treatment also helps the clinician understand the client's social and cultural setting in which they are living. Clinicians' understanding of the client's background, values, and priorities is integral to providing client-centered, culturally responsive care.

Culturally Responsive Care

The nature of work for a SLP is innately personal, involving the areas of communication, which focuses the lens of how we perceive and interact with the world. As such, it is not possible to provide appropriate or adequate care to our clients without considering their culture, including family, language, social history, and values, to name a few components. In order to do so, it is important to consider the terms *cultural competence* and *cultural responsiveness.* For years, speech-language pathology students and clinicians have been provided nominal training in *cultural competence.* While important, this particular phrase implies that a clinician is able to fully appreciate and understand all cultures that they encounter. Realistically, it is (a) not possible for a clinician to know everything about any culture, and (b) regardless of how much information is gathered, no clinician is able to experience any culture but their own. A more current and reflective term is *cultural responsiveness.* This term indicates that a clinician has cultural awareness and puts in the time and effort needed to understand a client and their family in order to provide the best, most appropriate care for them. Campinha-Bacote (2002) developed the "Process of Cultural Competence in the Delivery of Healthcare Services," which provides a clear explanation of this. In her model, Campinha-Bacote proposes that cultural competence is an ongoing process, rather than a state, in which the clinician integrates cultural awareness, cultural knowledge, cultural skill, cultural encounters, and cultural desires. It behooves the treating clinician to examine these constructs and engage in the practice of persistently becoming culturally competent, which will afford the clinician the opportunity to provide culturally responsive care (Campinha-Bacote, 2002).

It is essential to the care of each client to employ culturally responsive care in assessment and treatment. Unfortunately, the current state of our field has limited options for assessments, normative data, and intervention programs that consider cultural diversity. Particularly in recent years, there is a strong push to turn the field in this direction to best serve all clients, beginning with SLP graduate education and in recruiting more diverse graduate students in order to further enhance the diversity of clinicians within the field. Increasingly, more resources are now available to help clinicians along this journey.

Terminating Services

Determining time for discharge can be a complicated task in the outpatient setting. Discharge is planned based on the client achieving set goals or due to a plateau in progress. In some situations, a client may be discharged due to comorbidities, sudden decline in function, or new injury or illness. Planned discharge, however, involves reassessing function (formal or informal) and preparing the client for discharge. In some further unfortunate cases, discharge may be planned due to exhaustion of insurance benefits. It is part of the SLP's responsibilities to know the client's insurance benefits at the start of care so that they can plan for expected termination and prepare the client for this end. It may be possible in some cases to appeal an insurance denial for continued services based on medical necessity; these cases should be considered individually as they arise.

Being discharged from outpatient rehabilitation can be a frightening point in a client's recovery. At this point, the client has potentially been on the rehabilitation journey for some time. Following outpatient care, the client is often not moving on to another level of service, but rather, they are going on to live in their previous or new home environments and carry on their recovery through their home programs. At time of discharge, the SLP must provide the client with education on their progress in treatment, must develop an understandable and sustainable home program, and must ensure that the appropriate supports are in place for successful transition. It is not unusual for clients and their families to be resistant to discharge. They may feel they are not ready, that there is still progress to be made, or overall concern that they are being discharged before they have returned back to baseline. To alleviate some of these concerns and ease the transition, clinicians can set realistic expectations and collaborate when setting goals. Discussing progress toward goals, particularly when nearing discharge, can help the client see the ways in which they are ready for discharge. Clients also feel comforted if reassured that they can request a referral to return to services from their primary care provider should their symptoms or illness persist or worsen. If appropriate, the clinician can provide a work email address or phone contact number for the client or family members to reach out with questions. With the pervasive use of patient portals connected with electronic medical records, clients have the opportunity to reach out through these channels to ask questions or discuss potential return to therapy. Successful termination of services is marked by clients and their families understanding their current level of functioning, the discharge recommendations, with acceptance of the recommendations and agreement to follow through.

General Modalities of Outpatient Treatment

There are a variety of models in which outpatient treatment is provided for clients requiring speech-language services. Clients may participate in individual therapy sessions, which remains the predominant model in adult rehabilitation settings, or may be seen as part of an organized group or intensive program. The use of teletherapy rehabilitation has become increasingly popular for delivering some speech-language pathology services.

Individual Therapy Sessions

Individual therapy provides the opportunity for a highly customized, client-centered approach to treatment. The clinician and the client have the opportunity to establish highly customized and functional goals and to use their time together with great efficiency. For therapies that focus on needed practice, individual therapy assures that the client has enough time to acquire the skill, repeat it to gain proficiency, and receive constant feedback and gain self-awareness of performance and/or potential opportunities for improvement.

A common format for a 1-hr individual therapy session includes a brief social interaction, a review of the client's progress and practice of skills since the previous session, training new skills or expanding on previously learned material, feedback and evaluation time, and an assignment for home practice. If the client needs considerable assistance, it is important to include a family member in therapy.

As previously stated, the range of evidence-based therapies for the various types of communication or swallowing disorders is vast, and typically well examined in graduate programs. An excellent resource that should be familiar to every SLP is the ASHA Practice Portal (ASHA, n.d.). The practice portal includes a variety of tools, evidence-based resources, and client education materials organized by disorder type. This tool, and other databases, can help the clinician make important decisions about treatment.

Group Therapy Sessions

Group therapy may be offered as a complement to individual therapy (e.g., a place to practice learned skills) or as a primary approach to treatment. The obvious benefit of group therapy is that clients are afforded the benefit of learning from one another and can practice skills and compensations in a more dynamic interactive setting. For group therapy to be billable, each member must be working toward a targeted goal with skilled treatment provided by a clinician. The group is only the setting in which the intervention is provided. Group therapy requires significant planning to assure that all the group members' needs are being met and that all group members participate in the session.

Group therapy has been utilized for areas such as aphasia interventions and cognitive skills groups, to name a few. Aphasia groups can facilitate interventions within true conversational context and elicit more varied and natural responses and interactions (Fama et al., 2016). There are even some specific evidence-based group approaches. For example, the Rusk Institute has developed the Problem-Solving Group Protocol. In this protocol, groups of individuals participate in 24 sessions targeting self-regulation and motivation as well as "clear thinking" through modeling, role-playing, worksheets, and daily logs (Rath et al., 2003). Other cognitive skills groups include executive skills groups and community skills groups.

One may also consider posttreatment communication or cognitive groups, which focus on carryover and maintenance of skills in a more natural but safe setting versus targeting specific goals. These groups are not billable but can provide much-needed supportive communication environments for clients after discharge. These groups also provide opportunities for individuals with similar communication challenges to connect and build community. Examples of these could be aphasia book clubs (see Box 6–1),

---

Box 6–1. Group Therapy Highlight: Aphasia Book Clubs

Aphasia book clubs can be found in outpatient or community settings and are designed to support language skills within the context of a group of peers. Book clubs typically engage three or more participants who meet on a regular basis. A moderator, typically an SLP, may select a book—or support the group in selecting a book—based on length, appropriateness for adults, reading level, and the ability to facilitate discussions based on the topics. Aphasia book clubs can provide similar social support as a support group, with a more structured framework that also promotes cognitive and communication skills. A typical book club includes assigning a certain number of chapters or pages to complete before each meeting. The facilitator can utilize visual aids, vocabulary lists, summaries, and discussion questions to support comprehension, recall, and expression. Cognitive and linguistic benefits of aphasia book clubs may include:

- reading comprehension,
- auditory comprehension within group discussion,
- verbal and/or written expression of plot points or opinions,
- recall of plot details and characters,
- synthesis of information, and
- social communication.

Aphasia book clubs also go beyond engaging in book topics and cognitive-linguistic skills. Group members often will participate in a "check-in" with one another to build social rapport. Regular meetings of individuals with similar experiences can foster a sense of community. There is no particular format that an aphasia book club needs to follow; provided that the book club is designed to facilitate engagement with the material and other members of the group, participation can increase social engagement and reduce social isolation (Knollman-Porter & Julian, 2019).

---

monthly voice maintenance groups, social communication groups, and other venues facilitated by SLPs outside the context of targeted individual goals. The SPEAK OUT! model for treatment of voice disorders in Parkinson's disease is followed by participation in the "Loud Crowd," a weekly community group session to promote generalization and maintenance of learned skills (The Parkinson's Voice Project).

Group therapy can offer opportunities that cannot be found in individual therapy; however, it may not be appropriate for all clients depending on severity and presentation of impairments. Establishing a therapy group in an outpatient clinic requires the support of administration and demonstrated interest by clients in the area that would be appropriate for the group.

Day Rehabilitation

Both individual and group therapy may be provided within the context of the day rehabilitation setting. Day rehabilitation, frequently referred to as "day rehab" is a distinct type of ongoing rehabilitation program. Care in day rehab is coordinated between disciplines, similar to the care provided in inpatient rehabilitation facilities (Chapter 3), but it is provided in an outpatient environment, meaning the client lives at home and attends therapy each day for a specified "block" of time. Clients who are medically stable enough to be at home but who still require an intensive, coordinated therapy program are often considered good candidates for day rehab.

In a day rehab program, a client typically attends three to five times a week and may receive therapy for a longer period of time. For example, a client may participate in day rehab for several months, or longer, provided they continue to make gains and require the intensity of a day rehab program. Day rehab clients must participate in at least two, and often three, therapy disciplines (e.g., physical therapy, occupational therapy, and/or speech-language pathology). As opposed to the traditional outpatient setting, where therapy appointments are scheduled independently, therapy services for day rehab clients are coordinated. For example, the client may attend day rehab for a 3-hr block (e.g., 9:00 a.m. until 12:00 p.m.) and participate in an hour of each therapy discipline with a team of collaborating physical therapy, occupational therapy, and SLP clinicians. Therapy may involve individual sessions, as well as group sessions, with each client working toward their own identified goal areas to promote independence and return to premorbid activities. Additionally, therapy may take place "outside" the therapy room and may involve community activities or outings to practice independence and specific skills in everyday locations, such as the grocery store, the library, or a coffee shop.

Specialty Clinics

The field of speech pathology covers an extensive list of conditions and disorders. As a result, new SLPs leave their graduate programs as generalists in their field. In most outpatient clinics, this generalist background serves clinicians well, as they may encounter any of the diagnoses they have prepared for. There are, however, some areas within speech pathology that are best served by clinicians who have specialized skills and knowledge within the area. These clinicians often complete their clinical fellowship year in clinics such as these or are otherwise trained in the field. Some of these areas include augmentative and alternative communication, voice and airway disorders, and swallowing disorders. Other clinics may specialize in specific medical diagnoses such as amyotrophic lateral sclerosis, concussion, or memory clinics (dementia). If a client were to present with a particular disorder or condition, they may be best served by a specialty clinic. The clinicians in specialty clinics work with a narrow subset of conditions and are therefore well-versed in all possible treatments, the latest research for the conditions, and may also have equipment and resources specific to those conditions. For example, a client with laryngectomy often requires a clinic that can assess, fit, place, and replace tracheoesophageal voice prostheses. Most clients can be served in a general clinic where they present. In some cases, the generalist may refer their client to a specialty clinic for severe or complicated cases. In other cases, the client may receive services in an interdisciplinary outpatient clinic that includes all disciplines that are relevant to the specific diagnosis and client needs.

Intensive Therapy Programs

In some situations, there is benefit in an intensive experience of treatment. Intensive treatments for persons with aphasia and other language disorders are increasingly utilized. Intensive programs typically provide clients with both individual and group sessions, a variety of activities focused on functional recovery, and extensive practice in real-world settings. There is support for intensive therapy in aphasia (an example of an Intensive Comprehensive Aphasia Program is highlighted in Box 6–2) and in certain other treatment areas within the SLP's scope of practice (e.g., Lee Silverman Voice Treatment [LSVT] for individuals with Parkinson's disease; LSVT Global, 2022).

Box 6–2. Intensive Therapy Highlight:
Intensive Comprehensive Aphasia Programs

Rachel Pittman

The most common approaches to aphasia treatment in the outpatient setting are the traditional rehabilitation model that may involve one to three visits per week, each visit lasting 30 to 60 min, and the intensive model, which is described later. Determining which treatment model (or combination of treatment models) works best for clients is paramount. This section describes one approach to intensive therapy called an intensive comprehensive aphasia program (ICAP). An ICAP is defined as a service delivery model that provides a minimum of 3 hr of daily treatment over a specified period of at least 2 weeks to a cohort of participants who begin and end the program at the same time (Rose et al., 2013). Since the goal for clients participating in an ICAP is to maximize communication potential and enhance life participation (Persad et al., 2013), ICAPs are often interprofessional in nature so that clients not only receive speech-language pathology intervention, but they participate in many other services as well. Those other services include occupational therapy, physical therapy, nutrition counseling, music therapy, adaptive sports programs, family and caregiver educational programming, and other programs.

Given the stated goal of maximizing communication and enhancing life participation, ICAPs are rooted in the WHO's International Classification of Functioning, Disability and Health known as the WHO-ICF framework (WHO, 2001). For context, the WHO-ICF framework views disabilities through a biopsychosocial lens that incorporates elements of a medical model and a social model (see Chapter 3 for additional information regarding the WHO-ICF framework as it applies to various rehabilitation settings). Figure 6–1, as introduced in Chapter 3, shows that when using the ICF framework, a disability is viewed as the outcome of interactions between health conditions, in this case aphasia, and contextual factors such as environmental and personal factors.

ICAPs are also grounded in the Life Participation Approach to Aphasia (Chapey et al., 2000), which is a service-delivery approach whose core values serve to guide assessment, treatment, and research in aphasia. Those core values are the following:

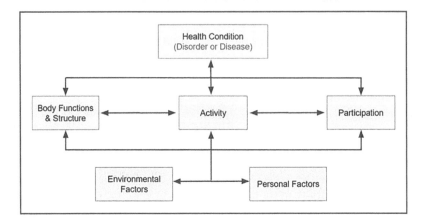

FIGURE 6–1. *Source:* Adaptation of the International Classification of Functioning, Disability, and Health (ICF) Framework. https://www.who .int/standards/classifications/international-classification-of-functioning-disability-and-health

1. The explicit goal is enhancement of life participation.
2. Everyone affected by aphasia is entitled to service.
3. Success measures include documented life enhancement changes.
4. Both personal and environmental factors are intervention targets.
5. Emphasis is on availability of services as needed at all stages of aphasia. (Chapey et al., 2000, p. 6)

Given the influence of the WHO-ICF and LPAA frameworks, ICAPs are structured such that they are comprehensive and interprofessional in scope, utilizing individual and group therapy and client and family education, and outcomes are often defined by each domain of the WHO-ICF framework. An example of one program's ICAP weekly schedule is shown in Table 6–1 in order to illustrate its comprehensive and interprofessional nature.

Outcomes of ICAPs can be described in many ways and according to the four WHO-ICF domains, including reporting changes in impairment-based measures such as a change in score on a traditional aphasia battery such as the Western Aphasia Battery—Revised (WAB-R; Kertesz, 2007) and/or nonverbal assessments of cognition such as the Cognitive Linguistic Quick Test—Plus (CLQT+; Helm-Estabrooks, 2017). Other ways to assess outcomes include changes on participation,

TABLE 6-1

Sample Weekly Treatment Schedule for an Intensive Comprehensive Aphasia Program (ICAP)

Weeks 2–5: ICAP Treatment Schedule

Time	Monday	Tuesday	Wednesday	Thursday	Friday
8:30–9:00 a.m.	No activities	Arrive at IHP	Arrive at IHP	Arrive at IHP	Arrive at IHP
9:00–10:00 a.m.		Individual SLP Session	Individual SLP Session	Individual SLP Session	Individual SLP Session
10:00–11:00 a.m.		Individual SLP Session	Small Group SLP Session	Individual SLP Session	Individual SLP Session
11:00 a.m.–12:00 p.m.		Occupational Therapy Group	Occupational Therapy Group	Physician Assistant Studies Student Group	Occupational Therapy Group and Lunch
12:00–1:00 p.m.		Travel to SRH	Travel to SRH	Travel to SRH	
1:00–2:00 p.m.		Social Lunch	Social Lunch	Social Lunch	Travel to SRH
2:00–3:00 p.m.		Adaptive Sports	Wellness	Adaptive Sports	Wellness
3:00–4:00 p.m.		Transition Time and Music Therapy	Large Group SLP Session	Transition Time and Music Therapy	Large Group SLP Session
4:00–5:00 p.m.		Swim Group	End at 4:00 p.m.	End at 4:00 p.m.	Harmonica Group

Note: IHP, MGH Institute of Health Professions; SLP, speech-language pathology; SRH, Spaulding Rehabilitation Hospital.

Source: Adapted from "Outcomes of an Interprofessional Intensive Comprehensive Aphasia Program's First Five Years," by M. Nicholas, R. Pittmann, S. Pennington, L. T. Connor, D. Ambrosi, L. Brady Wagner, . . . M. Savastano, 2021, *Topics in Stroke Rehabilitation*, pp. 1–17 (https://doi.org/10.1080/107493 57.2021.1970452). Copyright © 2022 Taylor & Francis Group.

environment, person, and caregiver measures. Improvement and changes in one's participation in life are often reported through changes in Stroke Impact Scale (Duncan et al., 1999) score, Canadian Occupational Performance Measure (Law et al., 2014), and the like. Outcomes in the domains of environment and person are often reported through changes on scores in measures such as the Medical-Outcomes Study (Sherbourne & Stewart, 1991) as well as the Communication Confidence Rating Scale for Aphasia (Babbitt et al., 2011). Caregiver-reported changes are reported through satisfaction surveys as well as through qualitative interviews.

Teletherapy

In addition to in-person therapy, teletherapy is an increasingly utilized modality for outpatient care. Teletherapy is only appropriate when the quality of service provided matches the quality that in-person services would provide. Appropriateness of teletherapy should be determined on a case-by-case basis, considering diagnosis, client's comfort with technology, and client's ability to participate without in-person support.

There are different ways in which to provide teletherapy services. Synchronous services involve meeting with the client in real time via telecommunications, video, or telephone, and providing services directly. These services look very similar to in-person services, utilizing screen sharing and emailed materials to support interventions. Asynchronous services include assigning the client with work, often via app-based treatment activities (e.g., Constant Therapy [2022] or Tactus Therapy [2022]) and providing feedback and strategies. Studies investigating efficacy of teletherapy are increasing with the telepractice boom following the start of the COVID-19 pandemic. For example, Gauch and colleagues (2022) completed a review of quality-of-life outcomes following aphasia telepractice. Their findings suggest telepractice in aphasia treatment can improve quality of life with both synchronous and asynchronous treatments.

In many ways, teletherapy has enhanced access to care for clients who may otherwise be unable to receive services, whether related to geographic location, problems with transportation, mobility limitations, or fatigue. There are, however, challenges associated with teletherapy. These include poor internet access, unexpected technical difficulties, and difficulty adapting available diagnostic and therapeutic materials. Given the many variables discussed here, careful consideration should be taken before incorporating tele-therapy into a given client's treatment plan.

Conclusion

This chapter considers the structure and variety of settings in which outpatient and ongoing therapy services are provided, as well as the responsibilities of an SLP working in these settings. Some clients receive outpatient care as they move through the care continuum (e.g., moving from an acute-care hospital to an inpatient rehabilitation facility to ongoing outpatient services), while other clients may present directly for outpatient services after referral from their primary care provider due to a change in speech, language, cognitive, or swallowing status, or from self-referral. As a result, chart review and outreach to previous providers is an important component for developing continuity of care. In the outpatient evaluation, clinicians have the benefit of having more time than they may have in other settings. The use of full standardized assessments is generally more typical here than in inpatient levels of care. In treatment, the focus of care is centered on the client's participation in their home, work, community, or school settings. In many cases, the clients are already within these settings while they are in therapy. Because outpatient services are provided in this context, episodes of care can be long, lasting months, and perhaps recurring. The relationships between the client and the outpatient therapist can be ongoing throughout the client's recovery or disease process. As a partner in their recovery, the outpatient therapist must engage family and social support systems into therapy and be certain to consider and utilize the client's culture into setting goals and treatment planning.

References

American Medical Association. (1999). *CPT (Current Procedural Terminology)*. https://www.ama-assn.org/amaone/cpt-current-procedural-terminology

American Speech-Language-Hearing Association. (n.d.). *The practice portal*. https://www.asha.org/practice-portal/

Babbitt, E. M., Heinemann, A. W., Semik, P., & Cherney, L. R. (2011). Psychometric properties of the communication confidence rating scale for aphasia (CCRSA): Phase 2. *Aphasiology, 25*(6–7), 727–735.

Bovend'Eerdt, T. J., Botell, R. E., & Wade, D. T. (2009). Writing SMART rehabilitation goals and achieving goal attainment scaling: A practical guide. *Clinical Rehabilitation, 23*(4), 352–361. https://doi.org/10.1177/0269215508101741

Campinha-Bacote, J. (2002). The process of cultural competence in the delivery of healthcare services: A model of care. *Journal of Transcultural Nursing, 13*(3), 181–184.

Chapey, R., Duchan, J. F., Elman, R. J., Garcia, L. J., Kagan, A., Lyon, J. G., & Simmons Mackie, N. (2000). Life participation approach to aphasia: A statement of values for the future. *The ASHA Leader, 5*(3), 4–6.

Constant Therapy Health. (2022). *The Learning Corp.* https://constanttherapyhealth.com/

Duncan, P. W., Wallace, D., Lai, S. M., Johnson, D., Embretson, S., & Laster, L. J. (1999). The stroke impact scale version 2.0: Evaluation of reliability, validity, and sensitivity to change. *Stroke, 30*(10), 2131–2140.

Edmonds, L. A., Nadeau, S. E., & Kiran, S. (2009). Effect of Verb Network Strengthening Treatment (VNeST) on lexical retrieval of content words in sentences in persons with aphasia. *Aphasiology, 23*(3), 402–424.

Fama, M. E., Baron, C. R., Hatfield, B., & Turkeltaub, P. E. (2016). Group therapy as a social context for aphasia recovery: A pilot, observational study in an acute rehabilitation hospital. *Topics in Stroke Rehabilitation, 23*(4), 276–283. https://doi.org/10.1080/10749357.2016.1155277

Gauch, M., Leinweber, J., Plath, A., Spelter, B., & Corsten, S. (2022). Quality of life outcomes from aphasia telepractice: A scoping review. *Aphasiology,* 1-25.

Goodglass, H., Kaplan, E., & Barressi, B. (2000). *Boston Diagnostic Aphasia Examination, Third Edition (BDAE-3).* Pro-Ed.

Helm-Estabrooks, N. (2017). *Cognitive-linguistic quick test–plus (CLQT+).* Pearson.

Helm-Estabrooks, N., & Nicholas, M.(2000). *Sentence production program for aphasia.* Pro-Ed.

Kaplan, E., Goodglas, H., & Weintraub, S. (2001). *Boston Naming Test-2 (BNT-2).* SpringerLink.

Kertesz, A. (2007). *Western Aphasia Battery—Revised.* Pearson.

Knollman-Porter, K., & Julian, S. K. (2019). Book club experiences, engagement, and reading support use by people with aphasia. *American Journal of Speech-Language Pathology, 28*(3), 1084–1098.

Law, M., Baptiste, S., Carswell, A., McColl, M. A., Polatajko, H., & Pollock, N. (2014). *The Canadian Occupational Performance Measure, Fifth edition.* CAOT Publications ACE.

LSVT Global. (2022). *LSVT Loud: Speech therapy for Parkinson's disease and similar conditions.* https://www.lsvtglobal.com/LSVTLoud

Miller, W. R., & Rollnick, S. (2013). *Motivational interviewing: Helping people to change* (3rd ed.). Guilford Press.

Nicholas, M., Pittmann, R., Pennington, S., Connor, L. T., Ambrosi, D., Brady Wagner, L., . . . Savastano, M. (2021). Outcomes of an interprofessional intensive comprehensive aphasia program's first five years. *Topics in Stroke Rehabilitation,* 1–17. https://doi.org/10.1080/10749357.2021.1970452

Persad, C., Wozniak, L., & Kostopoulos, E. (2013). Retrospective analysis of outcomes from two intensive comprehensive aphasia programs. *Topics in Stroke Rehabilitation, 20*(5), 388–397.

Randolph, C., Tierney, M. C., Mohr, E., & Chase, T. N. (1998). The repeatable battery for the assessment of neuropsychological status: Preliminary clinical validity. *Journal of Clinical and Experimental Neuropsychology, 20*(3), 310–319.

Rath, J. F., Simon, D., Langenbahn, D. M., Sherr, R. L., & Diller, L. (2003). Group treatment of problem-solving deficits in outpatients with traumatic brain injury: A randomised outcome study. *Neuropsychological Rehabilitation, 13*(4), 461–488.

Rogers, C. R. (1950). A current formulation of client-centered therapy. *Social Service Review, 24*(4), 442-450.

Rollnick, S., & Miller, W. R. (1995). What is motivational interviewing? *Behavioural and Cognitive Psychotherapy, 23*(4), 325–334.

Rose, M. L., Cherney, L. R., & Worrall, L. E. (2013). Intensive comprehensive aphasia programs: An international survey of practice. *Topics in Stroke Rehabilitation, 20*, 379–387.

Sherbourne, C. D., & Stewart, A. L. (1991). The MOS social support survey. *Social Science & Medicine, 32*(6), 705–714.

Sohlberg, M. M., & Mateer, C. A. (1987). Effectiveness of an attention-training program. *Journal of Clinical and Experimental Neuropsychology, 9*(2), 117–130.

Tactus Therapy. (2022). https://tactustherapy.com/

Tierney-Hendricks, C., Schliep, M. E., & Vallila-Rohter, S. (2022). Using an implementation framework to survey outcome measurement and treatment practices in aphasia. *American Journal of Speech-Language Pathology, 31*(3), 1133–1162. https://doi.org/10.1044/2021_AJSLP-21-00101

World Health Organization. (2001). *International classification of functioning, disability, and health (ICF)*. https://www.who.int/standards/classifications/international-classification-of-functioning-disability-and-health

World Health Organization. (2016). *ICD-10: International statistical classification of diseases and related health problems, 10th revision.* https://icd.who.int/browse10/2016/en#/

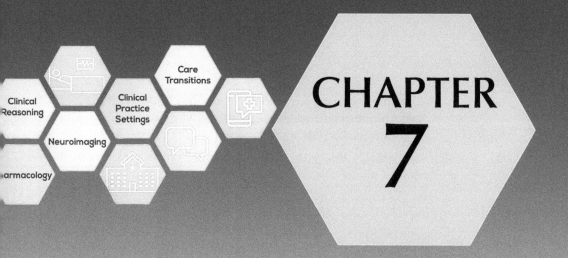

CHAPTER 7

Pediatric Medical Speech-Language Pathology

Kaitlyn Johnston Minchin

Chapter Objectives

Upon completion of this chapter, the reader will be able to:

- Describe common settings where pediatric medical speech-language pathology services are provided.
- List and discuss common pediatric medical speech-language pathology populations and conditions:
  - Define and discuss the prevalence of prematurity and congenital heart disease.
  - Describe possible impacts of prematurity on feeding/swallowing and cognitive-communication development.
  - Describe possible impacts of congenital heart disease on feeding/swallowing and cognitive-communication development.
  - List common airway and neurologic conditions that may impact feeding/swallowing and cognitive-communication development in children.

☐ Describe reasons for tracheostomy in children and list possible impacts on feeding/swallowing and/or cognitive-communication development.

▪ Describe SLP assessment and treatment considerations in the pediatric acute- and subacute-care settings.

▪ Discuss roles of the SLP alongside various team members in the pediatric medical setting.

▪ Describe impact of children with complex medical conditions on the pediatric health care system.

▪ Discuss role of families and caregivers in the pediatric medical setting.

▪ Compare and contrast palliative care in pediatric versus adult populations.

Introduction

*P*ediatric medical speech-language pathology is a specialized yet heterogeneous arena of speech-language pathology. It includes the near entirety of the traditional speech-language pathology scope of practice (i.e., feeding/swallowing, speech-language, and cognitive-communication) with a focus on children in medical settings and with overt medical conditions. Knowledge of medical speech-language pathology is meaningful across SLP settings (e.g., schools, hospitals, outpatient clinics, home health, early intervention) because children with medical needs are served across settings, but it is most concentrated in the pediatric critical- and acute-care hospital setting. It is also particularly prevalent in outpatient clinics in large academic medical settings, in pediatric rehabilitation or long-term care centers, and in home health and early intervention services. This chapter should be relevant to clinicians serving across settings, but it will particularly focus on the pediatric inpatient hospital setting. For an overview of the speech-language pathologist's (SLP) role and activities in acute care, please see Chapter 2.

Pediatric hospitals have become the de facto medical structure for serving children and families in the United States and around the world. There are more than 250 children's hospitals, and most specialty pediatric care is provided via these centers (Casimir, 2019). Staff, facilities, and processes are designed particularly for children and families. Many children's hospitals are home to a neonatal intensive care unit (NICU) for sick infants, a pediatric intensive care unit (PICU), acute-care unit(s), an emergency department, and outpatient services. Large children's hospitals typically have a variety of specialists available including, but not limited to, pediatric hospitalists, neonatologists, pediatric intensivists, pediatric surgeons, pediatric otorhinolaryngologists (ENT), pediatric neurologists, pediatric gastroenterologists, pediatric nephrologists, pediatric pulmonologists, pediatric hematologists/oncologists, and pediatric infectious disease providers. Children's hospitals also typically have a focus on psychosocial and whole family care and often employ certified child life specialists (CCLS) who help children and families process and cope with the challenges of hospitalization, illness, and disability. Outpatient care—including primary, specialty, and multidisciplinary care—is also provided through large children's hospital systems. Children's hospitals may be located (physically and organizationally) within larger health systems, including adult hospitals, but can alternatively be freestanding and separate. Children's hospitals tend to be found in large urban centers and are often associated with academic medical centers. SLP services are delivered in both inpatient and outpatient settings at these large centers.

SLPs who practice in the area of pediatric medical speech-language pathology need specialized training not only in medical conditions and health care systems but also in typical and atypical infant and child development as well as in more traditional swallowing and communication assessment and treatment. Critical thinking skills are vital as these children have highly complex diagnoses, comorbidities, and other challenges that require thoughtful diagnosis and treatment. SLPs must be able to communicate efficiently and effectively with other providers and professionals, as the SLP's role is deeply intertwined with other specialties, and SLPs make contributions to the larger medical plan of care. The American Speech-Language-Hearing Association (ASHA) provides guidelines on knowledge and skills for SLPs working with children and families in the NICU (ASHA, 2004).

Common Populations

Populations served by SLPs in pediatric medical settings are diverse, but a few specific populations are frequently seen. Children's hospitals usually care for individuals from birth to age 18 years, but it should be noted that some adults may be served in the pediatric medical setting, particularly those with congenital or childhood conditions (e.g., congenital heart disease). This section covers populations frequently encountered with the understanding that these patients can have multiple diagnoses and comorbidities.

Neonatal Population

Infants are a substantial portion of children treated by SLPs, and many children start their lives in the NICU. Approximately 8% to 15% of children born in the United States are admitted to the NICU (Braun et al., 2020; Harrison & Goodman, 2015). Many of these children are born prematurely, and others are sick term infants. Most infants in the NICU are admitted immediately or shortly after birth. Conditions requiring children to be admitted to the NICU often have feeding/swallowing and cognitive-communication impacts both in the NICU period and beyond (e.g., Caskey et al., 2014; Pados et al., 2021; Rand & Lahav, 2014; Zimmerman, 2018).

Children with prematurity are frequently admitted to the NICU. Term gestation of babies is typically considered to be 37 to 42 weeks gestation with some organizations separating the gestation further into early term (37 to 38 weeks gestation), full term (39 to 40 weeks gestation), late term (41 weeks gestation), and post term (42 weeks plus gestation) (American College of Obstetricians and Gynecologists [ACOG], 2013). Infants born before 37 weeks gestation are considered premature. Approximately 1 in 10 babies in the United States and worldwide are born prematurely (Centers for Disease Control and Prevention [CDC], 2021; World Health Organization [WHO], 2018). Preterm birth and complications related to preterm birth are the leading cause of death in children under the age of 5 years globally (WHO, 2018). Prematurity is often subdivided into categories such as extremely preterm (<28 weeks gestation), very preterm (28–32 weeks gestation), and moderate to late preterm (32–26 weeks gestation). At the time of this publication, viability was arguably considered to be in the 22- to 23-weeks gestation range (ACOG, 2017). Children with suspected gestational ages slightly younger than this have survived the neonatal period, and some have survived even with good neurodevelopmental outcomes as judged subjectively. However, many children born extremely premature do not survive their NICU stay; many have lifelong medical conditions and technology dependence. Reasons for preterm birth are varied and not always known.

Children born prematurely frequently need NICU support to help with a myriad of symptoms and needs including most often respiratory support, thermoregulation, infection control, and treatment of anatomic and physiologic anomalies. Prematurity impacts children across body systems. The respiratory system is impacted as premature infants' lungs are often too immature and underdeveloped to support breathing ex utero without support such as mechanical ventilation, continuous positive airway pressure (CPAP), or oxygen via a nasal cannula.

Fetuses receive nutrition via the placenta in utero (as well as via amniotic fluid to a lesser degree). Nutritional support for hospitalized infants may involve enteral nutrition such as expressed human milk or formula via feeding tube or by mouth and/or parenteral nutrition such as traditional intravenous (IV) fluids or total parenteral nutrition (TPN) (Figure 7–1). Most children receiving tube feeding in the NICU will have a nasogastric (NG) or orogastric (OG) tube, though some may have a gastrostomy tube (commonly

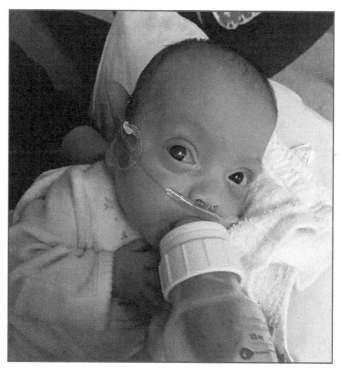

FIGURE 7–1. Neonate with history of extreme prematurity.

referred to as a "g-tube" or even a "button" in this setting given that many infants and children receive low-profile gastrostomy tubes). Additionally, the premature infant's gastrointestinal system is vulnerable to diseases and infections. Necrotizing enterocolitis (NEC) is the most common gastrointestinal disease in premature infants and involves intestinal tissue death that can lead to infant death. Etiologies for NEC likely involve poor perfusion to the intestines, bacteria, and/or viruses. Prematurity can greatly impact the neurologic system with neural immaturity and increased risk for brain bleeds. Most NICUs will offer serial head ultrasounds for the most premature infants to routinely assess for brain abnormalities. Intraventricular hemorrhage (IVH) is one of the most common acquired brain difficulties for premature neonates. IVHs are graded in severity (I–IV), and IVHs are associated with poor neurodevelopmental outcomes (Bolisetty et al., 2014). Children who are born prematurely often have cardiac challenges (see later section on Congenital Heart Disease for further discussion). For example, patent ductus arteriosus (PDA) is a heart defect more common in children born prematurely. If a PDA does not close on its own and is impacting a child's cardiopulmonary status, pharmaceutical or surgical intervention may be necessary. Children born prematurely may experience cardiopulmonary "events" often referred to colloquially as "A/B/D" (apnea/bradycardia/[oxygen] desaturation) events that are likely related to multisystem immaturity. During these "events," babies typically have abruptly decreased heart rate and oxygen saturations. Recovery from events can be "spontaneous" or can require interventions such as oxygen supplementation or tactile stimulation. Severity and frequency of events typically decrease as infants mature, and persistent events often impact discharge readiness (Eichenwald et al., 2016). Retinopathy of prematurity (ROP) is another common NICU condition that is closely monitored and treated. Numerous other body systems and processes can be impacted by prematurity, including renal function and thermoregulation.

Box 7–1. Special Focus: Case Study: Yousef, a Baby With Bronchopulmonary Dysplasia/Chronic Lung Disease

Yousef was born at 25 weeks gestation due to preterm labor of an unclear etiology. He was admitted to the NICU and spent several months receiving various forms of support including mechanical ventilation, CPAP, fluids, and enteral feeding. He had a Grade I Right IVH and Grade II Left IVH discovered on routine head ultrasound. Yousef was diagnosed with broncho-pulmonary dysplasia (BPD), a form of chronic lung disease (CLD), given his ongoing need for respiratory support as he matured. The SLP team met with Yousef's family when Yousef was 32 weeks corrected gestational age (CGA, also referred to as postmenstrual age [PMA]); these ages are of course different from chronologic age (CA), which is calculated as time since birth; in this case study, baby Yousef at 32 weeks PMA/CGA would be 7 weeks old CA since he was born at 25 weeks gestation age [GA]) to discuss oral stimulation techniques while Yousef was awaiting oral feeding readiness. When Yousef was 35 weeks and 2 days PMA, his respiratory status (requiring O_2 via low-flow nasal cannula) appeared reasonable for oral feeding, and the NICU team reconsulted the SLP service. Initial evaluation revealed readiness to feed cues with consistent awake/alert states around care times and feeding cues including bringing his hands to his mouth. Yousef's family preferred bottle feeding while in the hospital, and Yousef readily accepted his first bottle. However, he was observed to gulp vigorously and to not stop to take breathing breaks which resulted in A/B/D events with oral feeding. SLP interventions included (a) slowing the flow of the bottle nipple to increase coordination, (b) elevated side-lying positioning to maximize his respiratory comfort and coordination, and (c) careful coregulated pacing (in Yousef's case, "tilting" the bottle down when he showed stress cues or signs of needing a breath) to gently impose breathing breaks for Yousef. These interventions resulted in near elimination of A/B/D events. Yousef continued to progress in his oral feeding skills, and he also was weaned off oxygen support. He was discharged home taking all of his nutrition by mouth, and his mother began breast-feeding with the support of an International Board-Certified Lactation Consultant (IBCLC) after discharge. Yousef followed up with early intervention SLP services shortly after discharge to continue to assist with oral feeding skills and to provide support for developing speech-language skills as appropriate.

In addition to children born prematurely, the NICU is home to "sick term" infants and infants born prematurely with other medical conditions not overtly tied to prematurity. It should be noted that prematurity is still often a comorbid condition in children experiencing the conditions described later. Intrauterine growth restriction (IUGR) is a condition involving poor uterine growth, and it sometimes requires NICU care. Children may be admitted to the NICU with sepsis or concern for sepsis, a potentially dangerous bloodstream infection. Children with various known and unknown genetic syndromes (e.g., Trisomy 21, Trisomy 13, Prader-Willi syndrome) may be admitted to the NICU depending on their medical needs. Children with intrauterine drug exposure (IUDE) or neonatal abstinence syndrome (NAS) may also be admitted depending on their needs. Children who experienced hypoxic ischemic encephalopathy (HIE) which involves brain injury due to reduced oxygen to the brain (often during a difficult birth) are often admitted to the NICU. Children may experience respiratory distress syndrome (RDS) at or shortly after birth for a variety of reasons and may require NICU support. Meconium aspiration can be a cause for NICU admission, particularly in the most severe cases. Children with congenital anomalies such as congenital diaphragmatic hernia (CDH), omphalocele, gastroschisis, or esophageal atresia may require NICU care.

Best practices in the NICU involve focus on "developmental care," which is care that is mindful of the physical, emotional, and neuropsychologic vulnerabilities that infants and families in the NICU likely experience; this care seeks to reduce the negative impacts of the NICU in the short and long term. Developmental care is not always consistently defined or practiced, but core elements likely include protected sleep, pain and stress management and awareness, developmental activities of daily living, family-centered care, and a healing environment (Coughlin et al., 2009). Babies in the NICU experience a variety of prenatal and postnatal stressors that may have negative impacts, and trauma-informed care for both babies and families is vital in the NICU (Sanders & Hall, 2018).

Almost all these challenges can impact oral feeding. Oral feeding is a highly complex task for infants and requires precise coordination of the suck–swallow–breathe mechanism. It is therefore not surprising that many children with respiratory, gastrointestinal, and/or neurologic challenges struggle to orally feed safely and efficiently. For example, poor respiratory status makes it difficult to breathe and maintain stable vitals while feeding. Decreased gastrointestinal integrity can make toleration of enteral nutrition poor, which can lead to oral aversion or poor acceptance of oral feedings. Decreased alertness related to neural immaturity and/or insult can make it difficult for babies to stay awake and to engage in oral feeding. Specific conditions can also increase risks such as a PDA requiring ligation (surgical intervention) leading to increased risk for vocal fold paralysis, which could, in turn, cause poor airway closure and possible aspiration during oral feeding. Successful oral feeding is often one of the last requirements before children can discharge from the NICU. Infants in the NICU may begin oral feeding as early as 31 to 32 weeks PMA (also called CGA) if their physiologic stability and medical status allow. However, many children in the NICU are not offered oral feeding opportunities until much later PMAs (when they are older) given their medical status (e.g., not physiologically stable, not tolerating enteral nutrition). There are likely pros and cons to early oral feeding opportunities based on maximizing critical periods but also reducing stress which could negatively influence neurodevelopmental outcomes (Griffith et al., 2020). Cue-based feeds or oral feeds offered based on infant readiness and cues, rather than focusing on a specific volume, have shown improvements in time to oral feeding, length of stay, and parent involvement (e.g., Thomas et al., 2021). Children born prematurely frequently experience ongoing feeding and swallowing difficulties even after NICU discharge (e.g., Pados et al., 2021, identified up to 42% of formerly premature infants in their study with ongoing feeding/swallowing difficulties postdischarge).

Children with a history of prematurity are at increased risk for speech-language and cognitive-communication difficulties (e.g., Zambrana et al., 2021). Exact mechanisms for speech-language vulnerabilities in this population are not always clear, but there are numerous reasonable hypotheses such as neuroanatomic factors and/or structural changes, atypical functional brain organization, changes in early sensory experiences, changes in infant–caregiver relationship, and/or global cognitive difficulties that spill over into communication skills (Vandormael et al., 2019). Children born prematurely may also be at increased risk for autism spectrum disorder (ASD) (Crump et al., 2021), though some discussion exists regarding the differences in presentation and the validity of these autism diagnoses in children born prematurely when compared to children diagnosed with autism who were born full term (Johnson & Marlow, 2011; Pineda et al., 2015).

Box 7–2. Special Focus: Case Study: Addilyn, a Baby With Hypoxic Ischemic Encephalopathy

Addilyn was born at 40 weeks and 4 days gestation. A planned vaginal birth was converted to an emergent cesarean section given multiple fetal heart rate abnormalities during the pushing phase of labor. Her Apgar scores at birth were poor (0 at 1 min and 1 at 5 min). She had minimal respiratory effort or movement, and her skin color was pale/blue. Neonatal resuscitation efforts were begun immediately, and she was ultimately placed on mechanical ventilation and provided with therapeutic cooling due to concerns for HIE. A brain magnetic resonance image (MRI) later confirmed HIE with noted ischemic injury and restricted diffusion in both the cortex and the basal ganglia and thalamus. She was extubated several days later, and although she was breathing on her own, she continued to have very little movement or interactivity. She was being fed expressed human milk through a NG tube when the SLP was consulted to assess her feeding/swallowing skills. Initial assessment revealed that Addilyn had difficulty coming to and maintaining an awake/alert state and had inconsistent oral-motor reflexes. She did not consistently exhibit rooting or sucking. Therapeutic tastes of expressed human milk were offered. Repeated assessment and intervention were offered over a 2-week period. Addilyn slowly became more awake and engaged, and she eventually progressed to consuming small PO (by mouth) trials. Occasional coughing with oral feeding was noted, and given Addilyn's history, a videofluoroscopic swallowing study (VFSS) was recommended. The VFSS revealed that Addilyn's swallowing pattern was uncoordinated with an occasionally delayed swallow. However, she appeared to protect her airway during the VFSS, and PO trials continued. Unfortunately, Addilyn did not have the endurance to take close to full recommended volumes of milk by mouth. Addilyn was discharged from the NICU with a g-tube to support primary nutrition, and she was cared for by a home health SLP upon discharge. Addilyn also followed up with the NICU development outpatient clinic, and she began early intervention developmental therapy in the months following discharge and speech-language therapy before turning 1 year old.

Congenital Heart Disease

Congenital heart disease (CHD) impacts about 1 in 100 infants (CDC, 2022; Hoffman & Kaplan, 2002; Reller et al., 2008). CHD is present from birth and can range in severity. Approximately 20% of children with CHD have a known genetic syndrome (typically with extra-cardiac features) that is likely related to their cardiac disease, such as Trisomy 21, Turner syndrome, 22q11.2 deletion syndrome, and Williams syndrome (Eskedal et al., 2004; Ko, 2015). About one in four children with CHD require surgery within the first year of life (Oster et al., 2013). CHD can be separated into cyanotic and acyanotic congenital heart disease depending on if the heart defects reduce oxygen delivery to the rest of the body. Cyanotic CHD is also known as critical CHD (CCHD). See Table 7–1 for a sample of types of CHD lesions organized by severity. Children with the most severe forms of CHD often spend substantial time hospitalized and may require multiple surgeries to correct or palliate their heart disease. Large children's hospitals may have a pediatric cardiovascular intensive care unit (PCICU) where these children can be monitored closely. Children with CHD have known oral feeding challenges that may relate to a variety of factors including, but not limited to, delayed initiation of oral feeding, reduced stamina, oral aversion, medical complications, and/or negative impacts of prolonged exposure to the ICU environment (Jones et al., 2021). Additionally, while CHD is often diagnosed prenatally via ultrasound, postnatal diagnoses are not uncommon, and feeding difficulties can be a part of a constellation of symptoms leading to diagnosis. Speech-language delays and deficits have been well-documented in the CHD population (Turner et al., 2022). Etiology for impaired communication skills in this population likely involves multiple factors such as altered neurodevelopmental environment (e.g., reduced speech-language input due to hospitalizations, increased stress) and reduced cerebral blood flow because of heart disease and related interventions (e.g., Wernovsky, 2006).

TABLE 7–1	Examples of Congenital Heart Disease
Degree	**Examples**
Simple	Atrial septal defect (ASD), ventricular septal defect (VSD), isolated valve disease, patent ductus arteriosus (PDA), coarctation of the aorta (simple)
Moderate	Atrioventricular septal defect (AVSD), coarctation of the aorta (complex), total anomalous pulmonary vein return (TAPVR)
Complex	Tetralogy of Fallot, transposition of the great arteries (d-TGA), hypoplastic left heart syndrome (HLHS), triscuspid atresia, pulmonary atresia

Source: Based on "Heart Failure in Adults With Congenital Heart Disease: A Narrative Review," by E. Zengin, C. Sinning, C. Blaum, S. Blankenberg, C. Rickers, Y. von Kodolitsch, . . . V. Stoll, 2021, *Cardiovascular Diagnosis and Therapy, 11*(2), p. 529.

Box 7–3. Special Focus: Case Study: Townes, a Boy With Hypoplastic Left Heart Syndrome

Townes was born full term and appeared healthy immediately after birth. However, he quickly became cyanotic and exhibited poor feeding. An echocardiogram revealed that Townes had single ventricle physiology CHD, specifically hypoplastic left heart syndrome (HLHS). The left side of his heart was severely underdeveloped and unable to pump blood to the rest of his body. He was transferred from the community hospital where he was born to a larger academic children's hospital where he quickly underwent the first surgery in a planned three-stage palliation. After surgery, he exhibited poor endurance and limited PO intake, possibly related to oral aversion from repeated emesis in the weeks after surgery. He received most of his nutrition from a feeding tube until his second surgery around 6 months of age. He had increased energy and was more interested in eating after his second surgery, but sadly he had vocal fold paralysis after his second operation due to injury to the recurrent laryngeal nerve, which limited oral feeding safety. He worked with outpatient feeding therapy for years to develop compensatory measures including thickened liquids, drinking systems that limited sip size, and behavioral supports to allow for increased PO feeding. At 3 years of age, he went for a third palliative surgery and unfortunately had surgical complications that required a brief stint on extracorporeal membrane oxygen (ECMO; a form of cardiac and/or respiratory life support that performs the functions of the heart, lungs, or both outside of the patient's body). He subsequently had a stroke. After his stroke, he again worked with the inpatient and outpatient SLP teams to optimize feeding and speech-language skills. When he entered kindergarten, he was taking most of his nutrition by mouth and had an individualized education program (IEP) in place for academic and speech-language supports given his ongoing delays and impairments from his stroke. Unfortunately, his cardiac function had recently worsened, and his team was considering whether heart transplant would be in his best interest.

Gastroenterology and Growth

Infants and children are often admitted to the pediatric hospital or seen in outpatient clinics due to poor feeding of an unclear etiology, and this poor feeding is frequently accompanied by poor weight gain or even weight loss. SLPs are often involved in assessing the oral feeding and swallowing skills of these children to assist in diagnosis and treatment. Oral-motor feeding difficulties may play a role, such as an inefficient suck, due to reduced lingual movement. Sensory or learned neurobehavioral feeding difficulties such as oral aversion in the setting of severe reflux may play a role. Feeding refusals are often accompanied by an underlying gastroenterology challenge such as gastroesophageal reflux (GER), constipation, or allergies. Although SLPs typically defer to the primary medical team on medical management of these issues, oral-motor, sensory, and behavioral feeding difficulties are strongly linked to these conditions. SLPs may be the first to ask a physician or family about possible gastrointestinal discomfort as an etiology of poor feeding. Additionally, environmental factors such as caregivers not offering or not having access to enough food may play a role. Numerous other medical diagnoses or etiologies of poor feeding are possible (e.g., malignancy, neurologic event or disorder). Children experiencing treatment for cancer such as chemotherapy or radiation often experience feeding difficulties and poor oral intake. Pediatric SLPs may be involved in assessing and treating feeding/swallowing skills in children with cancer, especially given the importance of nutritional status in this population (Jacobs-Levine et al., 2006). SLPs can also be collaborators in treatment for children with eating disorders such as working with children with ARFID (avoidant/restrictive food intake disorder) in conjunction with other professionals. Often, etiologies for feeding difficulties (and thus interventions) are multifactorial and involve communication among multiple team members as well as very close collaboration with families and caregivers. It should also be noted that consistent weight gain and growth in early childhood are vital to brain development and positive life outcomes (Corbett & Drewett, 2004) and are therefore quite important to monitor and support. Growth charts are often used to measure weight, height, and head circumference. Percentile rankings on growth charts in and of themselves are not necessarily meaningful; the overall trajectory of growth over time is most closely monitored (Figure 7–2). Registered dieticians and physicians often calculate estimated goals for caloric intake based on child-specific factors such as weight and special diagnoses. It should also be noted that difficulties with infant/child feeding and subsequent poor weight gain can be emotionally charged and associated with increased stress for families (Silverman et al., 2021). "Failure to thrive" is a term used to describe poor weight gain and is gradually being eliminated in favor of terms such as poor weight gain or weight faltering (Tang et al., 2021). SLPs should be aware of the multifactorial nature of

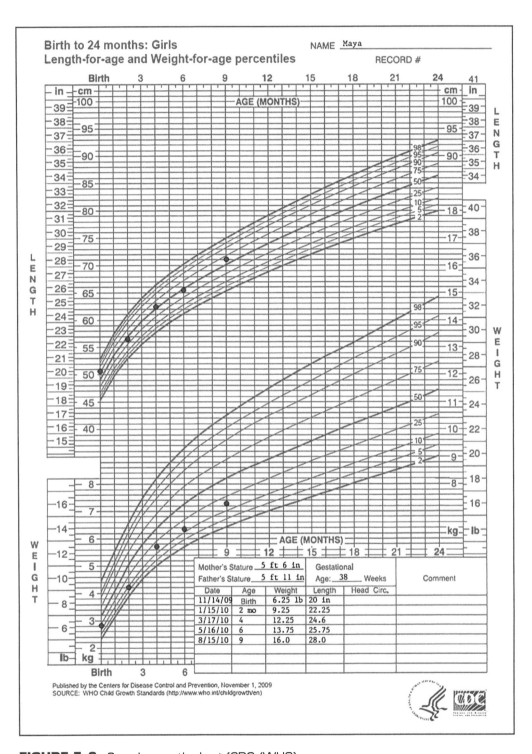

FIGURE 7-2. Sample growth chart (CDC/WHO).

feeding difficulties, particularly considering common and uncommon gastrointestinal diseases in young children and the important contribution of SLPs to their management.

Box 7–4. Special Focus: Case Study: Samuel, a Baby With Reflux and Oral Aversion

Samuel was born at 35 weeks gestation and initially was breastfed. He developed consistent emesis (vomiting) during and after feeds causing his primary care physician to (a) trial multiple different formulas and maternal diet adjustments, (b) send him for an ultrasound to look for pyloric stenosis, and (c) ultimately refer him to a pediatric gastroenterology specialist at a children's medical center. By the time Samuel went to his gastroenterology appointment, he had begun to refuse to eat and would only consume minuscule amounts of formula or breastmilk when he was in a very drowsy state. He was admitted to the children's hospital, and an SLP consult was part of the diagnostic process. SLP assessment revealed multiple aversive behaviors during feeding such as pulling away, grimacing, arching, and crying when presented with a bottle. The SLP and Samuel's family worked on creating positive associations with feeding for Samuel while the medical team switched him to an elemental formula (elemental formulas are formulas with proteins and nutrients broken down to their simplest forms—to "elements" or amino acids; they are often better tolerated by people with allergies and intolerances) and optimized reflux medications. Samuel returned to eating adequate volumes in the following weeks. He followed up with home health SLP services at discharge to ensure continued success.

Otorhinolaryngologic Anomalies

Many children who see SLPs in the pediatric medical setting experience otorhinolaryngologic anomalies, particularly airway anomalies that impact breathing, feeding, swallowing, and voice/speech production.

Sample Airway Anomalies

Laryngomalacia is a congenital "softening" of the laryngeal cartilages that is present from birth but does not always manifest itself functionally until a baby is slightly more mobile and active. It typically presents first as "noisy" breathing with audible inhalation, exhalation, or both. The laryngeal structures are floppy and can fall over (prolapse) into the airway, creating audible, sometimes stridorous, breathing sounds. Symptoms of laryngomalacia are often worse with feeding and may change with positioning. Laryngomalacia typically resolves on its own as a baby grows; most children see resolution of symptoms by 1 year of age. Most mild cases do not substantially impact daily life and require no intervention. More severe cases can impact breathing, weight gain, and/or feeding safely and efficiently. Laryngomalacia can affect the suck–swallow–breathe sequence, and multiple SLP clinical interventions may be beneficial, particularly positioning (e.g., Mills et al., 2021). Otolaryngologists may perform a supraglottoplasty procedure to shave off excess and floppy parts of the laryngeal cartilages in the most severe cases. Tracheomalacia and bronchomalacia involve the "softening" of the cartilage of the trachea and lower airway and can also impact breathing and feeding.

Vocal fold anomalies, particularly changes in vocal fold mobility, are frequently seen in the pediatric medical SLP setting. Vocal fold immobility can be bilateral or unilateral, and bilateral immobility may leave the glottis in an abducted (open) or nearly adducted (closed) position. Vocal folds may be partially mobile but unable to fully adduct, and laryngoscopy reveals a glottal gap. Respiratory stridor and a rough, weak, or absent cry can be one of the first signs of a vocal fold movement disorder in babies. The most severe cases may present as immediate respiratory distress and may require tracheostomy. The most common etiologies of vocal fold paralysis in this population are iatrogenic (e.g., injury to recurrent laryngeal nerve during cardiac surgery, forceps use during birth) and idiopathic (no apparent etiology), though there are also neurologic bases of vocal fold impairment (Daya et al., 2000). Impaired vocal fold mobility can have substantial impact on feeding/swallowing and oral communication given difficulties with respiration, airway closure during feeding, and phonation. SLP interventions for vocal fold immobility are varied and may include changes in viscosity such as thickening liquids or changes in positioning to allow maximal protection of the airway during swallowing. SLPs may also be part of multidisciplinary discussions regarding benefits of otolaryngology surgical intervention such as vocal fold augmentation or reinnervation.

A laryngeal cleft is an abnormal gap or opening near where the esophagus and larynx meet in the hypopharynx. Laryngeal clefts are graded in severity from Type 1 laryngeal clefts and deep interarytenoid notches that may have minimal impacts all the way to a Type 4 laryngeal cleft that requires immediate surgical repair at or near birth. Laryngeal clefts are associated with dysphagia and aspiration (Rahbar et al., 2006). Laryngeal clefts are congenital conditions related to embryonic challenges in the separation of the trachea and the esophagus during the first trimester in utero. Tracheoesophageal fistula (abnormal communication between the trachea and the esophagus below the level of the larynx) and esophageal atresia (lack of esophageal connection to the stomach) are other conditions that are related to embryonic defects of the trachea and the esophagus. SLPs may be involved in the feeding/swallowing assessment and treatment of these children as well, particularly postoperatively after repairs, as there can be iatrogenic complications such as oral aversion after esophageal atresia or vocal fold paralysis after tracheoesophageal fistula repair. Additionally, an H-type tracheoesophageal fistula can be difficult to diagnose and is often incidentally found on a VFSS when an infant presents with coughing and choking with oral feeds (Urik et al., 2021).

Sample Craniofacial Anomalies

Craniofacial structural abnormalities such as cleft lip and cleft palate are congenital conditions caused by defects in embryologic development and typically occur during the first trimester in utero. Craniofacial anomalies can occur alone such as an isolated cleft palate or part of a larger constellation of symptoms associated with a genetic syndrome or larger diagnosis (e.g., Apert syndrome, Crouzon syndrome, Goldenhar syndrome, 22q11.2 deletion syndrome also known as DiGeorge syndrome or velocardiofacial syndrome). SLPs care for children who have feeding/swallowing and communication impacts from craniofacial conditions. Children with cleft palate, a failure of palatal fusion resulting in a gap in the hard palate, are one of the most common craniofacial populations managed by SLPs. Cleft palates can be unilateral or bilateral and range in severity; they may be accompanied by a cleft lip. Cleft palates impact oral feeding starting in infancy when most children are unable to produce suction for typical breast or bottle feeding given an inability to create a vacuum seal. Special bottle systems and feeding techniques are almost always necessary for children with cleft palates to feed effectively. Cleft palates are usually surgically repaired before or around 1 year of age. Children may also experience micrognathia (small mandible) or retrognathia (abnormal mandible positioning) that can impact breathing, feeding, and communicating. The most severe cases may require surgical intervention such as tracheostomy or mandibular distraction. Jaw abnormalities are sometimes part of a larger syndrome or diagnosis (e.g., Pierre Robin syndrome, Treacher Collins syndrome). Voice and resonance changes can arise in children with cleft palate, as a cleft can create velopharyngeal insufficiency (VPI), which results in unintentional nasal air escape during speech. VPI can also occur in the absence of clefts. VPI may be diagnosed via nasoendoscopy, and speech therapy and/or surgical intervention may be appropriate.

Pediatric Tracheostomy

A tracheostomy is an artificial airway placed in the neck below the vocal folds. Pediatric patients with tracheostomies can vary greatly from their adult counterparts. Indications for tracheostomy may be different. One indication for tracheostomy is the long-term need for mechanical ventilation. In the adult ICU population, long term typically means days or weeks, and early tracheostomy is common and routine (Vargas et al., 2015). However, most pediatric centers will leave children orally or nasally intubated for longer periods and are more hesitant to place tracheostomies, particularly in children who entered the ICU with no respiratory support needs (Watters, 2017; Wood et al., 2012). Children who receive tracheostomies due to the long-term need for mechanical ventilation may need ventilation for months or years, and pediatric patients with tracheostomies are more likely to have tracheostomies for an extended period of time or to not experience decannulation (Watters, 2017). Congenital (e.g., mass, vocal fold anomalies) or acquired (e.g., subglottic stenosis from prolonged intubation) upper airway obstruction is another common indication for pediatric tracheostomy as are neuromuscular conditions or neurologic conditions that cause difficulties with breathing or managing secretions. Most pediatric patients who receive tracheostomies are less than 1 year of age (Berry et al., 2009). Children with airway anomalies commonly need airway reconstruction surgery by ENT surgeons to safely be decannulated.

Quality of life and tracheostomy is an important intersection, particularly in the pediatric population where placement is longer, and children are typically very dependent on caregivers. Caregivers of children with tracheostomy experience increased stress (e.g., Chandran et al., 2021; Joseph et al., 2014; Winkler et al., 2006). Many children with tracheostomies have home nursing support, but time and expertise of services can be variable (Amar-Dolan et al., 2020; Mai et al., 2020). Adverse outcomes and events (e.g., accidental decannulation, airway obstruction, tracheostomy event-related mortality) in children, particularly infants and very young children, with tracheostomies are not uncommon (Edwards et al., 2010; Hebbar et al., 2021; Watters et al., 2016), but family training, protocols, and safety plans may decrease risks (McKeon et al., 2019).

The pediatric medical SLP is typically deeply involved in pediatric patients with tracheostomies given the profound impacts on feeding/swallowing and communication needs. Clinical and instrumental feeding/swallowing services are standard care for children with tracheostomies given the high incidence of dysphagia and aspiration (Luu et al., 2022; Pullens & Streppel, 2021; Streppel et al., 2019). Traditional speech-language therapy as well as intervention with a speaking valve (e.g., Passy Muir valve or PMV) is also vital, especially given documented changes in speech-language development in children with tracheostomies (Jiang & Morrison, 2003). Speaking valves may allow infants, children, and adults to cry, vocalize, and talk as developmentally appropriate; to have better smell and taste; to generate subglottic pressure for coughing and swallowing; and to manage secretions (Abraham, 2009; Eibling & Gross, 1996; Hull et al., 2005; O'Connor et al., 2019). Candidates for speaking valve placement need to be able to tolerate a cuff deflation and to be grossly medical stable. Children receiving mechanical ventilation via a tracheostomy can also be candidates in the appropriate circumstances (Brooks et al., 2020). Infant and pediatric speaking valve assessment and intervention are typically challenging, yet rewarding. Teasing apart behavioral versus physiologic tolerance in pediatric patients involves clinical expertise, input from ENT and pulmonology colleagues, and increasingly objective measures such as transtracheal pressure manometry (Brooks et al., 2020).

Box 7–5. Special Focus: Deja, a Girl With a Tracheostomy

Deja was a typically developing 10-year-old girl with scoliosis. After scoliosis surgery, she was unable to be extubated, and an airway evaluation was completed. Circumferential pharyngeal collapse and severe tracheomalacia were noted. Given this new onset of an airway obstruction (presumably triggered by manipulation of the spine and excess pressure on the airway with her scoliosis), Deja was given a tracheostomy. She woke up in the ICU and was unable to talk. She had an NG feeding tube. She was receiving mechanical ventilation via her tracheostomy. SLP involvement initially focused on augmentative and alternative communication (AAC) supports such as a whiteboard and marker as well as communication buttons to share quick messages. When the ENT and ICU team agreed that Deja was medically stable, an in-line with the ventilator speaking valve assessment was completed. Deja tolerated cuff deflation on the ventilator, and some of her first words were "thank you for giving me my voice back." Clinical evaluation of swallowing was insufficient and inconclusive given Deja's history. A fiberoptic endoscopic evaluation of swallowing (FEES) was completed given the need to visualize laryngeal structures and difficulties moving Deja off the ICU for a VFSS. Severe dysphagia with aspiration of all consistencies and signs of poor laryngeal sensation were noted. Deja then began several weeks of intensive rehabilitation while hospitalized. She completed daily physical, occupational, and speech therapy sessions. SLP intervention focused on speaking valve use (to promote communication, swallowing, and upper airway airflow), therapeutic PO trials and swallowing exercises, and functional communication tasks. Repeat instrumental swallowing assessment revealed a swallow that was grossly within normal limits. Deja was discharged from the hospital wearing a speaking valve during all waking hours and consuming all nutrition by mouth.

Congenital and Acquired Neurologic Impairment

Infants and children with neurologic challenges comprise a sizable portion of the pediatric medical SLP's caseload. Many of the acquired neurologic conditions seen in the adult hospital setting are also seen in pediatrics, but there are variations in presentation and frequency. Traumatic brain injuries of varying severity are assessed and treated as are anoxic brain injuries that may happen prior to hospitalization or in the course of patient care (e.g., after a cardiac arrest). Pediatric stroke is less common than stroke in adults, but certain populations experience stroke more frequently, including intraventricular hemorrhage in premature infants and ischemic stroke in children receiving ECMO therapy (e.g., Le Guennec et al., 2018). Pediatric brain tumors can cause a variety of speech-language, cognitive-communication, and feeding/swallowing difficulties depending on location and tumor size. Pediatric brain tumors are one of the most common forms of childhood cancer, and the posterior fossa region of the brain is particularly impacted in children (Lannering et al., 1990). Congenital brain abnormalities such as agenesis of the corpus callosum and cerebellar hypoplasia can also impact development and care. Chiari malformations are skull-base abnormalities that can be acquired or congenital and can impact swallowing. Children with seizures (typically coexisting with other diagnoses) are frequently served by the pediatric medical SLP; in children actively experiencing seizures, it is vital to understand that communication and swallowing skills are likely continually changing and may vary greatly across points of assessment and treatment.

ASD along with other neurodevelopmental disorders and differences is frequently seen as a diagnosis by children in the medical setting. Children with autism may or may not have other medical diagnoses. As previously mentioned, children born prematurely are more likely to be diagnosed with ASD (Crump et al., 2021); however, presentation may not be identical to children who were born full term (Pineda et al., 2015). ASD can be accompanied by challenges with feeding (Sharp et al., 2013).

Box 7–6. Special Focus: Antonio, a Boy With Medulloblastoma

Antonio was diagnosed with medulloblastoma in the posterior fossa region at 4 years of age. After resection of the primary brain tumor, he experienced posterior fossa syndrome, which is a range of neurologic symptoms that occur in up to 40% of patients (Wells et al., 2010) after posterior fossa region brain tumor removal. A hallmark symptom of posterior fossa syndrome (also known as cerebellar mutism) is complete (or partial) loss of spoken language; hypotonia, ataxia, dysphagia, and emotional lability are other common symptoms (Gudrunardottir et al., 2011; Kirk et al., 1995). Antonio's SLP assessment and intervention varied throughout his medical course, beginning with a preoperative assessment prior to his tumor resection and continuing all the way through his chemotherapy and radiation treatment regimen. Antonio communicated using unaided AAC for several weeks after resection due to his complete loss of spoken language. He slowly regained spoken language skills but had moderate ataxic dysarthria. Speech and language skills slowly improved with time. Poor oral-motor skills and a delayed swallow resulted in aspiration of multiple liquid consistencies necessitating placement of a NG tube. As his overall status improved, his ability to swallow liquids safely improved. Impacts of chemotherapy led to substantial sensory feeding difficulties overlaid on his dysphagia. Antonio continued to work with an SLP for over a year after his posterior fossa mass resection.

Other Populations

Numerous other conditions and populations are served by the pediatric medical SLP. This section highlights a few of these conditions and populations.

Children are frequently admitted to the hospital with respiratory illnesses such as influenza or respiratory syncytial virus (RSV). These illnesses can cause feeding problems that are typically temporary (Cooper et al., 2003). The etiology of feeding difficulties in respiratory illnesses is likely multifactorial and may involve difficulties coordinating respiration and swallowing, general malaise resulting in poor intake, inability to safely or efficiently consume adequate oral intake given the level of respiratory support needed, and oral aversion from numerous invasive oral procedures (e.g., intubation, deep suctioning). It is common for SLPs to assist with feeding and swallowing safety, comfort, and efficiency in children admitted to the hospital, particularly during "respiratory season." Debates are ongoing regarding safety and efficiency of feeding in children receiving intensive forms of respiratory support via high-flow nasal cannula (HFNC) and nasal CPAP, and best practices involve individualized assessment and treatment (Dodrill et al., 2016; Ferrara et al., 2017; Hirst et al., 2017).

Children with functional disorders are often seen in the pediatric medical SLP setting. Functional disorders (also referred to as functional neurologic disorders, previously referred to as conversion disorders) typically involve neurologic symptoms that are not clearly explainable by a specific disease process or medical diagnosis. Swallowing and speech difficulties are often symptoms associated with functional neurologic disorders (Barnett et al., 2019). Functional disorders can cause great impairment, patient and family stress, and disability. Risk factors for functional disorders may include mental health difficulties and known comorbid neurologic or physiologic impairment (Carson et al., 2016). Children with functional disorders require careful assessment that documents consistency and severity of symptoms. Thoughtful attention to language used to describe functional neurologic disorders with children is vital (Kozlowksa et al., 2021). Current best practices involve intensive rehabilitation efforts for patients with neurologic impairment of an unclear etiology (Baker et al., 2021). Collaboration with multiple disciplines such as other therapy services, psychiatry, and/or neuropsychology can also be beneficial (Baker et al., 2021).

Fictitious disorder imposed by another (FDIA; previously known as Munchausen syndrome by proxy) is a condition in which a caregiver (often mother) acts as if a child has a medical condition that is nonexistent, creates conditions that cause a medical condition, or both. FDIA can be considered a form of child abuse that involves maltreatment, unnecessary and possibly painful medical assessments and treatments, and even death (Faedda et al., 2018). FDIA can be very difficult to diagnose and is complicated to treat. FDIA red flags may include observations and investigations inconsistent with caregiver report, atypical presentations of a disorder, symptoms that occur only in a caregiver's presence, and multiple hospitalizations (Faedda et al., 2018). SLPs should be aware of the possibility of FDIA.

Feeding/swallowing and cognitive-communication difficulties in the medical setting are frequently iatrogenic, that is, caused directly by medical or surgical intervention. For example, children who are orally or nasally intubated are unable to verbally communicate. SLPs may be involved in providing communication supports (often AAC) for children experiencing iatrogenic communication impairment (Costello et al., 2010). Current ICU best practices are more broadly focused on reducing negative long-term impacts of ICU care (e.g., ICU Liberation, ABCDEF bundle as described by Ely, 2017), and these initiatives may involve SLP services (Altschuler et al., 2018; Betters et al., 2022). Delirium prevention and management are also increasingly important to SLPs and care teams, especially given that delirium is an independent predictor of mortality (Ely et al., 2004; Traube et al., 2017). See Chapter 2 for more information on ICU liberation best practices and the SLP's role.

Box 7–7. Special Focus: Lali, a Teenager With Spinal Cord Injury

Lali was 14 years old when a motor vehicle crash left her with a high-level cervical spinal cord injury. She found herself not only orally intubated in the ICU and unable to talk but also unable to move or have sensation below her neck. Her communication options were limited. The SLP team was consulted to assess and treat Lali's communication challenges. Lali was able to use head nods for yes/no with a partner-assisted scanning letter board to ask questions and to make requests (including for TV shows to watch in the ICU). She also participated in a care conference using multimodal AAC. Lali later received a tracheostomy and used a speaking valve and leak speech to verbally communicate. When later asked about her experience with the letter board and partner-assisted scanning, she responded, "I can't believe I did that . . . but I really wanted to watch Netflix!"

Comorbidities

It should be noted that the previously discussed patient populations are presented as separate, discrete groups when in the actual hospital setting these conditions are highly comorbid, and populations frequently overlap. For example, an infant with prenatally diagnosed CHD may be born prematurely and require prolonged intubation leading to an iatrogenic airway stenosis requiring tracheostomy and mechanical ventilation. Following cardiac surgery, this infant may require cannulation to ECMO with a secondary impact of stroke. After surgery and stroke, the infant may repeatedly have emesis related to poor gastrointestinal tolerance of enteral nutrition leading to oral aversion and poor weight gain/growth. Although this example may seem extreme, comorbidities are the rule and not the exception.

Special Considerations

The pediatric medical SLP world shares many features with the adult medical SLP world, but there are also numerous differences. This section highlights considerations in feeding/swallowing and speech-language-cognitive assessment and treatment (particularly in pediatric critical and acute care) as well as a particular focus on children with complex medical conditions, the impact of ongoing development, and managing limited evidence bases.

*Feeding and Swallowing Assessment
and Treatment Considerations*

As outlined in previous chapters, thoughtful assessment (and then treatment) in the acute-care setting requires thorough chart review; agility in evaluation and treatment planning as patients change quickly with need to continually adapt to new diagnoses, interventions, skills, and goals of care; and a strong understanding of a patient's overall medical course and plan of care. Clinical swallow evaluations for infants and children require knowledge of typical development and variations in typical development. Fetuses typically begin sucking and swallowing amniotic fluid in utero. Early infant feeding (breastfeeding and/or bottle feeding) is particularly reliant on rooting, sucking, and swallowing reflexes that diminish between 4 and 6 months of age. The transition to solids is partially cultural but typically begins around 6 months of age, and breastfeeding and/or bottle feeding continue for some time. Several changes in the anatomy and physiology of the swallowing mechanism in the early years occur, such as growth of the oral cavity and descent of the larynx (Arvedson et al., 2019). Additionally, completion of a clinical swallow evaluation of a young child in a medical setting typically requires creativity and sensitivity (e.g., encouraging a toddler to participate in a cranial nerve exam). Instrumental swallowing assessments such as FEES and VFSS (or modified barium swallow [MBS]) are important in pediatrics. Considerations for pediatric FEES include the ability to assess breastfeeding (SLPs are unable to assess breastfeeding during a VFSS), providers necessary to be present (e.g., SLPs do not perform FEES independently in many children's hospitals; it is common clinical practice for the pediatric ENT to pass the scope and the SLP to interpret and manage the study), and participation of children who are uncomfortable with nasoendoscopy. VFSS is likely the most common instrumental swallowing assessment in pediatrics. VFSS considerations include participation in an unfamiliar task (e.g., drinking barium) in an unfamiliar environment, reducing radiation exposure (particularly in radiation-sensitive pediatric populations such as ataxia telangiectasia), and standardization. Although standardization of the VFSS is considered beneficial and feasible in adults (e.g., MBSimP as described in Martin-Harris et al., 2008), standardization in pediatrics is much more difficult given the diversity of patients, differences in developmental stages, and challenges with participation, though some recommendations exist (e.g., BaByVFSSImP as described in Martin-Harris et al., 2020). Families are frequently encouraged to bring children's preferred foods, drinks, and utensils (e.g., favorite sippy cup) to a VFSS to maximize participation. Interestingly, providers sometimes request a VFSS with a particular interest in the role of enlarged tonsils on the oropharyngeal swallow, typically in children who may be candidates for tonsillectomy. Ultrasound is also an emerging mode of swallowing assessment, particularly for assessment of breastfeeding (e.g., Geddes et al., 2010), but it is not commonly used in clinical practice.

Dysphagia treatment considerations in children must include developmental status, family and caregiver involvement, and current goals of care and setting. Children in the inpatient setting frequently need dysphagia assessment and treatment to progress to the next level of care (e.g., home, inpatient rehab). Treatment can be (re)habilitative, compensatory, and/or diagnostic. Diagnostic treatment sessions are common in the inpatient acute setting as patients' skills and abilities are typically highly dynamic in this setting. Assessment and treatment frequency in the pediatric inpatient setting is highly individualized and based on patient needs and status. "PO trials with SLP only" is a common recommendation for the most fragile patients during the early stages of oral feeding establishment (or reestablishment), and these patients are typically seen most frequently to help the patient progress effectively through the plan of care. Compensatory strategies and feeding techniques are common in the pediatric medical SLP setting; examples of interventions include changes in bottle flow rate (through choice of a particular nipple) or changes in infant feeding positioning such as right side-lying positioning in the setting of left vocal fold paralysis.

Speech-Language and Cognitive-Communication Assessment and Treatment Considerations

Speech-language and cognitive-communication assessment and treatment in the pediatric acute-care setting is often informal and uses primarily criterion-referenced measures. Many institutions have developed an outline of criterion-referenced tasks based on developmental stages and current status of the patient. Items typically include questions or tasks related to attention, orientation, memory, executive functioning, speech, language, and literacy. Some standardized measures are valuable and used as adjuvant assessment tools in the acute-care setting, such as the Children's Orientation and Amnesia Test (COAT; Ewing-Cobbs et al., 1990) and the Pediatric Test of Brain Injury (PTBI; Hotz et al., 2010). Treatment can be (re)habilitative, compensatory, or diagnostic; intervention is frequently a combination of all three. Treatment objectives and frequency are typically dynamic and strongly related to the patient's overall plan of care (e.g., is the patient able to communicate with providers and family members as developmentally appropriate? Does current documentation of the child's speech-language skills support discharge recommendations?). Even in the acute-care setting, pediatric treatment is typically play based and focused on functional tasks and meaningful activities (e.g., contacting the nurse, sharing a message with a loved one). AAC services are provided in the acute-care setting but typically relate to new-onset difficulties and patient–provider communication. AAC in the ICU has been reported to decrease patient frustration, to decrease ventilator days, and to increase patient engagement in adult studies (Patak et al., 2006; Radtke et al., 2011); AAC in the pediatric hospital setting has been shown to have meaningful outcomes as well (Costello et al., 2010).

Children With Complex Medical Conditions

Children's hospitals are for all children, but children's hospitals are not used at the same frequency or intensity by all children. A small group of children with complex medical needs tends to dominate children's hospital use. Sometimes referred to as children with medical complexity (CMC), this group of children comprises a very small portion of the pediatric population overall (<1% by most measures) but proportionately use a higher volume of resources—30%–60% resource use by some measures including overall child health care spending, inpatient hospital spending, pharmacy spending, physician charges, and hospital admission days (Berry et al., 2013; Cohen et al., 2012; Neff et al., 2004). CMC often have multisystem disease, may be technology dependent, and often have rare or severe challenges. The discussion around the medical and surgical management of this population has become more prominent in the literature as our ability to save and care for children with high needs improves (e.g., children born extremely premature increasingly survive, often with lifelong medical challenges; children in the ICU have improved mortality outcomes but possibly increased disability rates). Complex care programs, particularly for CMC, are becoming increasingly common at large children's hospitals. The goal of these programs is to coordinate care and decrease unnecessary hospital resource use for both families and institutions (Cohen et al., 2010; White et al., 2017). Complex care programs typically require patients to have multiple specialty services involved in their care, which is typically reflective of multisystem disease, a history of multiple hospital admissions, and/or technology dependence. Given the complex needs of these patients and their prevalence in the pediatric medical setting, it is vital for pediatric medical SLPs to have a deep understanding of the interactions between multiple body systems across various diseases and disabilities, the experiences of families and caregivers of children with complex medical conditions, and the roles of multidisciplinary team members.

Box 7–8. Special Focus: Case Study:
Li Jie, a Boy With Complex Needs

Li Jie was adopted from China at 3 years of age. He had a known CHD condition called tetralogy of Fallot with pulmonary atresia. Shortly after his adoption, he underwent cardiac surgery that resulted in several complications including time on ECMO, pneumonia with lung damage and subsequent need for tracheostomy with mechanical ventilation, renal disease, feeding difficulties, and a stroke. His status was tenuous, and small changes in his medical status would greatly impact each body system. For example, if his renal function decreased, he would have increased overall fluid retention that would lead to difficulties in breathing requiring increased oxygen requirements. Increased oxygen requirements and work of breathing would impact oral feeding and tube feeding. Additionally, constipation brought on by thickening agents would lead to increased abdominal pressure and decreased respiratory status. Li Jie was admitted to the hospital for months. When he was finally discharged, Li Jie had follow-up appointments with numerous specialty services (cardiology, cardiothoracic surgery, neurology, pulmonology, otorhinolaryngology, nephrology, infectious diseases, and orthopedics) and was receiving home health and home rehabilitation therapy services. Li Jie was followed by the complex care team while inpatient and after discharge, not only to assist with coordinating his care but also to facilitate communication among teams about the interactions between each body system and related interventions. Li Jie's family considered the complex care team to be the "quarterback" of Li Jie's team. Complex care teams have been demonstrated to reduce hospitalization length of stay and outpatient visits in patients with complex needs (Cohen et al., 2010).

Acquired Versus Congenital/Developmental Conditions

A hallmark of pediatric medical care is understanding how acquired and congenital medical conditions interact with development. One needs to understand not only typical and atypical development but also how those developmental trajectories can be interrupted by expected and unexpected events such as acquired medical conditions. For example, a 14-month-old toddler may have a stroke leading to aphasia and apraxia; not only must one consider the immediate reduced expressive and receptive language abilities (e.g., no longer saying single words, no longer using differentiated gestures to communicate) as well as motor speech skills (e.g., changes in speech sounds and prosody), but one also must consider how this will impact the acquisition of speech-language skills as the child grows (e.g., development of multiword utterances, expansion of speech sound inventory). Consider also a 2-month-old baby who is the victim of a severe mixed traumatic-anoxic brain injury with a particular insult to the cortex. The baby may retain functional rooting, sucking, and swallowing reflexes and may be able to take a bottle or breastfeed shortly after injury. However, as the baby grows and as feeding and swallowing become a cortex-mediated behavior, it may appear that the child is "losing" the skill given the damage to the cortex, when it is an unfortunate conglomeration of acquired injury interacting with the developmental timetable. Figure 7–3 illustrates this concept of disrupted development impacting not only current skills but also likely trajectory.

Also, an understanding and knowledge of typical infant and child development cannot be underestimated. Typical development has wide ranges of normal and expected behaviors and events. Understanding what truly deviates from the typical or even the difference between deviance and difference can drastically impact patient care. SLP students and SLPs interested in the pediatric medical field would be wise to study typical infant and child development.

Managing Limited Evidence Base

Given the heterogeneous nature of the pediatric medical SLP arena, it is not surprising that the literature base for evidence-based practice can feel limited. It is common for SLPs to consider applying evidence-based assessment and intervention practices validated for

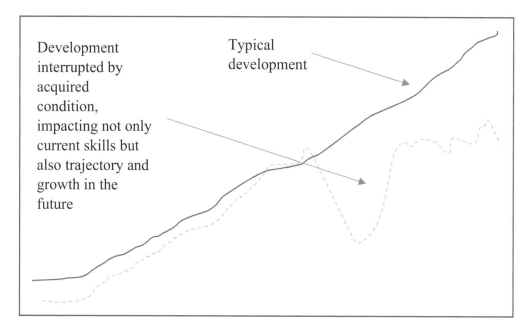

FIGURE 7–3. Developmental trajectory disruption.

adults to children. SLPs may use evaluation and treatment protocols validated for children with a particular disorder, with infants diagnosed with the same condition. Considerations for the appropriate application of research literature may include comparison of anatomy and physiology of the studied population versus treatment population, comparison of cognitive-communication status, and comparison of disease process. For example, the Yale Swallow Protocol is a well-supported, valid, and reliable screening measure for dysphagia in certain adult populations that includes exclusion criteria, a brief cognitive screen that includes orientation questions, a limited oral mechanism evaluation, and a 3-oz water swallow challenge (Leder & Suiter, 2014; Suiter & Leder, 2008; Suiter et al., 2014). Although some studies of the Yale Swallow Protocol have included older children and adolescents (Suiter et al., 2009), the literature on and considerations for children, particularly young children, is limited (Delaney, 2015). One might want to consider applying principles from the Yale Swallow Protocol evidence base into a clinical swallow evaluation for a preschool-age child with a respiratory illness postextubation given that the preschooler likely has similar enough anatomy/physiology to an adult, can likely engage in orientation assessment (though "what is the date?" may need to be replaced by a question such as "is it winter or summer?"), and appears to have a diagnosis and treatment course that is similar enough to an adult course. Evidence directly related to the patient population and specific patient condition is of course ideal in conjunction with family and patient values and clinical expertise (Sackett et al., 2000). However, it is very common for the pediatric medical SLP to find situations for which no formal evidence base exists. Critical thinking skills are therefore vital—as are practicing SLPs willing to engage in clinical research.

Collaborative Care

Collaborative care is vital in the pediatric medical SLP setting, particularly in acute care. It is common for pediatric medical SLPs to interact with physicians, advanced practice providers (APP), registered nurses, nursing assistants, CCLS, physical therapists, occupational therapists, radiology technologists, respiratory therapists, registered dieticians, lactation consultants, and others in a single day in the pediatric acute-care setting. An understanding of the role, scope, and expertise of each discipline allows for efficient and effective communication. Ultimately, this results in better outcomes for patients and their families.

In the inpatient pediatric medical setting, a patient who is admitted to the hospital is typically cared for by a specific primary medical team (e.g., pediatric hospitalists, pediatric ENTs, pediatric neurology, pediatric critical care, or pediatric neurosurgery). This team provides leadership and accountability and manages orders and referrals to other "consulting" teams and providers and to nursing staff who care for the patients at bedside daily. Children in the ICU are receiving a higher level of care ("critical care"), and intensivists are usually, but not always, the primary medical team in the ICU. Other teams will manage patients on acute-care units. SLP services are typically requested by a "consult" in the electronic medical record by the primary team. However, other consulting teams may also request SLP services for a child. The inpatient SLP team is typically expected to respond to all SLP consults or orders within 24 hr. SLPs will then document assessment and treatment sessions in the medical record. Prompt communication that considers a child's overall medical care and course is vital to ensuring quality care. SLPs must consider the urgency and importance of direct communication in addition to documenting in the medical record for each patient and situation (e.g., are the SLP recommendations vital to discharge or holding up discharge? Do the SLP recommendations need immediate action by a primary or consulting team? Are the SLP services more of an adjuvant to the plan of care and therefore do not require the immediate care of the primary medical team?).

Academic medical centers have residency training programs for a variety of professionals, particularly for physicians and providers such as nurse practitioners. Children's hospitals often have a pediatrics residency program that staffs a large portion of the pediatric and pediatric subspeciality provider teams. Pediatric residency follows medical school and is 3 years in length; pediatrics residents rotate throughout various teams (e.g., pediatric hospitalists, pediatric emergency room) and provide care under the supervision of attending providers and fellows. Pediatric fellowship programs follow a residency program such as a pediatric residency or a surgical residency and are even more specialized. Medical students may also be care providers at some institutions. Advanced practice providers are usually nurse practitioners or physician assistants and may also be part of care teams. Attending providers are physicians and have completed all training and are ultimately responsible for care and the supervision of the trainee providers. It is beneficial to understand that there is a degree of hierarchy in this system and that it may be judicious to discuss various aspects of patient care with different "levels" of providers, but ultimately all team members are responsible for patient care.

Collaborative care is also important in outpatient pediatric medical care. In addition to siloed SLP or medical specialist outpatient appointments, large children's hospitals have multidisciplinary outpatient clinics for special populations. In these clinics, children see not only one specialist but a whole team in one visit, which often includes an SLP. Teams typically conference about patients before and after clinic visits to maximize streamlined and integrated care. For example, Trisomy 21 clinic may include a developmental pediatrician who specializes in Trisomy 21, cardiology, nutrition, occupational therapy, speech-language pathology, and physical therapy; complex aerodigestive clinic might include gastroenterology, pulmonology, ENT, dietician, respiratory therapy, and speech-language pathology. Additionally, the input of the outpatient community or hospital-based SLP is strongly considered by the specialist medical team in decision-making, regardless of mode of outpatient care.

In addition to collaborative care involving providers and other professionals, patients, families, and caregivers are the main collaborators. Family-centered care is medical care that views patients and families as partners and involved in decisions. Family-centered care is individualized and takes into consideration family contextual factors including goals, culture, and values. Patients treated in the pediatric medical setting are largely minors, and this greatly impacts their care. Families are partners and important stakeholders in the pediatric setting. Families are diverse in their presentation and needs. Families may include biological, adoptive, or foster parents; legal guardians such as the state or other relatives; other caregivers and important adults; siblings and other children in the family unit; and more. A respect for and understanding of dynamic and diverse family systems is vital in this setting. "Educating" family and caregivers is also a vital part of the pediatric SLP's role in the medical SLP setting; however, it is important to view families being "educated" as partners and co-directors of care and not as students or subordinates to the professional/SLP.

Additionally, it should be noted that this chapter largely comes from the perspective of the medical model of disease and disability; however, this is not the only model, and models of care are not necessarily mutually exclusive (e.g., consider the WHO ICF model that attempts to merge a medical and social model [World Health Organization, 2007]). Children may experience challenges that for some families or practices are labeled as disabilities or disorders, wherein for other children and families, these challenges are largely seen as differences with the environment supporting the child's success (for further reading and reflection, consider exploring neurodiversity perspectives on autism). One cannot make assumptions about how a family may perceive a child's differences, and a thoughtful, individualized approach is best.

Palliative Care in Pediatrics

Pediatric palliative care is focused on supporting infants and children with serious medical conditions along with their families. Palliative care emphasizes maximizing quality of life, managing symptoms, minimizing suffering, and providing clear communication across disciplines regarding goals of care. Children receiving palliative care services may have genetic conditions, cancer, neuromuscular disease, progressive or stable complex conditions, or other needs that warrant specialty care. See Table 7–2 for examples of case management for children receiving palliative care services. Palliative care can be provided across the continuum of care including inpatient acute/critical care, outpatient clinics, and home or hospice settings. Hospice care is palliative care specifically provided for patients with a life expectancy of less than 6 months. Hospice care for adults is focused almost exclusively on symptom management and comfort since forgoing curative or life-prolonging therapies is typically required for admission into hospice care. However, since the passage of the Patient Protection and Affordable Care Act in 2010, hospice care and curative and life-prolonging therapies can be provided concurrently for children (Lindley, 2011).

Most large children's hospitals employ palliative care teams whose members include pediatricians with subspecialty training in hospice and palliative medicine, social workers, spiritual care workers, case management service providers, and team members from other disciplines. SLPs are increasingly involved in the care of patients receiving pediatric palliative care services. SLPs provide dysphagia and communication services to children and families receiving palliative care with emphasis on family and patient goals, consideration of not only "risks" and safety of feeding, but also comfort and pleasure and focus on communication interventions that support patient–provider and patient–family relationships (Krikheli et al., 2021).

Conclusion

Pediatric medical SLPs have the privilege of caring for an interesting and heterogeneous group of infants, children, and families. Frequently seen populations and conditions include, but are not limited to, prematurity, congenital anomalies including CHD, airway challenges, craniofacial differences, and neurologic conditions. Children with medical needs are becoming increasingly complex

TABLE 7–2 Examples of Pediatric Palliative Care

Current Status	Diagnosis/ Conditions	Prognosis	Possible Palliative Care Supports
Prenatal consult, fetus is 24 weeks' gestation	Prenatal diagnosis of Trisomy 13	Trisomy 13 is typically associated with severe intellectual disabilities and physical abnormalities; most children do not survive the first year of life without medical technology	Family preparation for birth, discussion regarding curative versus comfort measures, communication support with multiple specialty teams
Outpatient clinic consult, inpatient continuity visits, 18-year-old boy	Duchenne muscular dystrophy	Life-limiting neuromuscular progressive condition, young adulthood is average life expectancy	Support family and patient goals, management of symptoms and pain, emotional and spiritual support, discussion of advanced directives
Outpatient clinic visit, inpatient continuity visits, 14-month-old girl	Extreme prematurity, neurologic impairment, respiratory difficulties with tracheostomy need, feeding difficulties with g-tube need	Ongoing complex challenges associated with multiple medical conditions and high vulnerability for illness, potential for shortened life span	Support family and patient goals, management of care, continuity of care, symptom management
Outpatient clinic visits, inpatient continuity visits, hospice care, 3-year-old girl	Atypical teratoid rhabdoid tumor	Aggressive brain tumor with poor neurologic prognosis and high likelihood of mortality	Support patient and family goals, pain management, continuity of care, hospice care, bereavement support

and are served across settings, particularly in the children's hospital setting. Pediatric medical speech-language pathology requires critical thinking, a strong understanding of the relations between typical and atypical development, an appreciation for diverse families and models of care, and a deep commitment to collaboration.

References

Abraham, S. S. (2009). Perspectives on the pediatric larynx with tracheotomy. In M. Fried & A. Ferlito (Eds.), *The larynx* (Chap. 32). Plural Publishing.

Altschuler, T., Klein, D., & Scully, A. C. (2018). *Get moving with AAC* [ASHA Oral Presentation]. Presented in Boston, MA. https://www.patientprovidercommunication.org/files/Talking%20Early%20Mobility.No%20Pics.pdf

Amar-Dolan, L. G., Horn, M. H., O'Connell, B., Parsons, S. K., Roussin, C. J., Weinstock, P. H., & Graham, R. J. (2020). "This is how hard it is." Family experience of hospital-to-home transition with a tracheostomy. *Annals of the American Thoracic Society, 17*(7), 860–868.

American College of Obstetricians and Gynecologists. (2013, Reaffirmed 2022). ACOG Committee Opinion No. 579: Definition of term pregnancy. *Obstetrics and Gynecology, 122*(5), 1139–1140.

American College of Obstetricians and Gynecologists & Society for Maternal-Fetal Medicine. (2017). Obstetric Care Consensus No. 6: Periviable birth. *Obstetrics and Gynecology, 130*(4), e187–e199. https://doi.org/10.1097/AOG.0000000000002352

American Speech-Language-Hearing Association. (2004). *Knowledge and skills needed by speech-language pathologists providing services to infants and families in the NICU environment* [Knowledge and skills]. https://www.asha.org/policy

Arvedson, J. C., Brodsky, L., & Lefton-Greif, M. A. (Eds.). (2019). *Pediatric swallowing and feeding: Assessment and management.* Plural Publishing.

Baker, J., Barnett, C., Cavalli, L., Dietrich, M., Dixon, L., Duffy, J. R., . . . McWhirter, L. (2021). Management of functional communication, swallowing, cough and related disorders: Consensus recommendations for speech and language therapy. *Journal of Neurology, Neurosurgery & Psychiatry, 92*(10), 1112–1125.

Barnett, C., Armes, J., & Smith, C. (2019). Speech, language and swallowing impairments in functional neurological disorder: A scoping review. *International Journal of Language & Communication Disorders, 54*(3), 309–320.

Berry, J. G., Graham, D. A., Graham, R. J., Zhou, J., Putney, H. L., O'Brien, J. E., . . . Goldmann, D. A. (2009). Predictors of clinical outcomes and hospital resource use of children after tracheotomy. *Pediatrics, 124*(2), 563–572.

Berry, J. G., Hall, M., Hall, D. E., Kuo, D. Z., Cohen, E., Agrawal, R., . . . Neff, J. (2013). Inpatient growth and resource use in 28 children's hospitals: A longitudinal, multi-institutional study. *JAMA Pediatrics, 167*(2), 170–177. https://doi.org/10.1001/jamapediatrics.2013.432.

Betters, K. A., Tandon, R. S., & Minchin, K. J. (2022). Caregiver perceptions of an early mobility and communication protocol in the pediatric ICU [Preprint]. *Journal of Pediatric Rehabilitation Medicine,* 1–7.

Bolisetty, S., Dhawan, A., Abdel-Latif, M., Bajuk, B., Stack, J., Oei, J. L., & Lui, K. (2014). Intraventricular hemorrhage and neurodevelopmental outcomes in extreme preterm infants. *Pediatrics, 133*(1), 55–62.

Braun, D., Braun, E., Chiu, V., Burgos, A. E., Gupta, M., Volodarskiy, M., & Getahun, D. (2020). Trends in neonatal intensive care unit utilization in a large integrated health care system. *JAMA Network Open, 3*(6), e205239.

Brooks, L., Figueroa, J., Edwards, T., Reeder, W., McBrayer, S., & Landry, A. (2020). Passy Muir valve tolerance in medically complex infants and children: Are there predictors for success? *Laryngoscope, 130*(11), E632–E639.

Carson, A., Hallett, M., & Stone, J. (2016). Assessment of patients with functional neurologic disorders. *Handbook of Clinical Neurology, 139*, 169-188.

Casimir, G. (2019). Why children's hospitals are unique and so essential. *Frontiers in Pediatrics, 7*, 305. https://doi.org/10.3389/fped.2019.00305

Caskey, M., Stephens, B., Tucker, R., & Vohr, B. (2014). Adult talk in the NICU with preterm infants and developmental outcomes. *Pediatrics, 133*(3), e578–e584.

Centers for Disease Control and Prevention. (2021). *Preterm birth*. https://www.cdc.gov/reproductivehealth/maternalinfanthealth/pretermbirth.htm

Centers for Disease Control and Prevention. (2022). *Data and statistics on congenital heart defects*. https://www.cdc.gov/ncbddd/heartdefects/data.html

Chandran, A., Sikka, K., Thakar, A., Lodha, R., Irugu, D. V. K., Kumar, R., & Sharma, S. C. (2021). The impact of pediatric tracheostomy on the quality of life of caregivers. *International Journal of Pediatric Otorhinolaryngology, 149*, 110854.

Cohen, E., Berry, J. G., Camacho, X., Anderson, G., Wodchis, W., & Guttmann, A. (2012). Patterns and costs of health care use of children with medical complexity. *Pediatrics, 130*(6), e1463–e1470.

Cohen, E., Friedman, J. N., Mahant, S., Adams, S., Jovcevska, V., & Rosenbaum, P. (2010). The impact of a complex care clinic in a children's hospital. *Child: Care, Health and Development, 36*(4), 574–582.

Cooper, A. C., Banasiak, N. C., & Allen, P. J. (2003). Management and prevention strategies for respiratory syncytial virus (RSV) bronchiolitis in infants and young children: A review of evidence-based practice interventions. *Pediatric Nursing, 29*(6).

Corbett, S. S., & Drewett, R. F. (2004). To what extent is failure to thrive in infancy associated with poorer cognitive development? A review and meta-analysis. *Journal of Child Psychology and Psychiatry, 45*(3), 641–654.

Costello, J. M., Patak, L., & Pritchard, J. (2010). Communication vulnerable patients in the pediatric ICU: Enhancing care through augmentative and alternative communication. *Journal of Pediatric Rehabilitation Medicine, 3*(4), 289–301.

Coughlin, M., Gibbins, S., & Hoath, S. (2009). Core measures for developmentally supportive care in neonatal intensive care units: Theory, precedence and practice. *Journal of Advanced Nursing, 65*(10), 2239–2248.

Crump, C., Sundquist, J., & Sundquist, K. (2021). Preterm or early term birth and risk of autism. *Pediatrics, 148*(3).

Daya, H., Hosni, A., Bejar-Solar, I., Evans, J. N., & Bailey, C. M. (2000). Pediatric vocal fold paralysis: A long-term retrospective study. *Archives of Otolaryngology–Head & Neck Surgery, 126*(1), 21–25.

Delaney, A. L. (2015). Special considerations for the pediatric population relating to a swallow screen versus clinical swallow or instrumental evaluation. *Perspectives on Swallowing and Swallowing Disorders (Dysphagia), 24*(1), 26–33.

Dodrill, P., Gosa, M., Thoyre, S., Shaker, C., Pados, B., Park, J., . . . Hernandez, K. (2016). First, do no harm: A response to "oral alimentation in neonatal and adult populations requiring high-flow oxygen via nasal cannula." *Dysphagia, 31*(6), 781–782.

Edwards, J. D., Kun, S. S., & Keens, T. G. (2010). Outcomes and causes of death in children on home mechanical ventilation via tracheostomy: An institutional and literature review. *Journal of Pediatrics, 157*(6), 955-959.e2. https://doi.org/10.1016/j.jpeds.2010.06.012

Eibling, D. E., & Gross, R. D. (1996). Subglottic air pressure: A key component of swallowing efficiency. *Annals of Otology, Rhinology & Laryngology, 105*(4), 253–258.

Eichenwald, E. C. & Committee on Fetus and Newborn, American Academy of Pediatrics. (2016). Apnea of prematurity. *Pediatrics, 137*(1). https://doi.org/10.1542/peds.2015-3757

Ely, E. W. (2017). The ABCDEF bundle: Science and philosophy of how ICU liberation serves patients and families. *Critical Care Medicine, 45*(2), 321.

Ely, E. W., Shintani, A., Truman, B., Speroff, T., Gordon, S. M., Harrell Jr, F. E., . . . Dittus, R. S. (2004). Delirium as a predictor of mortality in mechanically ventilated patients in the intensive care unit. *JAMA, 291*(14), 1753–1762.

Eskedal, L., Hagemo, P., Eskild, A., Aamodt, G., Seiler, K. S., & Thaulow, E. (2004). A population-based study of extra-cardiac anomalies in children with congenital cardiac malformations. *Cardiology in the Young, 14*(6), 600–607.

Ewing-Cobbs, L., Levin, H. S., Fletcher, J. M., Miner, M. E., & Eisenberg, H. M. (1990). The children's orientation and amnesia test: Relationship to severity of acute head injury and to recovery of memory. *Neurosurgery, 27*(5), 683–691.

Faedda, N., Baglioni, V., Natalucci, G., Ardizzone, I., Camuffo, M., Cerutti, R., & Guidetti, V. (2018). Don't judge a book by its cover: Factitious disorder imposed on children-report on 2 cases. *Frontiers in Pediatrics, 6*, 110.

Ferrara, L., Bidiwala, A., Sher, I., Pirzada, M., Barlev, D., Islam, S., . . . Hanna, N. (2017). Effect of nasal continuous positive airway pressure on the pharyngeal swallow in neonates. *Journal of Perinatology,* *37*(4), 398–403.

Geddes, D. T., Chadwick, L. M., Kent, J. C., Garbin, C. P., & Hartmann, P. E. (2010). Ultrasound imaging of infant swallowing during breast-feeding. *Dysphagia, 25*(3), 183–191.

Griffith, T., White-Traut, R., Janusek, L. W., & Harris-Haman, P. A. (2020). A behavioral epigenetics model to predict oral feeding skills in pre-term infants. *Advances in Neonatal Care, 20*(5), 392–400.

Gudrunardottir, T., Sehested, A., Juhler, M., & Schmiegelow, K. (2011). Cerebellar mutism. *Child's Nervous System, 27*(3), 355–363.

Harrison, W., & Goodman, D. (2015). Epidemiologic trends in neonatal intensive care, 2007–2012. *JAMA Pediatrics, 169*(9), 855–862.

Hebbar, K. B., Kasi, A. S., Vielkind, M., McCracken, C. E., Ivie, C. C., Prickett, K. K., & Simon, D. M. (2021). Mortality and outcomes of pediatric tracheostomy dependent patients. *Frontiers in Pediatrics, 9,* 661512. https://doi.org/10.3389/fped.2021.661512

Hirst, K., Dodrill, P., & Gosa, M. (2017). Noninvasive respiratory support and feeding in the neonate. *Perspectives of the ASHA Special Interest Groups, 2*(13), 82–92.

Hoffman, J. I., & Kaplan, S. (2002). The incidence of congenital heart disease. *Journal of the American College of Cardiology, 39*(12), 1890–1900.

Hotz, G., Helm-Estabrooks, N., Wolf Nelson, N., & Plante, E. (2010). *Pediatric Test of Brain Injury (PTBI).* Brookes Publishing.

Hull, E. M., Dumas, H. M., Crowley, R. A., & Kharasch, V. S. (2005). Tracheostomy speaking valves for children: Tolerance and clinical benefits. *Pediatric Rehabilitation, 8*(3), 214–219.

Jacobs-Levine, A. W., Ringwald-Smith, K., & Zoerink, S. (2006). Food for thought: Dysphagia treatment in pediatric patients with cancer: It takes collaboration. *Perspectives on Swallowing and Swallowing Disorders (Dysphagia), 15*(2), 26–30.

Jiang, D., & Morrison, G. A. J. (2003). The influence of long-term tracheostomy on speech and language development in children. *International Journal of Pediatric Otorhinolaryngology, 67,* S217–S220.

Johnson, S., & Marlow, N. (2011). Preterm birth and childhood psychiatric disorders. *Pediatric Research, 69*(8), 11–18.

Jones, C. E., Desai, H., Fogel, J. L., Negrin, K. A., Torzone, A., Willette, S., . . . Butler, S. C. (2021). Disruptions in the development of feeding for infants with congenital heart disease. *Cardiology in the Young, 31*(4), 589–596.

Joseph, R. A., Goodfellow, L. M., & Simko, L. M. (2014). Parental quality of life: Caring for an infant or toddler with a tracheostomy at home. *Neonatal Network, 33*(2), 86–94.

Kirk, E. A., Howard, V. C., & Scott, C. A. (1995). Description of posterior fossa syndrome in children after posterior fossa brain tumor surgery. *Journal of Pediatric Oncology Nursing, 12*(4), 181–187.

Ko, J. M. (2015). Genetic syndromes associated with congenital heart disease. *Korean Circulation Journal, 45*(5), 357–361.

Kozlowska, K., Sawchuk, T., Waugh, J. L., Helgeland, H., Baker, J., Scher, S., & Fobian, A. D. (2021). Changing the culture of care for children and adolescents with functional neurological disorder. *Epilepsy & Behavior Reports, 16,* 100486.

Krikheli, L., Erickson, S., Carey, L. B., Carey-Sargeant, C. L., & Mathisen, B. A. (2021). Speech-language pathologists in pediatric palliative care: An international study of perceptions and experiences. *American Journal of Speech-Language Pathology, 30*(1), 150–168.

Lannering, B., Marky, I., Lundberg, A., & Olsson, E. (1990). Long-term sequelae after pediatric brain tumors: Their effect on disability and quality of life. *Medical and Pediatric Oncology, 18*(4), 304–310.

Le Guennec, L., Cholet, C., Huang, F., Schmidt, M., Bréchot, N., Hékimian, G., . . . Luyt, C. E. (2018). Ischemic and hemorrhagic brain injury during venoarterial-extracorporeal membrane oxygenation. *Annals of Intensive Care, 8*(1), 1–10.

Leder, S. B., & Suiter, D. M. (2014). Yale Swallow Protocol administration and interpretation: Passing and failing. In S. B. Leder & D. M. Suiter (Eds.), *The Yale Swallow Protocol* (pp. 105–109). Springer.

Lindley, L. C. (2011). Health care reform and concurrent curative care for terminally ill children: A policy analysis. *Journal of Hospice and Palliative Nursing, 13*(2), 81.

Luu, K., Belsky, M. A., Dharmarajan, H., Kaffenberger, T., McCoy, J. L., Cangilla, K., . . . Padia, R. (2022). Dysphagia in pediatric patients with tracheostomy. *Annals of Otology, Rhinology & Laryngology, 131*(5), 457–462.

Mai, K., Davis, R. K., Hamilton, S., Robertson-James, C., Calaman, S., & Turchi, R. M. (2020). Identifying caregiver needs for children with a tracheostomy living at home. *Clinical Pediatrics, 59*(13), 1169–1181.

Martin-Harris, B., Brodsky, M. B., Michel, Y., Castell, D. O., Schleicher, M., Sandidge, J., . . . Blair, J. (2008). MBS measurement tool for swallow impairment—MBSImP: Establishing a standard. *Dysphagia, 23*(4), 392–405.

Martin-Harris, B., Carson, K. A., Pinto, J. M., & Lefton-Greif, M. A. (2020). BaByVFSSImP a novel measurement tool for videofluoroscopic assessment of swallowing impairment in bottle-fed babies: Establishing a standard. *Dysphagia, 35*(1), 90–98.

McKeon, M., Kohn, J., Munhall, D., Wells, S., Blanchette, S., Santiago, R., . . . Watters, K. (2019). Association of a multidisciplinary care approach with the quality of care after pediatric tracheostomy. *JAMA Otolaryngology–Head & Neck Surgery, 145*(11), 1035–1042. https://doi.org/10.1001/jamaoto.2019.2500

Mills, N., Keesing, M., Geddes, D., & Mirjalili, S. A. (2021). Flexible endoscopic evaluation of swallowing in breastfeeding infants with laryngomalacia: Observed clinical and endoscopic changes with alteration of infant positioning at the breast. *Annals of Otology, Rhinology & Laryngology, 130*(7), 653–665.

Neff, J. M., Sharp, V. L., Muldoon, J., Graham, J., & Myers, K. (2004). Profile of medical charges for children by health status group and severity level in a Washington State Health Plan. *Health Services Research, 39*(1), 73–90.

O'Connor, L. R., Morris, N. R., & Paratz, J. (2019). Physiological and clinical outcomes associated with use of one-way speaking valves on tracheostomised patients: A systematic review. *Heart & Lung, 48*(4), 356–364.

Oster, M. E., Lee, K. A., Honein, M. A., Riehle-Colarusso, T., Shin, M., & Correa, A. (2013). Temporal trends in survival among infants with critical congenital heart defects. *Pediatrics, 131*(5), e1502–e1508.

Pados, B. F., Hill, R. R., Yamasaki, J. T., Litt, J. S., & Lee, C. S. (2021). Prevalence of problematic feeding in young children born prematurely: A meta-analysis. *BMC Pediatrics, 21*(1), 1–15.

Patak, L., Gawlinski, A., Fung, N. I., Doering, L., Berg, J., & Henneman, E. A. (2006). Communication boards in critical care: Patients' views. *Applied Nursing Research, 19*(4), 182–190.

Patient Protection and Affordable Care Act of 2010, Pub. L. No. 111–148, 124 Stat. 119 (2010).

Pineda, R., Melchior, K., Oberle, S., Inder, T., & Rogers, C. (2015). Assessment of autism symptoms during the neonatal period: Is there early evidence of autism risk? *American Journal of Occupational Therapy, 69*(4), 6904220010p1–6904220010p11.

Pullens, B., & Streppel, M. (2021, June). Swallowing problems in children with a tracheostomy. *Seminars in Pediatric Surgery, 30*(3), 151053.

Radtke, J. V., Baumann, B. M., Garrett, K. L., & Happ, M. B. (2011). Listening to the voiceless patient: Case reports in assisted communication in the intensive care unit. *Journal of Palliative Medicine, 14*(6), 791–795.

Rahbar, R., Rouillon, I., Roger, G., Lin, A., Nuss, R. C., Denoyelle, F., . . . Garabedian, E. N. (2006). The presentation and management of laryngeal cleft: A 10-year experience. *Archives of Otolaryngology–Head & Neck Surgery, 132*(12), 1335–1341.

Rand, K., & Lahav, A. (2014). Impact of the NICU environment on language deprivation in preterm infants. *Acta Paediatrica, 103*(3), 243–248.

Reller, M. D., Strickland, M. J., Riehle-Colarusso, T., Mahle, W. T., & Correa, A. (2008). Prevalence of congenital heart defects in metropolitan Atlanta, 1998–2005. *Journal of Pediatrics, 153*(6), 807–813.

Sackett, D. L., Straus, S. E., & Richardson, W. S. (2000). *Evidence-based medicine: How to practice and teach EBM*. Churchill Livingstone.

Sanders, M. R., & Hall, S. L. (2018). Trauma-informed care in the newborn intensive care unit: Promoting safety, security and connectedness. *Journal of Perinatology, 38*(1), 3–10.

Sharp, W. G., Berry, R. C., McCracken, C., Nuhu, N. N., Marvel, E., Saulnier, C. A., . . . Jaquess, D. L. (2013). Feeding problems and nutrient intake in children with autism spectrum disorders: A meta-analysis and comprehensive review of the literature. *Journal of Autism and Developmental Disorders, 43*(9), 2159–2173.

Silverman, A. H., Erato, G., & Goday, P. (2021). The relationship between chronic paediatric feeding disorders and caregiver stress. *Journal of Child Health Care, 25*(1), 69–80.

Streppel, M., Veder, L. L., Pullens, B., & Joosten, K. F. (2019). Swallowing problems in children with a tracheostomy tube. *International Journal of Pediatric Otorhinolaryngology, 124*, 30–33.

Suiter, D. M., & Leder, S. B. (2008). Clinical utility of the 3-ounce water swallow test. *Dysphagia, 23*(3), 244–250.

Suiter, D. M., Leder, S. B., & Karas, D. E. (2009). The 3-ounce (90-cc) water swallow challenge: A screening test for children with suspected oropharyngeal dysphagia. *Otolaryngology–Head and Neck Surgery*, *140*(2), 187–190.

Suiter, D. M., Sloggy, J., & Leder, S. B. (2014). Validation of the Yale Swallow Protocol: A prospective double-blinded videofluoroscopic study. *Dysphagia*, *29*(2), 199–203.

Tang, M. N., Adolphe, S., Rogers, S. R., & Frank, D. A. (2021). Failure to thrive or growth faltering: Medical, developmental/behavioral, nutritional, and social dimensions. *Pediatrics in Review*, *42*(11), 590–603.

Thomas, T., Goodman, R., Jacob, A., & Grabher, D. (2021). Implementation of cue-based feeding to improve preterm infant feeding outcomes and promote parents' involvement. *Journal of Obstetric, Gynecologic & Neonatal Nursing*, *50*(3), 328–339.

Traube, C., Silver, G., Gerber, L. M., Kaur, S., Mauer, E. A., Kerson, A., . . . Greenwald, B. M. (2017). Delirium and mortality in critically ill children: Epidemiology and outcomes of pediatric delirium. *Critical Care Medicine*, *45*(5), 891.

Turner, T., El Tobgy, N., Russell, K., Day, C., Cheung, K., Proven, S., & Ricci, M. F. (2022, May 5). Language abilities in preschool children with critical CHD: A systematic review. *Cardiology in the Young*, 1–11.

Urík, M., Tuma, J., Jančíková, J., Bezděková, D., Urbanová, P., Dohnalová, L., . . . Jabandžiev, P. (2021). Videofluoroscopic swallow study in diagnostics of H-type tracheoesophageal fistula in children. *Ear, Nose & Throat Journal*, 01455613211021580.

Vandormael, C., Schoenhals, L., Hüppi, P. S., Filippa, M., & Borradori Tolsa, C. (2019). Language in preterm born children: Atypical development and effects of early interventions on neuroplasticity. *Neural Plasticity*, 2019, 6873270.

Vargas, M., Sutherasan, Y., Antonelli, M., Brunetti, I., Corcione, A., Laffey, J. G., . . . Pelosi, P. (2015). Tracheostomy procedures in the intensive care unit: An international survey. *Critical Care*, *19*(1), 1–10.

Watters, K., O'Neill, M., Zhu, H., Graham, R. J., Hall, M., & Berry, J. (2016). Two-year mortality, complications, and healthcare use in children with Medicaid following tracheostomy. *Laryngoscope*, *126*(11), 2611–2617. https://doi.org/10.1002/lary.25972

Watters, K. F. (2017). Tracheostomy in infants and children. *Respiratory Care*, *62*(6), 799–825.

Wells, E. M., Khademian, Z. P., Walsh, K. S., Vezina, G., Sposto, R., Keating, R. F., & Packer, R. J. (2010). Postoperative cerebellar mutism syndrome following treatment of medulloblastoma: Neuroradiographic features and origin. *Journal of Neurosurgery: Pediatrics*, *5*(4), 329–334.

Wernovsky, G. (2006). Current insights regarding neurological and developmental abnormalities in children and young adults with complex congenital cardiac disease. *Cardiology in the Young*, *16*(S1), 92–104.

White, C. M., Thomson, J. E., Statile, A. M., Auger, K. A., Unaka, N., Carroll, M., . . . Brady, P. W. (2017). Development of a new care model for hospitalized children with medical complexity. *Hospital Pediatrics*, 7(7), 410–414.

Winkler, M. F., Ross, V. M., Piamjariyakul, U., Gajewski, B., & Smith, C. E. (2006). Technology dependence in home care: Impact on patients and their family caregivers. *Nutrition in Clinical Practice*, 21(6), 544–556.

Wood, D., McShane, P., & Davis, P. (2012). Tracheostomy in children admitted to paediatric intensive care. *Archives of Disease in Childhood*, 97(10), 866–869.

World Health Organization. (2007). *International classification of functioning, disability, and health: Children & youth version: ICF-CY*.

World Health Organization. (2018). *Preterm birth*. https://www.who.int/news-room/fact-sheets/detail/preterm-birth

Zambrana, I. M., Vollrath, M. E., Jacobsson, B., Sengpiel, V., & Ystrom, E. (2021). Preterm birth and risk for language delays before school entry: A sibling-control study. *Development and Psychopathology*, 33(1), 47–52.

Zengin, E., Sinning, C., Blaum, C., Blankenberg, S., Rickers, C., von Kodolitsch, Y., . . . Stoll, V. M. (2021). Heart failure in adults with congenital heart disease: A narrative review. *Cardiovascular Diagnosis and Therapy*, 11(2), 529.

Zimmerman, E. (2018). Do infants born very premature and who have very low birth weight catch up with their full term peers in their language abilities by early school age? *Journal of Speech, Language, and Hearing Research*, 61(1), 53–65.

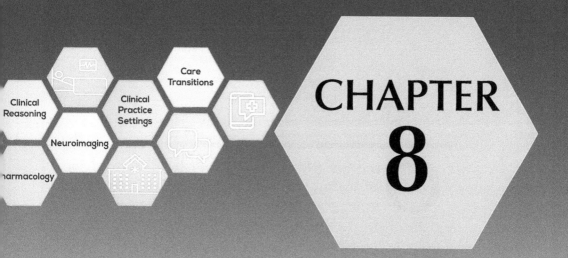

CHAPTER
8

Pharmacology in Medical Speech-Language Pathology

Abigail T. Burka

Chapter Objectives

Upon completion of this chapter, the reader will be able to:

- Recognize principles of pharmacology including pharmacokinetics and pharmacodynamics.
- Describe medication dosage forms as well as principles for the modification of dosage forms.
- Identify common adverse effects of medications relevant to the SLP including:
  - Delirium
  - Language Processing
  - Dysarthria
  - Dysphonia
  - Dysphagia
  - Xerostomia
- Locate reputable sources of medication information relevant to the practice of an SLP.

Chapter Overview

Over four billion prescriptions are dispensed annually in the United States, with the majority of adults taking some form of prescription medication, nonprescription medication, or dietary supplement. Awareness of the principles of pharmacology is essential for the speech-language pathologist in order for them to collaborate as members of the interprofessional healthcare team, regardless of their chosen practice setting. This chapter will focus on outlining terminology used when describing pharmacology as well as providing practical application in regards to identifying potential adverse effects of medications applicable to the practice of the speech-language pathologist. It will also provide recommendations for modifying medication dosage forms for those with swallowing difficulties as well as sources of reputable medication information.

Principles of Pharmacology

As members of the interprofessional health care team, speech-language pathologists (SLPs) greatly benefit from foundational knowledge in pharmacology. Many medications have the potential to affect the ability of the patient to communicate by affecting either cognitive functioning, motor speech abilities, or both. These alterations can be the results of known therapeutic functions of the medication or an adverse drug reaction (ADR). SLPs play an essential role in assessing cognitive and/or language functions and the ability to swallow oral medications, all of which are vital to maintaining medication adherence.

Pharmacology is the study of substances that interact with the living body through chemical processes. These processes can be therapeutic or toxic in nature, with both intended and unintended effects. Historically, medications used for therapeutic purposes have often been small molecules that are well-absorbed through the gastrointestinal tract. However, new therapeutic classes are increasingly being developed, which are protein-based biologic agents requiring administration via intravenous or subcutaneous injection. For the purposes of this chapter, we focus on the intended therapeutic application of certain classes of medications (or drugs) as well as their potential adverse effects that a SLP might encounter in their practice.

Pharmacology has several subdomains of study that are relevant to the practice of a SLP: pharmacodynamics and pharmacokinetics. Pharmacodynamics is the study of a drug's molecular, biochemical, or physiological effects or actions on the organism. Pharmacodynamics is driven by the action of the drug on specific receptors in the body. Although drugs are designed to act on an intended therapeutic target, some medications may also act on other receptors as well, leading to adverse effects, also known as side effects. The effects of medications are often dose-dependent in both intended therapeutic response as well as unintended adverse effects, where the effects of the medication change in direct response to changes in dose. This particularly affects older patients or those with reduced ability to eliminate medications, such as patients with liver or kidney disease.

Pharmacokinetics is the study of a drug's movement within the body through absorption, distribution, metabolism, and elimination. Although there are numerous pharmacokinetic principles, the two most clinically significant are clearance and volume of distribution. These drive medication dosing choices through the choice of medication dose and administration frequency. Medications may be delivered in numerous dosage forms to optimize their effectiveness. Choice of dosage form may depend on the intended route of administration, duration of action needed (immediate versus extended release), as well as economic considerations.

Absorption is the process of delivering the drug from the administration vehicle (tablet, capsule, ointment, etc.) into the blood. Medication absorption varies between drugs and can be influenced by the site of administration and drug formulation. Enteral routes of administration are the most common routes and rely on the gastrointestinal tract for absorption. Most oral medications are absorbed in the duodenum. Many oral medications undergo hepatic first-pass metabolism, where medications absorbed from the gastrointestinal tract enter the liver's portal vein, where the hepatic metabolism reduces drug concentrations before reaching systemic circulation. Not all medications can be absorbed orally, such as proteins like insulin or monoclonal antibodies. Other medications that undergo extensive first-pass metabolism must be administered via a parenteral route. Drugs administered via parenteral routes of administration do not rely on the gastrointestinal tract for absorption or undergo hepatic first-pass metabolism. One example of this is lidocaine, which is typically administered topically or intravenously due to its extensive first-pass metabolism.

Medications administered parenterally are often higher in cost than oral equivalents. Please refer to Table 8–1 for common routes of medication administration.

TABLE 8-1	Common Routes of Medication Administration

Enteral Routes of Administration

Administration Site (abbreviation)	Absorption	Hepatic First-Pass Metabolism	Example Medications
Oral (PO)	Variable (often in duodenum)	Yes	Numerous examples, such as ibuprofen tablets or capsules (Advil) for pain relief
Sublingual (SL)	Variable	No	Buprenorphine/naloxone (Suboxone) film for opioid dependence
Buccal	Variable	No	Fentanyl lozenge (Actiq) for severe pain
Rectal (PR)	Variable	Reduced	Promethazine (Phenergan) suppository for nausea and vomiting

Parenteral Routes of Administration

Administration Site (abbreviation)	Absorption	Hepatic First-Pass Metabolism	Example Medications
Intravenous (IV)	Complete	No	Numerous examples, such as antibiotics to treat systemic infections
Intramuscular (IM)	Usually complete	No	Cyanocobalamin (Vitamin B12) for anemia
Subcutaneous (SC or SQ)	Variable, but usually complete	No	Insulin for diabetes
Inhalational (INH)	Variable	No	Fluticasone (Flovent) for asthma
Transdermal (TD)	Variable	No	Nicotine TD patch for tobacco dependence
Intrathecal (IT)	Complete	No	Certain chemotherapies for malignancies in the central nervous system
Intraventricular	Complete	No	Certain antibiotics for infections in the central nervous system
Intra-arterial	Complete	No	Radioactive dyes for imaging procedures

Distribution is the process by which a drug leaves systemic circulation and enters the interstitium and cellular tissues. The volume of distribution, expressed in liters per kilogram (L/kg), represents a drug's propensity to leave the blood and enter tissue. Drugs with very high volumes of distribution have much higher concentrations in extravascular tissue than in the blood. Conversely, drugs with very low volumes of distribution have minimal distribution outside of the plasma compartment. A medication's volume of distribution determines its loading dose. Additionally, it influences the maintenance dose of a drug, along with clearance.

Metabolism is the process by which drugs are chemically altered in the body. Metabolism is necessary to transform medications in order to increase their solubility and allow them to be eliminated from the body. However, it can also be used to transform medications into active forms or metabolites. While the liver performs most metabolic activities, other organs and tissues including the lungs, intestines, kidneys, and blood also contain metabolic enzymes. Metabolism occurs in two phases: Phase I and Phase II. Cytochrome P450 enzymes involved in Phase I oxidative metabolism are involved in many drug–drug interactions, through either the inhibition or induction of activity.

Excretion is the process by which a drug or its metabolites are removed from the body. The major route of elimination for most drugs is the kidneys. Polar drugs, such as metformin, are filtered into the urine and do not undergo reabsorption. Urine pH can affect filtration. The other major route of elimination is the bile, where the liver actively secretes drugs. Some drugs may be reabsorbed and undergo enterohepatic recirculation, while others are eliminated through the feces. Other routes of elimination include the lungs, breast milk, sweat, saliva, and tears.

Drug Development and Regulation Processes

Developing and marketing a new medication is an extensive process that may take a decade or more. In the United States, the Food and Drug Administration (FDA) is the federal agency tasked with ensuring the safety, efficacy, and security of human and veterinary drugs, biological products, and medical devices, among other responsibilities. Drug candidates for potential approval by the FDA move from preclinical testing in lab models through four phases of human testing for full approval. Please refer to Table 8–2 for an overview of the FDA approval process (FDA, 2017). Once preclinical trials are completed, the manufacturer submits an Investigational New Drug Application prior to beginning human trials.

TABLE 8–2	Overview of the U.S. Food and Drug Administration Drug Approval Process		
Clinical Trial Phase	**Marketing**	**Patient Population**	**Clinical Testing**
Preclinical	Premarket	Animal	Safety; Pharmacokinetics and pharmacodynamics
Phase I	Premarket	Healthy human volunteer	Pharmacokinetics and pharmacodynamics Safety Dose finding
Phase II	Premarket	Human volunteers with disease/ condition	Clinical efficacy ± dose finding Placebo/active control
Phase III	Premarket	Human volunteers with disease/ condition	Clinical efficacy Placebo/active control
Phase IV	Postmarket	Patients with disease/conditions	Postmarketing surveillance

Source: From *The FDA's Drug Review Process: Ensuring Drugs Are Safe and Effective*, by the U.S. Food and Drug Administration, November 2017 (https://www.fda.gov/drugs/information-consumers-and-patients-drugs/fdas-drug-review-process-ensuring-drugs-are-safe-and-effective).

In Phase I human tests, a small group of healthy volunteers receive the drug. Basic pharmacokinetic and pharmacodynamic tests are performed in order to find human doses. In Phase II tests, a slightly larger group of volunteers with the targeted disease or disorder receive the drug, where pharmacokinetic and pharmacodynamic tests are repeated to further refine doses. In Phase III trials, large groups of volunteers with the targeted disease or disorder are recruited. The drug is usually compared with a placebo or active control. If the drug meets the Phase III trial's safety and efficacy endpoints, the manufacturer applies for a New Drug Application. Following FDA approval, the manufacturer conducts Phase IV or postmarketing surveillance to ensure that the drug is safe.

Some notable exceptions to FDA oversight over the medication process are dietary and nutritional supplements. Products that are marketed as dietary or nutritional supplements are regulated by the FDA as foods. These products undergo the same FDA approval process or have the same labeling requirements as prescription or over-the-counter medications, even if they have pharmaceutical-like effects. Some products may have drug–drug or drug–nutrient interactions with medications mediated through cytochrome P450 enzymes. Documenting dietary and nutritional supplements as well as other over-the-counter products should be a part of any complete patient or medication history.

Although the medication approval process is closely regulated by the FDA, patients may still experience adverse drug events (ADEs). An ADE is when someone is harmed by a medication, which can include both ADRs and medication errors. A few classes of medications are notably responsible for the majority of ADEs, including anticoagulants (blood thinners), diabetes medications (particularly insulins), opioid analgesics, and anticonvulsants (anti-seizure medications). Older adults are the population most likely to be hospitalized due to an ADE. Although an ADE can be from either error or intrinsic medication activity, the World Health Organization defines an ADR as "a response to a drug that is noxious and unintended and occurs at doses normally used in man for the prophylaxis, diagnosis or therapy of disease, or for modification of physiological function" (World Health Organization, 2002). ADRs can arise out of the intended pharmacologic action of the medication or an idiosyncratic or even an allergic reaction to the medication. Examples of each include hypoglycemia from an excessive dose of insulin or development of a rash following penicillin administration. MedWatch, the FDA's medical product safety reporting program, receives reports from the public and publishes safety alerts for FDA-regulated products (FDA, 2022a).

Medication Effects Relevant to the Speech-Language Pathologist

The lists of medications in the following sections contain medications that are commonly prescribed and have well-defined adverse effect profiles. As a general principle, medications that are intended to act in the central nervous system (CNS) tend to have therapeutic and adverse effect profiles of relevance to the SLP. These lists are not exhaustive, and the SLP is encouraged to check the medication's package insert or another reputable source of drug information from the section at the end of the chapter if there are questions about therapeutic or adverse effects of medications. Unless otherwise noted, medications are listed by the generic name, with brand names that are still commonly utilized following in parentheses.

Anticholinergic Medications

Acetylcholine is the primary neurotransmitter of the autonomic nervous system. Acetylcholine is synthesized in nerve terminals by acetyl coenzyme A and choline. It stimulates postsynaptic cholinergic neurons before being broken down by acetylcholinesterase. Many parasympathetic postganglionic and some sympathetic postganglionic fibers are cholinergic. Cholinergic receptors can be further broken down into muscarinic and nicotinic receptors. In the CNS, acetylcholine is the primary neurotransmitter responsible for attention and memory. Thus, medications affecting the synthesis, storage, release, activity, or metabolism of acetylcholine can have far-reaching effects in both peripheral and CNS function. Medications that promote the effects of acetylcholine through enhanced release or prevention of its metabolism are called cholinergic, while medications that block the effects of acetylcholine are considered to be anticholinergic, or more specifically antimuscarinic since the actions are usually specific to the muscarinic receptors. As with many ADRs, older individuals are usually more susceptible to adverse effects. These are often remembered using common phrases that date back centuries to the toxidrome of belladonna, a strong anticholinergic (Migirov & Datta, 2021). Please refer to Table 8–3 for a list of phrases and their corresponding anticholinergic adverse effects of medications.

TABLE 8–3	Anticholinergic Effects of Medications
Symptom	**Clinical Effect**
Mad as a hatter	Delirium
Blind as a bat	Mydriasis
Dry as a bone	Anhydrosis, xerostomia
Hot as a hare	Fever
Bloated as a toad	Constipation
The heart runs alone	Tachycardia
Full as a flask	Urinary retention
Red as a beet	Cutaneous vasodilation

Source: Adapted from Migirov, A., & Datta, A. R. Physiology, Anticholinergic Reaction. [Updated 2021 Aug 9]. In: StatPearls [Internet]. Treasure Island (FL): StatPearls Publishing; 2022 Jan–. Available from: https://www.ncbi.nlm.nih.gov/books/NBK546589/

Although some medications with cholinergic and anticholinergic properties are purposefully designed to act directly for therapeutic purposes, many others have unintended, indirect activities due to the ubiquity of cholinergic neurons throughout the body. Medications with indirect anticholinergic effects are much more common than those with cholinergic effects. Table 8–4 lists medication classes that have indirect anticholinergic effects.

Medications That Affect Cognitive Function

Various medications can affect cognitive function in ways that make it difficult for persons to function to their usual degree. In particular, medications may cause excessive drowsiness, sleepiness, or somnolence which may negatively affect a SLP's ability to perform communication and swallowing assessments or the patient's ability to function independently in activities of daily living. Additionally,

TABLE 8–4	Common Medications With Strong Anticholinergic Properties	
Medication Class	**Common Therapeutic Use**	**Representative Medications**
Antidepressants	Treatment of depression	Amitriptyline, desipramine, nortriptyline, paroxetine (Paxil)
Antiemetics	Treatment of nausea and vomiting	Prochlorperazine, promethazine (Phenergan)
Antihistamines (first-generation)	Treatment of allergic reactions	Chlorpheniramine, diphenhydramine (Benadryl), doxylamine (Tylenol PM), hydroxyzine (Vistaril), hyoscyamine
Antimuscarinics	Urinary incontinence	Darifenacin (Enablex), fesoterodine (Toviaz), oxybutynin (Ditropan), solifenacin (Vesicare), tolterodine (Detrol), trospium (Trosec)
Antiparkinsonian agents	Treatment of Parkinson's disease tremor	Benztropine (Cogentin), trihexyphenidyl
Antipsychotics/ neuroleptic agents	Treatment of psychosis	Chlorpromazine, clozapine (Clozapril), olanzapine (Zyprexa)
Antispasmodics	Treatment of gastrointestinal spasms	Atropine (non-ophthalmic), scopolamine (non-ophthalmic), belladonna alkaloids
Skeletal muscle relaxants	Treatment of muscle spasms	Cyclobenzaprine (Flexeril)

Source: Adapted from "American Geriatrics Society 2019 Updated AGS Beers Criteria for Potentially Inappropriate Medication Use in Older Adults," by the 2019 American Geriatrics Society Beers Criteria Update Expert Panel, 2019, *Journal of the American Geriatric Society, 67*(4), pp. 674–694. Please refer to the article's full text for a comprehensive list of medications with anticholinergic properties.

many of these medications have dose-dependent or additive effects on drowsiness when used in combination. Elderly patients or those with impaired renal or hepatic clearance are more likely to experience drowsiness or somnolence (American Geriatrics Society, 2019). Medications that may commonly cause excessive drowsiness are presented in Table 8–5.

Other medications may cause delirium, which is a disturbance of consciousness with reduced ability to focus, sustain, or shift attention. Delirium develops suddenly over the course of hours to days. Although the development of delirium is often multifactorial, including modifiable and nonmodifiable physiologic and environmental causes, the medication classes most often associated with the development of delirium can include benzodiazepines, anticholinergics, and opioid analgesics.

Some medications may affect cognitive function in the areas of cognitive and language processing efficiency. This can lead to difficulties in word finding. In particular, topiramate (Topamax), which is used for prevention of both seizures and migraines, has

TABLE 8–5	Select Medications That May Cause Drowsiness	
Medication Class	**Common Therapeutic Use/Mechanism of Action**	**Example Medications**
Opioids	Pain relief through agonism of mu receptor	Hydrocodone, oxycodone, morphine
Benzodiazepines	Relief of anxiety through agonism of GABA-A receptor	Alprazolam (Xanax), diazepam (Valium)
Antihistamines	Treatment of allergic reactions through blockade of histamine release	Diphenhydramine (Benadryl), cetirizine (Zyrtec)
Sedative-hypnotics	Induction of sleep through agonism of benzodiazepine receptor	Zolpidem (Ambien), eszopiclone (Lunesta), zaleplon (Sonata)
Skeletal muscle relaxants	Relief of muscle spasticity through various mechanisms of action	Baclofen, carisoprodol (Soma), methocarbamol (Robaxin)
Neuroleptics (antipsychotics)	Relief of psychosis through blockade of dopamine receptors	Haloperidol (Haldol), quetiapine (Seroquel), olanzapine (Zyprexa)

been associated with word-finding difficulties in 7.2% of patients (Mula et al., 2003). Table 8–6 lists select medications that may be associated with alterations in cognitive speed.

Other medications may affect speech production by causing dysarthria or slurring of speech. Dysarthria results from weakening of the muscles of the oral facial structures and larynx that control speech and voice production. Although it is most commonly caused by diseases or disorders of the brain or nervous system, medications that affect nerves or muscles may contribute to dysarthria. Please refer to Table 8–7 for medications that may contribute to dysarthria.

TABLE 8–6	Select Medications That Affect Cognitive Speed and Language Processing

Medication Class	Example Medications	Cognitive Domains
Antihistamines	Diphenhydramine (Benadryl), cetirizine (Zyrtec)	Attention
Anticonvulsants	Topiramate (Topamax)	Working memory, word finding, attention
Benzodiazepines	Alprazolam (Xanax), diazepam (Valium)	Working memory, long-term memory, aphasia

TABLE 8–7	Select Medications That Cause Dysarthria

Medication Class	Example Medications	Mechanism of Dysarthria
Antimanic agent	Lithium carbonate	Intracellular accumulation of lithium interferes with the propagation of action potentials
Antipsychotics, including atypical (second-generation)	Haloperidol (Haldol), quetiapine (Seroquel), olanzapine (Zyprexa)	Laryngeal dystonia
Benzodiazepines	Alprazolam (Xanax), diazepam (Valium)	Oversedation
Antidepressants: Tricyclics	Amitriptyline	Dyskinesis
Botulinum toxin	Botulinum toxin A (Botox)	Paralysis of affected muscles

Medications That Affect Voice Production

Dysphonia affects nearly one in three persons at some point in their lives. It is characterized by alterations in vocal quality, pitch, loudness, or effort that hinder communication. Although there can be numerous, non-medication-induced causes for dysphonia, which the SLP is most likely to be familiar with, medications can contribute to dysphonia (Stachler et al., 2018). Several medication classes are implicated in dysphonia; however, inhaled corticosteroids, which are utilized as first-line treatments for asthma and chronic obstructive pulmonary disease, may cause hoarseness in up to 58% of patients (Galvan & Guarderas, 2012). Table 8–8

TABLE 8–8	Select Medications That May Cause Dysphonia	
Medication Class	**Example Medications**	**Mechanism of Impact on Voice**
Angiotensin-converting enzyme inhibitors	Lisinopril, enalapril, benazepril	Cough
Antihistamines, diuretics, anticholinergics	Diphenhydramine (Benadryl), furosemide (Lasix), oxybutynin (Ditropan)	Drying effect on mucosa (usually dose-dependent)
Antipsychotics, including atypical (second-generation)	Haloperidol (Haldol), quetiapine (Seroquel), olanzapine (Zyprexa)	Laryngeal dystonia; vocal cord paresis and paralysis
Bisphosphonates	Alendronate (Fosamax), risedronate (Actonel)	Chemical laryngitis
Androgenic agents	Danazol (Danocrine), testosterone	Sex hormone production/ utilization alteration
Inhaled corticosteroids	Fluticasone (Flovent), budesonide (Pulmicort), momestasone (Asmanex Twisthaler)	Dose-dependent mucosal irritation, candidal or fungal laryngitis
Anticoagulants, phosphodiesterase-5 inhibitor	Warfarin (Coumadin), rivaroxaban (Xarelto), sildenafil (Viagra)	Vocal fold hematoma
Vinca alkaloids	Vinblastine, vincristine	Vocal cord paresis and paralysis

Source: Adapted from "Clinical Practice Guideline: Hoarseness (Dysphonia) (Update), by R. J. Stachler, D. O. Francis, S. R. Schwartz, C. C. Damask, G. P. Digoy, H. J. Krouse, . . . L. C. Nnacheta, 2018, *Otolaryngology–Head and Neck Surgery, 158*(1 Suppl.), pp. S1–S42.

contains select medication classes that are known to contribute to dysphonia.

Medications That Affect Esophageal Mechanics

Medications can contribute to dysphagia, or difficulty swallowing, through several mechanisms. Among them are direct mucosal injury, those that contribute to esophagitis, those that relax the lower esophageal sphincter tone, and those that cause inhibition or excitation of smooth muscle tone (Table 8–9). Alterations in saliva quantity or quality can also affect the food bolus and lead to dysphagia (Tutuian, 2010).

Medications with large tablet size or low pH (<3) are more likely to cause direct injury to the mucosa of the esophagus due to mechanical or chemical injuries. Medications well-known for esophageal mucosa injury include bisphosphonates, such as alendronate (Fosamax), ferrous sulfate, and immediate release forms of potassium chloride (Stochus & Allescher, 1993). Although some patients with preexisting dysphagia who are unable to swallow large tablets or capsules may need to crush tablets or open capsules, it is important to consult a reputable source of drug information before manipulating any dosage forms since doing so may

TABLE 8–9	Select Medications That May Reduce Lower Esophageal Sphincter Tone	
Medication Class	**Example Medications**	**Mechanism of Impact on Esophageal Motility**
Anticholinergics	Diphenhydramine (Benadryl), oxybutynin (Ditropan)	Inhibition of neurotransmission by acetylcholine
Tricyclic antidepressants	Amitriptyline, imipramine, nortriptyline	Inhibition of neurotransmission by acetylcholine
Nitrates	Nitroglycerine, isosorbide dinitrate, isosorbide mononitrate (Imdur)	Relaxation of smooth muscle by nitric oxide (NO)
Phosphodiesterase-5 enzyme inhibitors	Sildenafil (Viagra), tadalafil (Cialis), vardenafil (Levitra)	Relaxation of smooth muscle by inhibition of breakdown of NO via cGMP

Source: Adapted from "Drug-Induced Dysphagia," by B. Stochus and H. -D. Allescher, 1993, *Dysphagia, 8,* pp. 154–159.

remove important safety mechanisms against ulceration. Please refer to the section on drug information later in this chapter.

Other medications may contribute to dysphagia by altering the conduction of nerve signaling to the esophageal musculature (Table 8–10). Although the specifics of the innervation and musculature of the esophagus are beyond the scope of this chapter, the main neurotransmitters involved in swallowing include acetylcholine and nitric oxide (NO). Medications that affect levels of acetylcholine and NO may result in swallowing difficulties. Primary among these are medications with anticholinergic properties, which impair neurotransmission via cholinergic and muscarinic neurons. Medications with anticholinergic effects include antihistamines, antidepressants, antipsychotics, and agents used for urinary incontinence. Medications that act on the NO pathway relax smooth muscles. They are primarily used to treat angina (cardiac nitrates) as well as erectile dysfunction and pulmonary artery hypertension

TABLE 8–10   Select Medications That May Affect Esophageal Motility

Medication Class	Example Medications	Mechanism of Impact on Esophageal Motility
Anticholinergics	Diphenhydramine (Benadryl), oxybutynin (Ditropan)	Inhibition of neurotransmission by acetylcholine
Tricyclic antidepressants	Amitriptyline, imipramine, nortriptyline	Inhibition of neurotransmission by acetylcholine
Nitrates	Nitroglycerine, isosorbide dinitrate, isosorbide mononitrate (Imdur)	Relaxation of smooth muscle by nitric oxide (NO)
Phosphodiesterase-5 enzyme inhibitors	Sildenafil (Viagra), tadalafil (Cialis), vardenafil (Levitra)	Relaxation of smooth muscle by inhibition of breakdown of NO via cGMP
Cholinergic agonists	Atropine, pilocarpine	Enhancement of neurotransmission by acetylcholine

Source: Adapted from Wolff, A., Joshi, R. K., Ekström, J., Aframian, D., Pedersen, A. M. L., Proctor, G., Narayana, N., et al. (2016). A Guide to Medications Inducing Salivary Gland Dysfunction, Xerostomia, and Subjective Sialorrhea: A Systematic Review Sponsored by the World Workshop on Oral Medicine VI. *Drugs in R&Amp;D, 17*(1), 1–28. https://doi.org/10.1007/s40268-016-0153-9

(phosphodiesterase-5 enzyme inhibitors). Other medications may cause dysphagia by enhancing neurotransmission by excessive cholinergic action. Direct cholinergic agents are primarily used topically for ophthalmic indications but may be used systemically to treat xerostomia in the case of pilocarpine or bradycardia for atropine.

Medications That Affect Salivation

Dry mouth is a commonly encountered problem in clinical practice. It can be separated into the subjective feeling of dry mouth (xerostomia) and the objective finding of decreased salivary production. Xerostomia and hyposalivation are often related, but patients with normal salivation rates can complain of xerostomia, and those with low salivation do not always experience xerostomia. Medication-induced dry mouth has multiple consequences, including dental caries, candidiasis, halitosis, as well as difficulties in chewing, speaking, and swallowing. Although the subjective feeling of dry mouth (xerostomia) is bothersome, hyposalivation drives the poor health outcomes associated with dry mouth (Wolff et al., 2017). Although dry mouth can be multifactorial, with age, medical conditions, and medication-related causes, this section focuses on medication-related causes of dry mouth. Table 8–11 contains medications that can contribute to dry mouth.

Modifications to Medication Dosage Forms

Although medication administration is not within the typical scope of practice of an SLP, a general familiarity of the principles governing the choice of medications and adverse effects of enteral administration are good to know. Patients may have need for alterations and/or modifications of medications to enable them to be taken orally. Potential reasons for this may include administration of medications via an enteral feeding tube, crushing medications for administration on top of food or in a beverage, or even changing the dosage form from a capsule or tablet to a liquid or sublingual tablet. Medications may also be converted from an enteral dosage form to a parenteral dosage form such as a patch or an injectable. Crushing oral tablets has the potential to alter the integrity and function of the medication. Crushing tablets or opening capsules prior to administration can increase or decrease serum concentrations substantially from reference ranges. Generally, medications that are extended or sustained release, film or enteric coated, or have the potential to irritate or ulcerate tissue should not be

Medication Class	Common Therapeutic Use/ Mechanism of Action	Medications
Antispasmodics	Treatment of gastrointestinal spasms	Atropine (non-ophthalmic), scopolamine (non-ophthalmic), belladonna alkaloids
Centrally acting anti-obesity products	Weight loss	Phenteramine (Adipex)
Alpha-2 agonist	Hypertension, attention deficity hyperactivity disorder (ADHD)	Clonidine (Catapres)
Calcium channel blockers	Hypertension, arrhythmias	Diltiazem (Cardizem)
Antimuscarinics	Urinary incontinence	Oxybutynin (Ditropan), tolterodine (Detrol), solifenacin (Vesicare)
Skeletal muscle relaxants, centrally acting	Muscle spasms	Baclofen, tinazidine (Zanaflex), cyclobenzaprine (Flexeril)
Bisphosphonates	Osteoporosis treatment	Alendronate (Fosamax)
Anti-epileptics	Prevention of seizures; analgesia	Gabapentin (Neurontin)
Analgesics	Pain relief	Buprenorphine (Subutex), butorphanol (Stadol)
Dopamine	Treatment of Parkinson's disease	Rotigotine (Neupro)
Antimanic agent	Treatment of bipolar disorder	Lithium carbonate
Antipsychotics	Treatment of psychosis, schizophrenia	Chlorpromazine, perphenazine, ziprasidone (Geodon), clozapine (Clozaril), olanzapine (Zyprexa), quetiapine (Seroquel), risperidone (Risperdal), paliperidone (Invega), aripiprazole (Abilify)
Sedative—hypnotics	Induction of sleep through agonism of benzodiazepine receptor	Zolpidem (Ambien)
Antidepressants—tricyclics	Treatment of depression	Imipramine, amitriptyline, nortriptyline
Antidepressants—selective serotonin reuptake inhibitors	Treatment of depression	Fluoxetine (Prozac), citalopram (Celexa), paroxetine (Paxil), sertraline (Zoloft), escitalopram (Lexapro)

TABLE 8–11 *continued*		
Medication Class	**Common Therapeutic Use/ Mechanism of Action**	**Medications**
Antidepressants— selective norepinephrine reuptake inhibitor	Treatment of depression	Venlafaxine (Effexor), duloxetine (Cymbalta)
Centrally acting sympathomimetics	Simulants used for ADHD, narcolepsy	Methylphenidate (Concerta, Ritalin), dexmethylphenidate (Focalin), lisdexamfetamine (Vyvanse)
Inhaled anticholinergics	Reduces respiratory secretions in asthma and chronic obstructive pulmonary disease	Tiotroprium (Spiriva), aclindinium (Tudorza)

Source: Adapted from "A Guide to Medications Inducing Salivary Gland Dysfunction, Xerostomia, and Subjective Sialorrhea: A Systematic Review Sponsored by the World Workshop on Oral Medicine VI," by A. Wolff, R. Kumar Joshi, J. Ekström, D. Aframian, A. M. L. Pedersen, G. Proctor, . . . C. Dawes, 2017, *Drugs in R&D, 17*(1), pp. 1–28.

crushed. Medications that pose environmental or health hazards to those preparing them, such as chemotherapeutic or teratogenic agents, should never be crushed.

Many oral medications can be administered via enteral feeding tubes in modified dosage forms. The stomach is the preferred site of administration for most enteral medications. Gastric feeding tubes are generally larger in diameter than jejunal tubes and are less prone to obstruction. When available, commercially prepared or compounded liquid formulations of medications are preferred for enteral feeding tube administration since they usually have fewer excipients (inert ingredients) and binders than tablets or capsules, which are crushed and dissolved prior to administration. Those excipients and binders may contribute to the obstruction of enteral tubes. However, liquid medications are often more expensive than comparable tablets or capsules and have limited availability. Many have artificial sweeteners added to increase palatability. Sorbitol in particular is associated with diarrhea when given in large doses.

Sometimes medications are opened, cut, or crushed for administration on top of or mixed with a soft food such as yogurt, pudding, or applesauce. Others are dissolved for administration into a beverage. When reviewing information regarding medication co-administration with food, the pH of the intended food or beverage should be accounted for. Acidic foods, like applesauce, can accelerate the dissolution of enteric coatings of certain medications.

Other medications should be administered with acidic foods. Some enteric coatings are readily visible along the outside of a tablet, while others coating smaller particles inside of tablets or capsules may not be. All medications that are extemporaneously prepared for enteral administration should be administered immediately after crushing or dissolving.

Sources of Drug Information

Consulting a reliable drug information source is key to making recommendations regarding choice of pharmacotherapy, available dosage forms, or modification of dosage forms. Although the internet provides a readily available source of information, it can be difficult to verify the accuracy of medical information retrieved from there. Subscription databases, such as Lexi-Comp, Micromedex, and Facts and Comparisons, offer extensive, professional-level drug information; however, they may be cost-prohibitive for practitioners without institutional access. High-quality, online, open-access drug-information resources include Epocrates (https://www.epocrates.com) and Medscape (https://www.medscape.com). These contain information on medication indications, dosing, administration, and drug–drug interactions appropriate for the practice of an SLP. Both Epocrates and Medscape have free mobile smartphone apps. The Institute for Safe Medication Practices maintains a periodically updated list of medications that should not be crushed due to their special pharmaceutical properties. This list is freely available online (Institute for Safe Medication Practices, 2020). Individual medication package inserts are also required to have administration recommendations. Package inserts can be found on the FDA's website (National Library of Medicine, 2022). Additionally, manufacturers are often able to provide unpublished information regarding administration data through their medication information services. Not all medications with the same active ingredient are therapeutically interchangeable. The interchangeability of brands and generic forms of medications is found in the FDA's Orange Book (FDA, 2022b).

Conclusions

As members of the interprofessional health care team, SLPs play an essential role in ensuring that patients are able to take medications safely through assessing swallowing and cognitive functions as well as by alerting other members of the patient care team to potential medication-related side effects.

References

American Geriatrics Society Beers Criteria Update Expert Panel. (2019). Updated AGS Beers Criteria for potentially inappropriate medication use in older adults. *Journal of the American Geriatrics Society, 67*(4), 674–694. https://doi.org/10.1111/jgs.15767

Galvan, C. A., & Guarderas, J. C. (2012). Practical considerations for dysphonia caused by inhaled corticosteroids. *Mayo Clinic Proceedings, 87*(9), 901–904.

Institute for Safe Medication Practices. (2020). *Oral dosage forms that should not be crushed.* https://www.ismp.org/recommendations/do-not-crush

Migirov, A., & Datta, A. R. (2021). Physiology, anticholinergic reaction. In *StatPearls* [Internet]. StatPearls Publishing.

Mula, M., Trimble, M. R., Thompson, P., & Sander, J. (2003). Topiramate and word-finding difficulties in patients with epilepsy. *Neurology, 60*(7), 1104–1107.

National Library of Medicine. (2022). *DailyMed.* https://dailymed.nlm.nih.gov/dailymed/index.cfm

Stachler, R. J., Francis, D. O., Schwartz, S. R., Damask, C. C., Digoy, G. P., Krouse, H. J., . . . Nnacheta, L. C. (2018). Clinical practice guideline: Hoarseness (dysphonia) (Update). *Otolaryngology–Head and Neck Surgery, 158*(1 Suppl.), S1–S42. https://doi.org/10.1177/01945998 17751030

Stochus, B., & Allescher, H.-D. (1993). Drug-induced dysphagia. *Dysphagia, 8,* 154–159.

Tutuian, R. (2010). Adverse effects of drugs on the esophagus. *Best Practice & Research Clinical Gastroenterology, 24,* 91–97.

U.S. Food and Drug Administration. (2017). *The FDA's drug review process: Ensuring drugs are safe and effective.* https://www.fda.gov/drugs/information-consumers-and-patients-drugs/fdas-drug-review-process-ensuring-drugs-are-safe-and-effective

U.S. Food and Drug Administration. (2022a). *MedWatch: The FDA safety information and adverse event reporting program.* https://www.fda.gov/safety/medwatch-fda-safety-information-and-adverse-event-reporting-program

U.S. Food and Drug Administration. (2022b). *Orange book: Approved drug products with therapeutic equivalence evaluations.* https://www.accessdata.fda.gov/scripts/cder/ob/index.cfm

Wolff, A., Kumar Joshi, R., Ekström, J., Aframian, D., Pedersen, A. M. L., Proctor, G., . . . Dawes, C. (2017). A guide to medications inducing salivary gland dysfunction, xerostomia, and subjective sialorrhea: A systematic review sponsored by the World Workshop on Oral Medicine VI. *Drugs in R&D, 17*(1), 1–28. https://doi.org/10.1007/s40 268-016-0153-9

World Health Organization. Quality Assurance and Safety of Medicines Team. (2002). *Safety of medicines: A guide to detecting and reporting adverse drug reactions: Why health professionals need to take action.* https://apps.who.int/iris/handle/10665/67378

CHAPTER
9

Care
Transitions

Clinical
Reasoning

Clinical
Practice
Settings

Neuroimaging

harmacology

Neuroimaging for Speech-Language Pathologists

Erin L. Meier and Jeffrey P. Johnson

Chapter Objectives

Upon completion of this chapter, readers should be able to:

- Describe basic technical and scientific properties underlying a variety of neuroimaging modalities.

- Describe clinical and research applications of neuroimaging tools with relevance to medical speech-language pathology.

- Appreciate and identify differences between various neuro-imaging techniques, including their relative strengths, weaknesses, and risks.

Chapter Overview

The goal of this chapter is to provide a survey of the neuroimaging modalities with which speech-language pathologists (SLPs) should be familiar, either because of their use in clinical care for patients with neurogenic communication or swallowing disorders or because of their increasing popularity as research tools in the communication sciences and disorders.

Introduction

Neuroimaging refers to the process of producing images (i.e., pictures or other graphical representations) of the physical structure or function of the brain and broader nervous system. These images are used to identify, diagnose, and monitor strokes, tumors, neurodegenerative conditions, and other abnormalities and illnesses involving the nervous system. Neuroimaging is also extensively utilized in research and has been critical to recent advances in our understanding of the neural bases of motor and cognitive functions. Before the development and widespread implementation of computed tomography (CT), positron emission tomography (PET), magnetic resonance imaging (MRI), and other tools described in this chapter, brain structure was studied via postmortem dissection. Similarly, relationships between brain structure and function were investigated via careful observation and documentation of behavioral changes in individuals with neurologic damage or disease, sometimes in conjunction with postmortem dissection of the same individuals' brains. These approaches yielded remarkable insights into brain–behavior relationships and led to foundational theories of cognitive processing, lateralization and localization of functions in the brain, and the nature of neural insult, recovery, and rehabilitation. Of course, these methods, which are still widely employed today, have certain limitations, chief among them being that they do not provide direct or indirect measures of neuroanatomy or physiology in living subjects.

However, thanks to critical advances in medical imaging technology over the past several decades, clinicians and researchers can now examine and analyze the nervous system in vivo. For instance,

CT and MRI are routinely used to obtain high-definition two-dimensional images or virtual three-dimensional models of the brain in living people in a matter of hours or even minutes. Additionally, *functional* neuroimaging techniques like electroencephalography (EEG), functional MRI (fMRI), and PET make it possible to measure the brain's response to different types of stimuli in real time, as indicated by changes in electrical signals, blood oxygenation levels, and other markers.

Why Does Neuroimaging Matter to the Speech-Language Pathologist?

While most SLPs are rarely, if ever, directly involved in obtaining or producing neuroimages themselves, there are several important reasons for the SLP to be familiar with commonly used imaging tools and techniques. These include, but are not limited to, the following:

- **SLPs working in medical settings often have access to patients' images and/or imaging reports.** These materials can be an excellent source of information regarding the nature, locus, severity, and/or progression of neurologic disease or insult, which can be helpful when formulating an assessment plan and communicating with a patient and/or their family or caregiver. Additionally, there is emerging evidence that certain neurophysiologic measures obtained from neuroimaging may help predict rehabilitation outcomes in disorders like aphasia; thus, it is likely that neuroimaging data will have a direct impact on clinical prognostics and treatment planning in the future.

- **SLPs are essential members of the larger health care team in medical settings, including acute and subacute hospital units, inpatient and outpatient rehabilitation centers, and long-term care or skilled nursing facilities.** With a working knowledge of neuroimaging techniques and related issues, SLPs can more effectively and efficiently communicate with colleagues from other disciplines and contribute during interdisciplinary patient care meetings.

- **SLPs are viewed as trusted sources of information by patients and their families.** Additionally, in light of limitations on third-party coverage for rehabilitation services, it is not uncommon for SLPs in medical settings to suggest that their patients participate in clinical research studies, which may well involve neuroimaging. As such, SLPs may be asked to clarify or explain the results of a patient's neuroimaging tests or provide an overview of the procedures involved in potential research opportunities, not to mention findings from neuroimaging-based studies that appear in popular media.

■ **As noted previously, neuroimaging is widely used in research on speech, language, hearing, and swallowing in adults and children (Figure 9–1), and these applications are not limited to traditional health care settings.** For example, neuroimaging tools are used to investigate specific language impairment, stuttering, dyslexia, autism spectrum disorder, and other developmental conditions typically managed in school-based settings. Thus, familiarity with neuroimaging techniques will prepare SLPs to consume, interpret, and incorporate relevant literature into their own practice, no matter the setting in which they work.

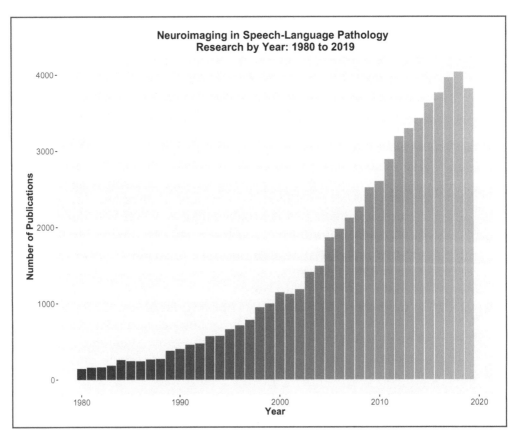

FIGURE 9–1. Neuroimaging-based research in the speech, language, hearing, and swallowing sciences from 1980 to 2019. Bars reflect the number of publications per year based on a *PubMed* search for the terms *speech, language, hearing,* or *swallowing* and either *neuroimaging* or *imaging.*

In summary, clinical SLPs working in medical settings should have at least a basic understanding of neuroimaging tools and their capabilities to provide high-quality, evidence-based assessment, treatment, and education services to patients and their families or caregivers. Furthermore, SLPs who work in *any* setting are likely to benefit from this information, as it will make them more skilled consumers of the literature in whichever area(s) of the field they practice.

Key Concepts

Before we delve into the specific tools and techniques that are commonly used to produce images of the brain and nervous system, it is important to first address several key concepts that will support readers' understanding of the capabilities of and differences between various imaging modalities, as well as their appreciation for the sample images presented in subsequent sections.

Structural Versus Functional Neuroimaging

First and foremost, neuroimaging techniques can be broadly classified as either **structural** or **functional** methods, depending on the type of information they provide (Table 9–1). Structural neuroimaging is, unsurprisingly, concerned with the physical structure (i.e., the anatomy) of the nervous system, especially the brain; thus, it is commonly used to examine the integrity of the brain and diagnose tumors, stroke, and other pathologic conditions affecting brain structure. In contrast, functional neuroimaging measures and depicts the timing, magnitude, and/or location of metabolic processes in the brain, as indicated by electrical impulses, blood flow and oxygenation levels, and other signals, depending on the imaging modality employed. As such, functional methods can be used to diagnose metabolic illnesses or plan surgery for patients with tumors or epilepsy by identifying areas of functionally critical brain tissue based on their involvement in cognitive-linguistic or memory tasks.

Whereas structural neuroimaging methods generate "pictures" of neuroanatomic structures, images produced via functional methods are actually graphical depictions of measured activity that can be represented as graphs, waveforms, colorful "blobs," or other formats. In some cases, such depictions of brain function may be overlaid on structural images to demonstrate the relationship between the measured activity and its approximate site of origin.

	Imaging Type		
TABLE 9–1	Overview of Neuroimaging and Brain-Mapping Modalities Addressed in This Chapter		

Modality	Structural	Functional	Current Uses
Computed tomography (CT)	✓		Routinely used in clinical diagnostic workups in hospital settings; still used in research although currently less so than structural MRI
Magnetic resonance imaging (MRI)	✓	✓	Certain sequences routinely used in clinical diagnostic workups in hospital settings; widely used in basic and clinical research
Single-photon emission computed tomography (SPECT)		✓	Used in follow-up diagnostic workups in hospital settings for certain conditions; used in basic and clinical research
Positron emission tomography (PET)		✓	Used in follow-up diagnostic workups in hospital settings for certain conditions; used in basic and clinical research
Electroencephalogram (EEG)		✓	Primarily used in basic and clinical research with a few clinical applications
Magnetoencephalography (MEG)		✓	Almost exclusively used in research
Functional near-infrared spectroscopy (fNIRS)		✓	Almost exclusively used in research
Wada test		✓*	Primarily used in surgical planning for seizure disorders
Electrical stimulation mapping (ESM)		✓*	Primarily used in surgical planning for seizure disorders; some use in basic science and clinical research
Electrocorticography (ECoG)		✓	Primarily used in surgical planning for seizure disorders; some use in basic science and clinical research
Transcranial magnetic stimulation (TMS)		✓*	Primarily used in surgical planning for seizure disorders; used in basic science and clinical research

Note: *These techniques are used to modulate brain function in order to measure how those manipulations affect cognitive or linguistic functions. Unlike other functional neuroimaging modalities, the instruments used for these procedures do not, in and of themselves, measure metabolic processes in the brain.

It bears mentioning that some of the tools described in this chapter are strictly used to obtain *either* structural or functional images, while others can be used to obtain both. For example, EEG equipment is used solely for functional neuroimaging, whereas an MRI scanner can be used for either structural or functional neuroimaging, depending on the settings selected by the operator.

Clinical Versus Research Applications of Neuroimaging

At the time of this writing, only some of the tools described in this chapter are used for standard clinical care among patient populations to whom SLPs are likely to provide services (see Table 9–1). Recently developed and more complex structural neuroimaging methods, such as diffusion tensor imaging (DTI), and many if not all functional neuroimaging methods (e.g., fMRI, EEG, transcranial magnetic stimulation [TMS], and functional near-infrared spectroscopy [fNIRS]) are *primarily*, if not exclusively, used for research. In the sections that follow, both clinical and research applications of neuroimaging modalities are discussed.

Image Orientation and Anatomic Planes

It is important to be familiar with the various orientations in which neuroimages are typically displayed and the anatomic planes along which they may be divided. With respect to orientation of the cerebrum, images are usually portrayed from one of the following perspectives: **anterior/rostral** (i.e., looking at the front); **posterior/caudal** (i.e., looking at the back); **superior/dorsal** (i.e., looking down from above); **inferior/ventral** (i.e., looking up from below); and **lateral** (i.e., looking at either the left side or right side) (Figure 9–2).

Neuroimages are also commonly viewed as "slices" along one of three anatomic planes: the **axial** or **transverse plane** runs horizontally and splits the image into superior and inferior sections; the **coronal plane** runs vertically from ear to ear and splits the image into anterior and posterior sections; and the **sagittal plane** runs vertically from front to back (i.e., from the nose to the back of the head) and splits the image into left and right sections (Figure 9–3).

Finally, images may be displayed according to **radiologic convention**, wherein the left side of the brain is shown on the right side of the image, and vice versa, or **neurologic convention**, in which the left side of the brain corresponds to the left side of the image, and vice versa. Note that most images in this chapter are presented in neurologic convention, and any exceptions are indicated in the figure captions.

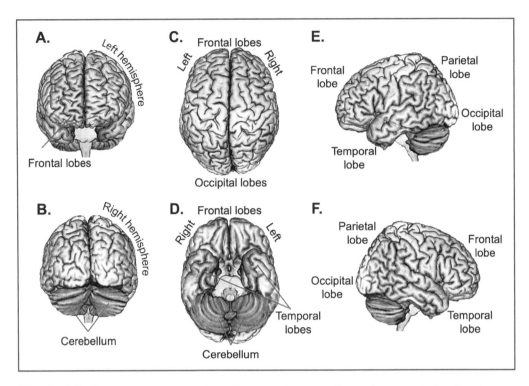

FIGURE 9–2. Standard orientations for neuroimages. Several anatomic landmarks are indicated to clarify the orientation of each figure. Anterior/rostral (**A**) and posterior/caudal (**B**) views depict the front and back of the brain, respectively; superior/dorsal (**C**) and inferior/ventral (**D**) views depict the top and bottom of the brain, respectively; lateral left (**E**) and lateral right (**F**) views depict the two hemispheres of the brain when viewed from either side. Note that in **A** and **D**, the left hemisphere appears on the right side of the figure and vice versa.

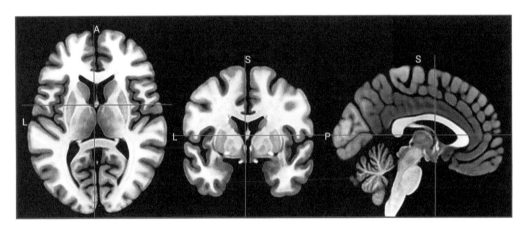

FIGURE 9–3. Standard neuroimaging planes. Neuroimaging software can be used to visualize different orientations of two-dimensional slices through the brain, including axial (*left*), coronal (*middle*), and sagittal (*right*) views. The red crosshairs pinpoint the same location in the brain in the three views. A = anterior (the front of the cerebrum), P = posterior (the back of the cerebrum), S = superior (the top of the cerebrum), and L = left hemisphere of the cerebrum.

Contrast

In neuroimaging, the term **contrast** most generally refers to differences in the magnitude of whatever property is measured in order to generate an image at various locations throughout the image itself. For example, some neuroimages are created by quantifying the extent to which x-rays either pass through or are absorbed (i.e., attenuated) by different types of tissues, as in CT. If an imaging modality can detect small variations in the property of interest (e.g., x-ray attenuation), those differences will be apparent in the resulting image, and the modality and/or image may be described as having "good" or "high" contrast. On the other hand, if a modality can only detect and depict drastic differences in the measured property, it can be described as having "low" contrast, and the resulting image would likely be less informative or appear less detailed than its high-contrast counterpart. In short, the better (or higher) the contrast of the modality, the clearer the images will be in terms of the distinction between tissues that vary on the property of interest.

Box 9–1 describes an alternative application of the term *contrast*, which is specifically used in the context of task-based functional neuroimaging methods that aim to identify the neural substrates of various behavioral processes.

Box 9–1. Cognitive Subtraction in Task-Based Imaging

As indicated in the main text, the term *contrast* can be used in different ways in neuroimaging. For task-based functional activation studies using fMRI, EEG, magnetoencephalography (MEG), or functional near-infrared spectroscopy (fNIRS), *contrast* refers to comparisons of brain activity for two different experimental conditions. Imagine that a researcher is interested in determining the areas of the brain that are activated when an individual makes decisions about semantic features of an item, a core aspect of semantic feature analysis treatment for aphasia (Boyle, 2010; Gilmore et al., 2020). One type of imaging experiment to assess this ability is a task in which a participant is shown a picture of an object (e.g., broccoli) and must determine via a yes/no button press whether a written semantic feature (e.g., *Is eaten*) applies to that item (Figure 9–4). In addition to semantic processing, this task involves other processes that are not of interest to the researcher (e.g.,

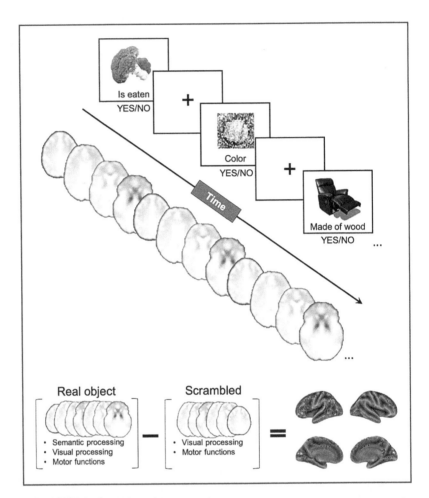

FIGURE 9–4. Experimental design utilizing cognitive subtraction. At top, experimental (i.e., real object) and control (i.e., scrambled object) trials from a semantic feature judgment fMRI task are shown. The fixation cross symbol denotes the interstimulus interval between trials. Over the course of the experiment, many brain volumes, which reflect the Blood-Oxygen-Level-Dependent fMRI signal, are collected. At bottom, a visualization of the subtraction (i.e., *contrast*) paradigm is provided, in which the scrambled trial signals are subtracted from the real object trial signals, yielding the fMRI activation map on the bottom right. Author-created image constructed using data from NIH/NIDCD P50DC012283 (Subproject PI: Swathi Kiran).

visual perception of the object, motor planning and execution for the button press). Therefore, the researcher designs a second task that engages these processes (i.e., a control condition), such as making judgments about the color of a scrambled, pixelated object. To isolate the semantic processes of interest, the researcher subtracts averaged activation from all control condition trials (i.e., the scrambled object condition) from all experimental trials (i.e., the real object condition). This is an example of **cognitive subtraction** that researchers use when designing task-based functional imaging experiments to study the neural correlates of specific sensorimotor, cognitive, or linguistic processes.

Spatial and Temporal Resolution

Spatial and temporal resolution are two additional concepts with which readers should be familiar to appreciate the contributions of and differences between various neuroimaging methods. A modality's *spatial resolution* refers to its capacity to discern between different locations in an image—you might think of it as how much a given modality can "zoom in" on the structures being imaged. A modality or technique with high spatial resolution can zoom in more than one with low spatial resolution and, therefore, produces more detailed images. Spatial resolution relates to the size of the sampling units used when an image is obtained; in two-dimensional images, these sampling units are called *pixels* (the name is derived from "picture elements"), and in three-dimensional (i.e., cross-sectional) images, they are called *voxels* (derived from "volume elements"). In general, the smaller the pixel or voxel size, the greater is the spatial resolution. Together with its contrast (described earlier), a modality's spatial resolution dictates how precisely distinct structures can be identified and differentiated from one another in an image.

Temporal resolution refers to the speed with which an imaging modality can detect a change in signal over time; more simply put, it describes a method's precision in determining *when* activity occurred or changed in the brain. As such, it is really only relevant to functional neuroimaging methods, which readers may recall are concerned with monitoring changes over time in metabolic activity. Temporal resolution depends on the sampling rate of the modality (i.e., how rapidly images can be acquired); as the sampling rate increases, so, too, does temporal resolution.

Neuroimaging methods differ in their spatial and temporal resolution, such that some are optimal for measuring the location of brain activity (e.g., PET) or the speed of brain activity (e.g., EEG), but not vice versa. Other modalities (e.g., fMRI) strike something of a balance between the two and have fairly good spatial *and* temporal resolution.

Neuroimaging Modalities

In this section, we provide an overview of the most common neuro-imaging modalities used in clinical practice and research. The following subsections describe the basic science, equipment, and processes involved in generating neuroimages for each modality, as well as their various advantages, disadvantages, and risks. Specific applications of each modality to disorders relevant to the medical SLP are described in a subsequent section (Clinical Applications of Neuroimaging Modalities).

Computed Tomography

Initially introduced in the 1970s, CT, also called computed axial tomography (CAT), rapidly became a widely accessible and commonly utilized imaging modality for assessing acute and chronic conditions. CT scanners essentially collect a series of x-ray images that are combined by a computer to produce a cross-sectional image (i.e., "slice") or a three-dimensional volume-based rendering (i.e., a computer-based model) of an organ or body part. In fact, the term *tomography* (or *tomographic imaging*) is not strictly limited to CT and refers to the procedure of building a single cohesive image from a series of sections or component images of an object, such as the brain.

During a CT scan, the patient lies on a table in the center of the scanner (Figure 9–5). X-rays (i.e., beams of ionizing radiation) are emitted from the x-ray tube, a component on one side of the scanner. The x-rays pass through the part of the patient's body under investigation and are received by specialized x-ray detectors on the other side. The scanner gantry (i.e., the part that surrounds the patient) rotates, and the process is repeated from multiple different angles. Modern scanners are designed to support helical (or spiral) scanning, in which the table holding the patient moves continuously through the center of the gantry while the x-ray tube and/or detectors rotate around the patient. An important benefit of helical scanning is that it can be completed rapidly, limiting potential discomfort and radiation exposure for the patient.

The fundamental concept underlying CT is *x-ray attenuation*, or the absorption/weakening of x-rays as they pass through the human body. The extent to which x-rays are attenuated varies depending on tissue density, so the strength of x-rays arriving at the detectors conveys information about the density of the intervening tissue. Dense tissue, such as bone, has relatively high attenuation and appears bright or white on the CT image; less

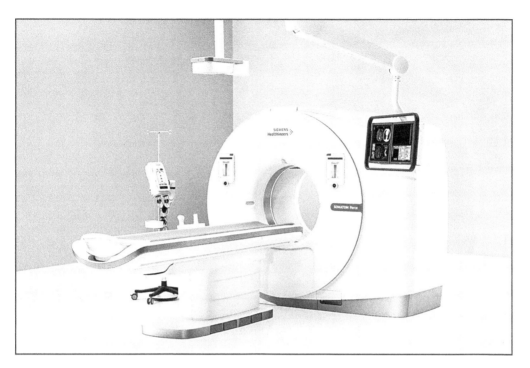

FIGURE 9–5. CT scanner. Courtesy of Siemens Medical Solutions USA, Inc.

dense material, like fat or cerebrospinal fluid, has lower attenuation and appears darker (Figure 9–6A). Abnormalities detected by CT can be either *hypodense* (i.e., less dense and, thus, darker than expected relative to the surrounding tissue) or *hyperdense* (i.e., denser and, thus, brighter than expected). A computer linked to the scanner receives information about the extent of x-ray attenuation at various locations in the body and combines it into a slice-by-slice reconstruction (i.e., image/rendering) of the scanned tissue, known as a *tomogram*.

In some cases, it is desirable to increase the contrast between tissue types to aid in differentiating structures or identifying pathologic formations on CT images. This can be achieved by administering a **contrast agent** to the patient. For brain scans, contrast agents are administered intravenously. Contrast agents have high x-ray attenuation properties and, therefore, appear white on the resulting images.

Computed Tomography Angiography

CT scanners can be used to visualize the cerebrovascular system via a technique called CT angiography (CTA), in which CT images are obtained while an intravenously administered contrast agent flows through the blood vessels that supply the brain with blood.

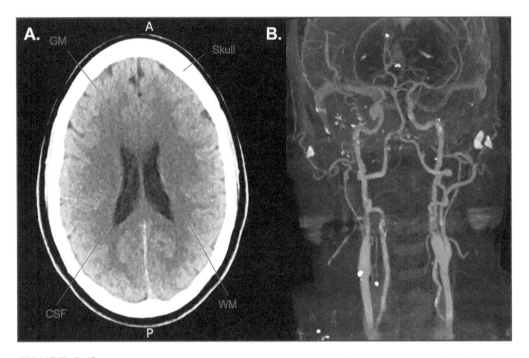

FIGURE 9–6. A. Axial slice of the brain, taken with a CT machine. Note that the skull appears bright white, the cerebrospinal fluid (CSF) appears dark, and the gray matter (GM) and white matter (WM) are different shades of gray due to differences in their density and attenuation properties. A = anterior, P = posterior. **B.** An example of CTA of the head/neck. The major blood vessels are clearly delineated due to administration of an intravenous contrast agent. Author-created image constructed using data from NIH/NIDCD R01DC005375, R01DC015466, and P50DC014664 (PI: Argye E. Hillis).

Unlike standard noncontrast CT, which is used to generate images of the brain, CTA produces images of the vasculature. Major blood vessels appear brighter/lighter than the surrounding tissue, due to the presence and high attenuation properties of the contrast agent (Figure 9–6B).

CTA should not be confused with conventional cerebral angiography, a more invasive procedure for visualizing blood vessels of the head and neck. During conventional angiography, a catheter is inserted into an artery—often, the femoral artery in the groin—and guided via x-ray to the vascular territory of interest. A contrast agent is administered, and x-rays are collected to monitor the movement of the agent through the cerebral vasculature. Due to the nature of the procedure, traditional angiography carries a small but serious risk of stroke or other complications should the catheter damage or puncture a blood vessel or dislodge a plaque causing an embolism (i.e., blockage). Nevertheless, cerebral angiography is highly regarded for its diagnostic precision and is considered by some to be the gold standard for assessing the gross integrity of the cerebrovascular system (Harrigan & Deveikis, 2013; Haussen & Nogueira, 2017).

Computed Tomography Perfusion

CT perfusion (CTP) is another application of CT that employs a contrast agent. Unlike CTA, which reveals the gross structure of major arteries and blood vessels, CTP measures the movement of blood through the cerebral microvasculature and its uptake by brain tissue (i.e., perfusion). Thus, CTP images reflect which areas of the brain have an adequate supply of blood and which may be undersupplied (i.e., *hypoperfused*), based on x-ray attenuation associated with the movement of the contrast agent through capillaries in the brain. CTP scans are used to quantify *cerebral blood volume*, or the volume of blood in a given portion of brain tissue. Areas with abnormally low cerebral blood volume appear darker on CTP images, as there is less perfusion, and, therefore, less flow of the contrast agent, to those areas than the surrounding tissue. Other perfusion metrics that can be derived from CTP include *cerebral blood flow* (i.e., the volume of blood moving through a given quantity of tissue over time) and *mean transit time* (i.e., the average amount of time it takes blood to move through a given portion of tissue).

Benefits, Advantages, Risks, and Disadvantages of Computed Tomography

Several important features have contributed to the widespread clinical use of CT for neuroimaging. These include its greater affordability and availability as compared to MRI, as well as the capacity for rapid image acquisition. CT is fairly versatile, supporting both perfusion imaging and angiography, the latter of which is a less invasive and lower risk procedure than conventional angiography (Vagal et al., 2016). Despite these advantages, a notable limitation of CT is that it is less sensitive than MRI for detecting certain conditions, such as acute ischemic stroke (Harrigan & Deveikis, 2013; Kidwell & Hsia, 2006).

An important advantage of CT is that, unlike MRI, it is perfectly safe for individuals with ferromagnetic material (such as pacemakers and other medical devices or surgical plates or screws) implanted in their body. Thus, it is often the scan of first choice for individuals whose medical history and contraindications for MRI are unknown, particularly when time is a factor, as in an acute stroke. However, CT has its own safety risks, chief among them being ionizing radiation exposure, which may elevate one's risk of developing cancer (Center for Devices and Radiological Health, 2019), with greater risks for children or those who have repeated or prolonged exposure. Another risk of CT is an adverse response to intravenous contrast agents, including allergic reaction and kidney dysfunction (Almandoz et al., 2011). Importantly, the risks associated with CT are somewhat mitigated by safety precautions and the design and scanning capabilities of modern CT machines, and tend to be outweighed by the immediate health benefits of the procedure in terms of the information it provides.

Finally, it is worth noting that CT is not strictly limited to clinical applications. It is also used in research that aims to examine relationships between brain structure and behavior, as described in Box 9–2.

Single-Proton Emission Computed Tomography and Positron Emission Tomography

Single-photon emission computed tomography (SPECT) and PET are two imaging modalities that fall within the broader category of nuclear medicine imaging. Catapulted forward by important scientific discoveries in the 1950s, nuclear medicine imaging capitalizes on the physical properties of the nuclei of atoms and the fact that radiation events occur when atomic nuclei are bombarded with particles. Today, SPECT and PET are used to diagnose and monitor a variety of diseases, including health conditions with concomitant communication disorders.

The general steps and physics involved in SPECT and PET scanning are the same. First, the patient receives an intravenous injection of a **radionuclide**, often commonly referred to as a **radiotracer**. Radionuclides are elements that have an unstable arrangement of protons and neutrons within the nucleus. Critical to SPECT and PET imaging, unstable nuclei transition to a more stable state by emitting particles and/or photons (i.e., small bundles of electromagnetic radiation) via a process called **radioactive decay**. SPECT is performed with radionuclides that decay by emitting photons of gamma rays, whereas PET is performed with radionuclides that decay by emitting a **positron** (i.e., a particle with the same mass as an electron but positively charged).

The way SPECT and PET work and the hardware of each type of imaging system are related to the properties of the radionuclides used. As the radiotracer travels throughout a person's body, gamma rays or positrons emitted during radioactive decay subsequently interact with and transfer energy to the surrounding tissues and

---

Box 9–2. Research Applications of
Structural Neuroimaging

In addition to being clinical workhorses, structural neuro-imaging modalities are also utilized for research purposes in the communication sciences and disorders. For example, structural images obtained via CT and MRI are frequently used in studies that employ techniques known as **voxel-based lesion-symptom mapping (VLSM)** (Bates et al., 2003) and **voxel-based morphometry (VBM)** (Wright et al., 1995).

VLSM aims to reveal brain–behavior relationships by aligning neuroimages from a group of patients with brain lesions (e.g., due to stroke) and determining the association between the presence of a lesion in a specific part of the brain and a particular clinical impairment (i.e., a symptom). For example, if some patients have lesions in brain area X and also have difficulty repeating spoken words, and other patients have neither damage to area X nor impaired speech repetition, this may be correlational evidence that area X plays a role in encoding phonologic information so that it can be reproduced.

VBM is used to calculate and compare the volume of cortical tissue at various locations throughout the brain. This can be used for a number of purposes, including identifying differences in gray or white matter volumes between patients with a particular disorder and healthy individuals, monitoring longitudinal changes in the brains of individuals with neurode-generative disorders, and identifying brain structural changes in response to treatment, including speech-language therapy.

As is true of many areas related to neuroimaging, VLSM and VBM have limitations, and researchers are constantly developing new and more advanced variations of these techniques to make them more reliable and informative research tools.

---

organs. These interactions produce the signals that SPECT or PET machines detect. The mechanisms of energy transfer in SPECT and PET imaging are quite complex.

In SPECT, as emitted photons travel through matter (i.e., body tissues and organs), interactions produce a path of secondary photons in the form of gamma rays. These gamma rays are detected by an Anger camera (named after its inventor) within the SPECT system. A special part of the Anger camera is the **scintillation detector**, which includes a compound that transforms ionizing radiation into visible light that can be measured. There are different arrangements of Anger cameras within SPECT systems. A single-headed Anger camera system has a single camera mounted on a moveable gantry so that it can be positioned over different parts of a patient's body. Dual- and triple-headed systems include more Anger cameras. The dual-headed configuration is most common for SPECT systems in hospitals (Figure 9–7). To obtain tomographic images, the Anger camera head(s) must be rotated around the patient's body to get images from many angles (also called *projections*). In SPECT, it is typical to perform a full 360° rotation around the patient's body, which can take many minutes.

In PET, positrons emitted as the radiotracer decays interact with electrons within body tissues, resulting in the ejection of a pair of high-energy photons, emitted at a 180° angle from each other. While the basic Anger camera components of SPECT and PET systems are the same, in a PET system, it is necessary to have radiation scintillation detectors at opposite ends of the 180° line in order to detect each of these photons at the same time. Thus, most PET systems have fixed detectors situated in opposing directions around the patient, usually in a circular, hexagonal, or octagonal configuration (Figure 9–8). Many PET sequences are faster than SPECT sequences since a gantry does not need to rotate around the patient or body part in PET imaging.

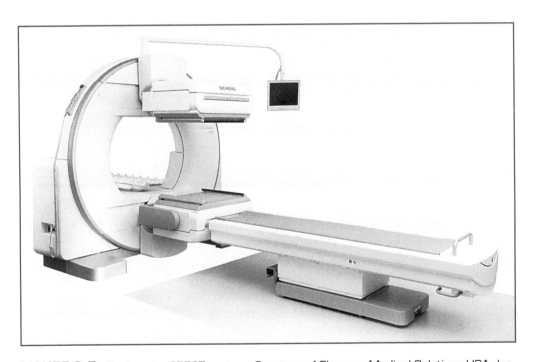

FIGURE 9–7. Dual-gantry SPECT system. Courtesy of Siemens Medical Solutions USA, Inc.

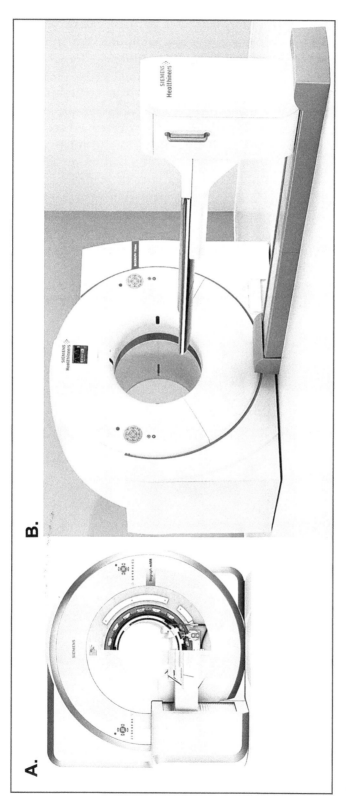

FIGURE 9–8. A. PET scanner with external housing partially removed to show the circular arrangement of scintillation radiation detectors. **B.** PET/CT machine. Courtesy of Siemens Medical Solutions USA, Inc.

The information detected by the camera within SPECT and PET systems is transmitted to a computer, which merges the information and uses it to generate an image. Like CT, SPECT and PET images are typically two-dimensional cross-sectional images or slices through an object. The slices are stacked together to obtain a three-dimensional representation of metabolic activity within the body. In these images, increased or decreased accumulation of the radiotracer within a given tissue or organ relative to surrounding tissues/organs can be indicative of pathology underlying certain diseases (see Clinical Applications of Neuroimaging Modalities). SPECT and PET images are displayed using a rainbow or spectrum color scale, often ranging from cool (e.g., blue) to hot (e.g., red) colors. The color of a given voxel (or location within the image) represents different values of the accumulated radionuclide in the body (Figure 9–9).

Certain radiotracers are ideal for detecting abnormalities in specific health conditions (e.g., malignant tumors in cancer,

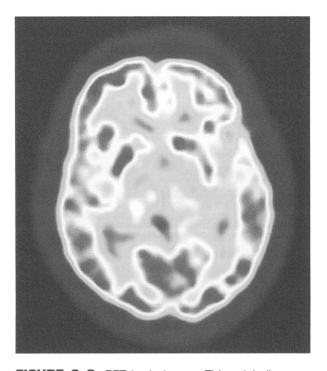

FIGURE 9–9. PET brain image. This axial slice was taken with PET using the radiotracer F-FDG. Warm-colored (e.g., red) areas indicate greater accumulation of the radiotracer and cool-colored (e.g., blue) areas indicate lower to no accumulation of the radiotracer. Figure in the public domain (https://commons.wikimedia.org/wiki/File:PET-image.jpg).

reduced blood flow in cerebrovascular disease). The most common radiotracer used in nuclear medicine imaging is F-fluorodeoxyglucose (^{F}-FDG or sometimes just F-FDG), but many other radiotracers exist. Scientists are currently developing new radiotracers targeted at metabolic pathology in different diseases.

Benefits, Advantages, Risks and Disadvantages of SPECT and PET

The main advantage of SPECT and PET is their ability to detect metabolic processes at high levels of granularity, at the molecular level. This detection ability is better even than other forms of functional imaging (e.g., functional magnetic resonance imaging [fMRI]). As with CT, tomographic imaging in SPECT and PET allows detection of organs with complex geometry that overlap with or are adjacent to other organs. In addition, gamma rays and positrons can reach tissues and organs that lie deep within the body. Specialized SPECT and PET systems also exist for imaging certain body parts, like the brain, breasts, and heart.

There are no outright contraindications for SPECT and PET imaging, yet a major limitation of both imaging modalities is that they are invasive techniques that require the injection of a radiotracer. The dosage of radiation is quite small, however, and precise dosimetry is used to determine the amount of radioactive material that must be injected to obtain adequate signal in the scan. Nonetheless, SPECT and PET scans are not recommended for women who are pregnant. In some rare cases, patients experience allergic reactions to an injected radiotracer. Furthermore, unlike CT, radiation is not restricted to a certain part of the patient's body in SPECT and PET.

SPECT and PET also provide poor anatomic/structural information. SPECT and PET both have worse spatial and temporal resolution than fMRI, and the spatial resolution of SPECT images is even worse than PET images. As such, other imaging modalities like CT and MRI can be combined with SPECT and PET to provide better information about the precise location of the SPECT/PET signal. While SPECT/CT scanners are still somewhat uncommon in hospital settings, most commercial PET systems sold to hospitals since the early 2000s are combined PET/CT scanners (see Figure 9–8B). PET/MRI scanners also exist, yet these types of scans are very costly for hospital systems. Therefore, combined PET/MRI systems are used mostly in biomedical research (Ehman et al., 2017). SPECT is less expensive than PET and combined PET/MRI. A trade-off, though, is that SPECT imaging of certain organs—like the brain—is more time-intensive than PET imaging (although some recent advances in detector technology have sped up SPECT acquisition times) (Slomka et al., 2019). Clinical SPECT and PET scans can take up to 60 min after the radiotracer has been absorbed, which makes these methods un-ideal for patients with poor tolerance for scanning or in emergency medicine (e.g., detection of acute stroke).

Despite the pervasive use of PET and SPECT imaging (see Clinical Applications of Neuroimaging Modalities), it is important to note that SLPs in most health care settings are unlikely to review SPECT and PET images in their daily practice. However, SLPs working in head and neck cancer centers or in other specialty clinics with specific populations (e.g., patients with Alzheimer's disease) are most likely to have access to SPECT/PET images. Most importantly, SLPs in such settings work in teams with other health care professionals adept at interpreting such images. Outside of clinical practice, PET and SPECT are widely used in neurogenic communication disorders research (e.g., stroke, Parkinson's disease, various forms of dementia), as well as voice and dysphagia research in patients with head and neck cancer.

Magnetic Resonance Imaging

In 1977, the first magnetic resonance image of the human body—a single slice through the torso showing the heart and lungs—was obtained with an MRI machine and took 4 hours to acquire. Since that time, MRI has rapidly evolved and is now widely used in countless areas of medicine to diagnose, assess, and monitor illness throughout the entire body.

MRI machines resemble CT and PET scanners (Figure 9–10), but the way MRI works is very different from these other modalities. MRI capitalizes on aspects of **nuclear magnetic resonance** (often referred to as just **magnetic resonance [MR]**) and involves measuring various properties of hydrogen atoms. Different types of brain tissues (e.g., gray matter, white matter, cerebrospinal fluid) contain different concentrations of water molecules and, thus, different concentrations of hydrogen atoms. A critical property of the hydrogen atom for MR is its **spin**, or the frequency at which it rotates around its axis. MRI scanners are tuned to the frequency of spinning hydrogen atoms (i.e., sometimes simply referred to as "spins").

To obtain an MR signal (i.e., the basis for an MR image) MRI scanners use superconducting magnets to generate a strong, static magnetic field (called the B_0 **field**). Outside of an MRI machine,

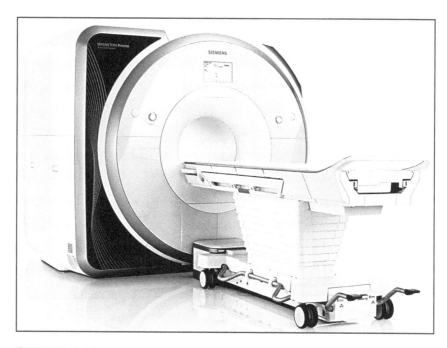

FIGURE 9–10. MRI machine. Courtesy of Siemens Medical Solutions USA, Inc.

hydrogen atoms align in different directions (Figure 9–11A). Inside of an MRI machine, however, the static B_0 field aligns the spins of the atoms (Figure 9–11B), such that they generally spin in a low energy state (Figure 9–11C), similar to a top spinning on its axis. During an MRI scan, special equipment in the MRI machine called **radiofrequency (RF) coils** emit pulses of **RF waves** (i.e., photons of energy that oscillate at the same frequency as hydrogen atomic spins). In a process called **excitation**, low-energy spins absorb energy from the RF pulses and jump to a high-energy state, falling down along their axes (Figure 9–11C).

After excitation, high-energy spins return to their low-energy state in a process called **relaxation.** During relaxation, hydrogen nuclei emit energy in the form of RF waves that are detected by special coils in the MRI scanner called **detector coils**. Changes in MR signal are determined by two relaxation components. **Longitudinal relaxation** occurs when spins return to their original state and is described by the time constant T1. Similar to bumper cars, spins in close proximity bump into each other, causing some spins to relax out of sync with others. This loss of spin coherence results in **transverse relaxation** and is captured by the time constant T2. Additionally, spatial inhomogeneity in the magnetic field causes

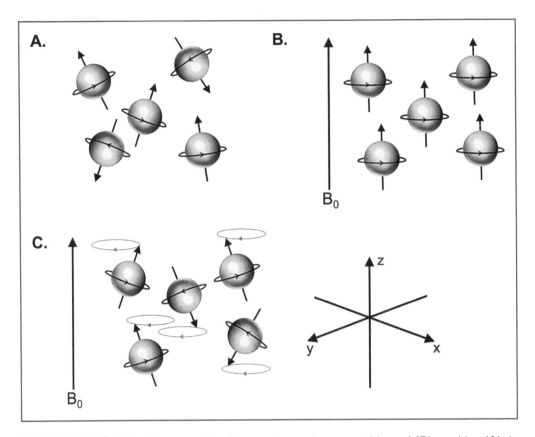

FIGURE 9–11. The alignment of hydrogen atoms shown outside an MRI machine (**A**), in the static field (B_0) of an MRI machine (**B**), and in either a low-energy state (oscillatory path shown in blue) or a high-energy state (oscillatory path shown in orange) following an excitation pulse (**C**). The spins of atomic nuclei can be described in terms of three-dimensional (x,y,z) space, where the z-direction corresponds to the direction of magnetization in the static B_0 field.

some spins to relax more rapidly than others. The timing of transverse relaxation due to combined spin–spin interactions and magnetic field inhomogeneities is described by the time constant T2*. The total magnetization of all atomic nuclei within a given volume at any moment is called the **net magnetization** and is determined by longitudinal magnetization and transverse magnetization.

T1 and T2 relaxations begin at approximately the same time after excitation from an RF pulse, yet their time courses are quite different. T1 is usually one order of magnitude greater than T2 (seconds compared to milliseconds). These time constants change with magnetic field strength; as the static magnetic field increases in strength, T1 becomes longer and T2 and T2* become shorter. These time constants also vary across different tissues as hydrogen atom concentrations are linked to the amount of water within a given tissue type. The timing of data acquisition during T1 and T2 relaxation determines the intensity of images for different tissue types.

Critically, MR signal alone does not generate an image because it does not provide information about *where* atomic spins are located in space. Thus, to obtain an image, another type of coil, called a **gradient coil**, is also necessary. During image acquisition, a given slice of an object (like the brain) is selected. Gradient coils apply RF pulses (sometimes referred to as *spatial gradients*) systematically over the entire slice within a given window of time, and this process is completed many times to cover the entire object. The timing and location of variations in the magnetic field induced by the spatial gradients provide essential spatial information. More specifically, the scanner's detector coils record the MR signal and spatial information across the scanned object, and the raw signal is ultimately reconstructed into an image that represents the distribution of changes in atomic spins over time in a given space.

Magnetic Resonance Imaging Pulse Sequences

The processes in the previous section describe the bases for the many different types of images that can be obtained using different MRI **pulse sequences**. Pulse sequences are programs comprising different patterns of RF pulses and applications of magnetic gradients that run by turning certain hardware within the scanner on or off. MR physicists have capitalized on the versatility of MRI by designing different pulse sequences that are capable of capturing various properties of hydrogen atomic spins. In MRI, images reflect intensity differences between different measured quantities (i.e., contrast) of hydrogen atoms. An important distinction between pulse sequences is whether they utilize static or motion contrast. **Static contrasts** are most sensitive to the number of atoms within a given tissue and/or the relaxation and resonance characteristics of atomic nuclei. As a result, brain tissues appear lighter or darker depending on specific parameters of the sequence, and different sequences are informative for understanding distinctive underlying pathologies. Common sequences that utilize static contrast are T1-weighted, T2-weighted, and fluid-attenuated inversion recovery (FLAIR) imaging sequences. On the other hand, **motion contrasts** take advantage of the dynamic nature of the human body; these contrasts are sensitive to the movement of hydrogen atoms that reflect metabolic processes in the body. Sequences that utilize motion contrasts include techniques that provide information about brain structure (e.g., MR angiography [MRA]) or brain function (e.g., diffusion-weighted imaging [DWI], perfusion-weighted imaging [PWI]). The most popular sequence in research using motion contrast is fMRI, described in greater detail in Box 9–3.

Box 9–3. Functional Magnetic Resonance Imaging

Although by no means the only indirect functional imaging modality used in research (see Box 9–4), fMRI is currently the most commonly used method to measure brain function. Similar to DWI and PWI, fMRI relies on motion contrast. Specifically, fMRI sequences utilize T2* contrast that is sensitive to the **deoxyhemoglobin** (i.e., hemoglobin without oxygen) in biological tissues. The amounts of deoxyhemoglobin and oxyhemoglobin present in brain tissue change with increased or decreased metabolic demands in response to neuronal firing. More specifically, neurons that are engaged by a cognitive, motor, or sensory process fire in response to a given stimulus. Firing neurons require more oxygen, which they extract from nearby blood vessels, and that results in increased deoxyhemoglobin. This in turn creates a need for more oxygen, so oxygen-rich oxyhemoglobin flows to the area, which results in an increase in MR signal in that area. Because of this process, fMRI MR signal is commonly referred to as the **blood-oxygenated-level-dependent (BOLD)** signal or contrast. Keep in mind that the BOLD signal is a direct measure of changes in blood oxygenation but an *indirect* measure of brain activity.

Because of the speed of neural processes and rapid changes in BOLD response, timing is critical in fMRI. Therefore, fMRI requires special, fast pulse sequences. The dynamic nature of fMRI also means that researchers must correct for certain data acquisition parameters (e.g., the order in which slices are acquired through the brain) and artifacts (e.g., patient motion). Published studies include sections describing such **data preprocessing** methods. Finally, researchers must design tasks that participants complete in the scanner so that data acquisition in the pulse sequence aligns with the conditions of interest in the task.

Today, most researchers use the concept of cognitive subtraction described previously to design tasks that isolate specific sensory, motor, or cognitive processes of interest. Published fMRI studies typically report the location and extent of brain activation for specific conditions of interest. Activation color maps represent brain activity averaged across an entire fMRI experiment (or **time series**) for those conditions. In recent years, however, researchers have moved away from reporting only activation, as there is a growing interest in understanding brain activity in terms of distributed networks of connections (see Box 9–5).

Box 9–4. Beyond fMRI: Other Indirect Measures of Brain Function Used in Research

Being able to tell what someone is thinking has fascinated scientists and popular media alike. Although neuroimaging by no means has such "mind reading" capacity, certain modalities can provide a window into which brain regions are recruited and when during a given task.

As explained earlier in the chapter, imaging modalities can be split into direct and indirect measures of brain function. fMRI is probably the most well-known indirect measure of brain activity among laypeople, yet other modalities that rely on blood-based measures exist. For example, in the 1980s and early 1990s, before the emergence of fMRI, PET measures of cerebral blood flow and volume were used to index brain activity while research participants completed different cognitive, sensory, or motor tasks. Task-based imaging studies with PET scanners are still done today, but such investigations are less common given the invasiveness of radiotracer injection.

A newer functional imaging method that takes advantage of the brain's optical properties and hemodynamic response is **functional near-infrared spectroscopy (fNIRS)**. In fNIRS, source optodes on the scalp or cap (Figure 9–12) emit near-

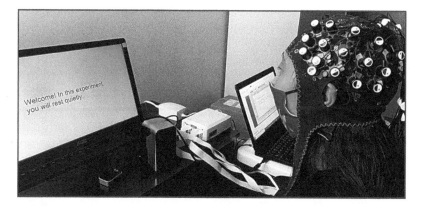

FIGURE 9–12. Setup of an example functional near-infrared spectroscopy (fNIRS) experiment. The participant is seated in front of a monitor that shows the experiment welcome screen. Source and detector optodes are affixed to the cap worn by the participant and are connected to the fNIRS device via cables. The device is also connected to the data acquisition computer, which is positioned out of the participant's line of sight during the experiment. Author-created image constructed using data from NIH/NIDCD RO1DC005375, RO1DC015466, and P50DC014664 (PI: Argye E. Hillis).

infrared light, which shines through the scalp and into the brain. Detector optodes measure the number of photons projected back from hemoglobin chromophores, and that signal ultimately is converted into signals that reflect changes in oxygenated or deoxygenated hemoglobin. In this way, the signal obtained in fNIRS is very similar to the BOLD response captured in fMRI. Unlike fMRI, though, fNIRS systems are relatively inexpensive, can be used in natural environments, and have no restrictions for use in any population, similar to EEG. Because of these characteristics, fNIRS has been used in infants and people with cochlear implants. Right now, fNIRS is used exclusively in research studies, but given its flexibility, it shows promise as a future clinical neuroimaging tool.

Box 9–5. From "Blobology" to Connectivity

From the beginning of functional imaging in the late 1980s, researchers have been interested in determining which areas of the brain are activated by specific tasks in healthy people and in clinical populations. This is still true today—many studies report activation maps such as those included in Figure 9–13A, which shows fMRI activity (indicated by the bright red and yellow "blobs") in a group of neurologically intact controls and a group of individuals with aphasia for the semantic feature judgment task referenced earlier in the chapter (Box 9–1 and Figure 9–4). As you can see in Figure 9–13A, the location of activity is distributed throughout the brain in both groups, with more activation in the left than the right hemisphere, as one would expect for a language task. While the activation extent (i.e., size) is smaller in patients than controls, the activation patterns (i.e., location of activity) are similar between groups.

Interpreting such activation results can be challenging. Can it be assumed that all neurons within activated regions are firing at the same time? Since so many regions are activated by the same task, can it be assumed that all areas are involved in the exact same processes? Since activity patterns are similar between patients and controls, can it be assumed that stroke did not alter brain function for these individuals with aphasia? The answer to all of these questions is a resounding no.

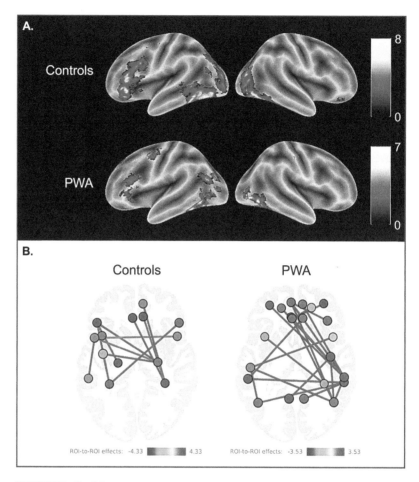

FIGURE 9–13. Functional activation versus connectivity. Activation maps (**A**) and functional connectivity results (**B**) are shown for neurologically intact older adults (i.e., controls) and people with chronic aphasia (PWA) while they participated in a semantic judgment fMRI experiment. The color bars at right in **A** and below the brain images in **B** indicate the statistical strength of the results. In **B**, brain regions of interest are indicated by the circles and the functional connections between regions are denoted by lines. Author-created image constructed using data from NIH/NIDCD P50DC012283 (Subproject PI: Swathi Kiran).

As SLPs and audiologists know, communication is incredibly complex, as are the underlying cognitive-linguistic, speech, and hearing processes that clinicians assess and treat. Because of this complexity, certain brain regions are implicated in particular processes that together comprise complex communication acts. As an example, the seemingly simple task of naming a pictured object aloud requires many steps: object perception (mediated by occipital cortex), object recognition (mediated by ventral temporo-occipital regions), retrieval of the item's semantic features (mediated by specific temporal, parietal, and frontal regions) and phonologic codes (mediated by other temporal, parietal, and frontal regions), and articulation (mediated by premotor and motor cortex). Successful picture naming requires these brain regions to communicate with each other, rather than function in isolation, by rapidly sending signals to each other at each stage of the naming process.

Similarly, the many brain regions activated by the semantic feature judgment task described previously support different aspects of the larger task, but it is impossible to tell from activation "blobs" which regions are communicating with each other and when. To address this issue, in recent years, researchers have moved away from studies of "blobology" to studies of **connectivity** (Poldrack, 2012). Connectivity studies allow researchers to investigate brain networks in terms of how a system of nodes (i.e., brain regions) communicate via anatomic (i.e., white matter tracts) or functional connections over time. The two types of brain function–based connectivity analyses are **functional connectivity** and **effective connectivity**. Functional connectivity describes regions that become activated at the same time. Effective connectivity describes how activity in one brain area changes activity in another brain area.

Connectivity analyses have revealed amazing things about the brain that activation studies alone could not. Case in point, functional connectivity patterns greatly differ between controls and people with aphasia in our semantic feature judgment task example, with individuals with aphasia appearing to recruit more, not fewer, connections than controls do (Figure 9–13B). Even more incredibly, connectivity analysis has uncovered the brain's **resting state**. Even when not engaged in a specific task, the brain is always active. A few years ago, researchers realized that certain parts of the brain are *consistently* active at the same time, even at rest (Fox & Raichle, 2007; Fox et al., 2005; Raichle, 2011; Raichle et al., 2001). These studies, and many others since, have demonstrated that the brain is organized in intrinsic networks. These networks have been linked to different sensorimotor and cognitive functions, and disrupted intrinsic connectivity is likely a critical clinical marker in certain populations.

Additional details regarding common MRI sequences used in clinical settings are provided later. Sequences utilizing other contrasts exist (Box 9–6), but as of now, these sequences are used relatively infrequently in most diseases with speech-language comorbidities.

Box 9–6. Other MRI Sequences

The sequences described in the Magnetic Resonance Imaging (MRI) section are performed most commonly in clinical hospital settings, yet they are not the only MR sequences available. Some older sequences have now been replaced by newer ones. For example, proton density (PD)–weighted sequences produce images that reflect the concentration of hydrogen atoms within tissues. At one time, PD-weighted sequences were used extensively for brain imaging in hospital settings, but for the most part, they have now been replaced by FLAIR sequences.

Other older sequences have been repurposed for new clinical applications. For example, **susceptibility-weighted imaging (SWI)** is sensitive to compounds that distort the local magnetic field and was first applied in the late 1990s to image the veins (Haacke et al., 2004; Reichenbach et al., 1997). Since then, SWI has been used to detect abnormalities in tissues (e.g., microhemorrhages, blood products due to hemorrhage or clot, calcium deposits) in a variety of disorders, including traumatic brain injury, brain tumors, and certain neurodegenerative diseases (Hakimi & Garg, 2016; Henriksen et al., 2016; Mutch et al., 2016; Schwarz et al., 2020).

MR physicists continue to develop and refine newer, advanced sequences that have promising future clinical applications. One such sequence is DTI, which we describe in greater detail in Box 9–7. Another promising new MR-based sequence is **MR spectroscopy**, which simply put, uses signals from hydrogen atom spins to detect concentrations of *metabolites* (i.e., metabolism by- or end-products) that reflect biochemical processes in the brain. MR spectroscopy has potential applications in many central nervous system disorders (Brody et al., 2015; Fink et al., 2015; Manias & Peet, 2018; Mutch et al., 2016; Öz et al., 2014; Shukla et al., 2017; Wintermark et al., 2015), some of which we reference in the Clinical Applications of Neuroimaging Modalities section.

Static Contrast Sequences

T1-Weighted Imaging. The contrast (i.e., intensity differences of tissues) of T1-weighted sequences is primarily determined by the longitudinal (T1) relaxation properties of biological tissues. Water has a long T1, so little signal is elicited from tissues that have high water content during this sequence. Therefore, in T1-weighted images, cerebrospinal fluid (CSF) appears dark. White matter and bone marrow, which have relatively low water concentration (and therefore short T1 values), appear bright white. Gray matter, which is intermixed with a rich blood supply, has T1 values that fall between the values of CSF and white matter and appears light gray. A robust, shorter sequence resulting in high-quality T1-weighted data is magnetization-prepared rapid acquisition with gradient echo (MPRAGE) imaging. MPRAGE sequences provide even sharper contrast between tissue types than traditional T1-weighted sequences and therefore are excellent scans for assessing anatomical changes in brain structure. An example of an MPRAGE image is shown in Figure 9–14A.

Sometimes, gadolinium contrast media is injected in the body to improve the clarity of biologic tissues in T1-weighted scans. Similar to contrast CT, gadolinium improves the visibility of blood vessels and perfusion within certain organs and pathologic conditions such as edema and brain tumors. Nonetheless, there has been recent debate over the safety of injectable gadolinium contrast

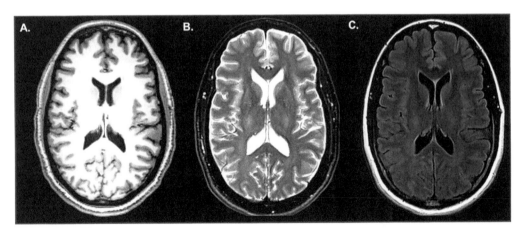

FIGURE 9–14. Axial slices from the same individual acquired from common static MRI contrasts, including T1-weighted magnetization-prepared rapid acquisition with gradient echo (MPRAGE) (**A**), T2-weighted (**B**), and fluid-attenuated inversion recovery (FLAIR) sequences (**C**). Author-created image constructed using data from NIH/NIDCD RO1DCO05375, RO1DCO15466, and P50DCO14664 (PI: Argye E. Hillis).

media (Choi & Moon, 2019; Kanda et al., 2014; Pinter et al., 2016; Ramalho & Ramalho, 2017), and its use has somewhat fallen out of favor in clinical settings.

T2-Weighted Imaging. The contrast of T2-weighted sequences is primarily determined by the transverse relaxation (T2) properties of tissue. Homogeneous tissues with high water content typically have longer T2 relaxation periods and therefore yield the most signal during a T2-weighted sequence. T2-weighted images look like the inverse of T1-weighted scans: CSF is bright white; white matter is very dark (due to having a short T2 value); and gray matter has a lighter gray appearance (due to an intermediate T2). Sample T2-weighted images are shown in Figure 9–14B.

Another common T2-weighted sequence is FLAIR. The acquisition parameters are closer to classic T2- than T1-weighted sequences, but FLAIR images look like a combination of the two. Like T1-weighted scans, CSF is attenuated and appears dark, but like T2-weighted images, white matter is a dark gray and gray matter is a lighter gray hue. Sample FLAIR images are shown in Figure 9–14C. T2-weighted and FLAIR images have clinical applications for detecting abnormalities (e.g., tumors or arteriovenous malformations) in fluid-filled areas of the brain. They are also sensitive to ischemic changes, white matter changes like demyelination (for example, due to multiple sclerosis), and edema (i.e., swelling) in the brain.

Motion Contrast Sequences

Magnetic Resonance Angiography. Like CTA, MRA provides information about the structure of major blood vessels. MRA of the head and/or neck is typically done in diseases with concomitant speech-language symptoms, but other body parts can also be scanned. Similar to CTA, MRA can be done with injected contrast, but it can also be done using endogenous contrast (based on intrinsic, naturally occurring properties in the body). Endogenous contrast in MRA is usually obtained by measuring either blood displacement over time or blood flow velocity using a specific pulse sequence.

Perfusion-Weighted Imaging. Like CT perfusion, the goal of MR-based PWI is to evaluate blood flow through the microvasculature (e.g., capillaries) of different types of tissues. Common clinical PWI sequences require intravenous injection of a contrast agent and rely on the relaxation properties of brain tissues. For example, in dynamic susceptibility contrast MR perfusion—a sequence frequently performed in clinical settings—the signal in each brain voxel reflects attenuation of the inherent T2/T2* properties of brain tissues by a contrast agent (e.g., gadolinium bolus) passing through the microvasculature. In other words, signal intensity over time is proportional to the amount of the contrast agent in capillary beds at any given moment. From this sequence, several different measures can be derived, including measures of regional cerebral blood volume, cerebral blood flow, and mean transit time, as in CT perfusion.

While most PWI sequences performed in hospital settings still require injection of contrast, a newer perfusion sequence, **arterial spin labeling (ASL)**, does not. In ASL, RF pulses magnetically "tag" certain water molecules in arterial blood. Subtraction of the signal from inflowing blood in tagged images from untagged control images provides a measure proportional to cerebral blood flow. Today, ASL sequences are still being optimized and take a long time to acquire; as such, they are mostly used in research rather than clinical settings.

Diffusion-Weighted Imaging. DWI is used to detect the direction and magnitude of the movement of water molecules in biologic tissues. The main principle behind DWI is that biologic tissues restrict the diffusion of water molecules within a medium to different degrees. In CSF, the movement of water molecules is completely **isotropic**, or unrestricted and, therefore, uniform in all directions. In gray matter, isotropic movement of water molecules is also observed but to a lesser extent than in CSF. In contrast, the movement of water molecules in white matter is **anisotropic**, meaning it has directional dependence; this is due to the density of neuronal cell bodies and axons constraining water molecule diffusion.

A DWI scan protocol usually involves, at a minimum, acquiring diffusion-weighted images along three directional planes (i.e., the *x*-, *y*- and *z*-planes) to generate a three-dimensional model of diffusion (O'Donnell & Westin, 2011). In clinical imaging, two images commonly reconstructed from a DWI sequence are **apparent diffusion coefficient (ADC)** (Figure 9–15A) and **trace** (Figure 9–15B) maps. These images are essentially the inverse of each other. In the trace image, CSF looks black; gray matter is a dark gray; and white matter is a lighter gray hue. In the ADC image, the unrestricted movement of water molecules in CSF makes the ventricles and cisterns appear bright white, and gray matter is a darker gray. The principles of diffusion that form the basis of DWI sequences also apply to DTI, a newer MRI sequence that, as of now, is used mostly in research (Box 9–7).

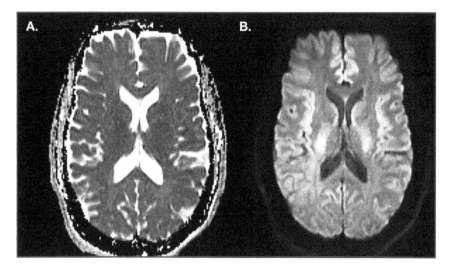

FIGURE 9–15. Axial slices from the same individual acquired from a diffusion-weighted imaging (DWI) sequence, including apparent diffusion coefficient (ADC) (**A**) and trace images (**B**). Author-created image constructed using data from NIH/NIDCD RO1DC005375, RO1DC015466, and P50DC014664 (PI: Argye E. Hillis).

Box 9–7. Diffusion Tensor Imaging

The principles behind DTI are similar to DWI. The critical exception is that DTI is a structural technique that provides information regarding the microstructure of different tissues, whereas DWI is a functional technique that measures diffusion over time. Currently, the macro-anatomic connections of white matter pathways that subserve speech and language can be defined and reconstructed in vivo with the use of DTI. Before the invention of DTI, neuroanatomists relied on postmortem dissections and animal models to understand the architecture of white matter tracts.

DTI captures the isotropic/anisotropic properties of white matter tissue through the calculation of a **diffusion tensor**, a mathematical model that describes the diffusion of water molecules in terms of its direction and magnitude. A diffusion tensor can be calculated from data acquired with at least six diffusion-weighted images. Equivalent diffusion in all directions (i.e., isotropic movement of water molecules) results in a spherical tensor, whereas diffusion restricted by tissues (i.e., anisotropic water molecule movement) results in an ellipsoidal tensor. Tensors (or DTI data) can be transformed into an array of measures that index the orientation of white matter fibers, as well as proxy measures of fiber integrity. Various DTI measures provide important information about certain neurologic conditions. For example, if a stroke destroys white matter tissue in a given area, there will no longer be axons to constrain the movement of water molecules in that space. Consequently, isotropy in the area will increase, and anisotropy will decrease, and, thus, these changes will be reflected in corresponding DTI metrics.

Metrics derived from DTI maps provide diffusivity information about white matter across the entire brain. DTI data can also be used to delineate established white matter tracts via a technique called **diffusion tensor tractography (DTT)**. DTT can produce a whole-brain *tractogram* that illustrates representations of white matter fibers called *streamlines* across the entire brain (Figure 9–16A). Canonical, large white

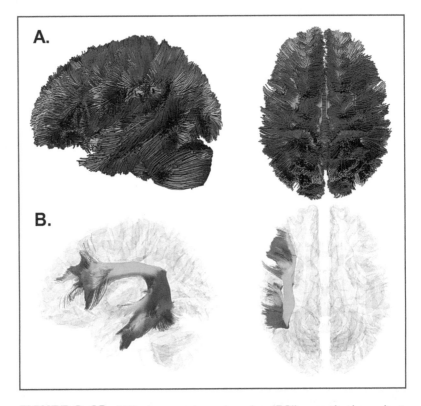

FIGURE 9–16. Diffusion spectrum imaging (DSI)–quantitative anisotropy (QA) images, including a whole-brain tractogram (**A**) and the left arcuate fasciculus (**B**) delineated in a neurologically intact healthy adult. Courtesy of Alexander M. Swiderski.

matter tracts, like the arcuate fasciculus, can also be delineated from a tractogram (Figure 9–16B). New diffusion models and tractography methods continue to be developed that improve our ability to accurately measure the structural integrity of white matter tracts in vivo in individuals with and without neurologic disorders.

Benefits, Advantages, Risks, and Disadvantages of Magnetic Resonance Imaging

MRI has many advantages over other imaging modalities. MRI has superior soft tissue contrast than CT, so it is easier to distinguish white and gray matter in many MR images than it is in CT scans. Unlike CT, SPECT, and PET, there is no exposure to ionizing radiation in MRI. As this section demonstrates, one of the major advantages of MRI is its versatility. Because there are so many different pulse sequences that can be used to measure different properties of biologic tissue, MRI is widely used in both clinical settings and research. In fact, many of the MRI sequences outlined in this section are included in standard clinical MRI workups when a patient is admitted to the hospital.

Like other imaging modalities, though, MRI has limitations. As referenced previously, the temporal resolution of fMRI and other MR-based motion contrasts is inferior to that of EEG and MEG. There are still fewer MRI machines than CT scanners in hospitals within the United States. MRI scans are also more expensive than CT scans. Furthermore, many MRI sequences have prolonged acquisition times (as compared to CT). Consequently, CT scans are typically first performed in an emergency situation, followed by MRI scan protocols. Because of longer scan times, MRI is not appropriate for critically ill patients or for patients who cannot tolerate lying flat for long periods of time.

The primary disadvantage of MRI is that safety is a major concern. Like any other magnet, the strong magnets used in MRI attract objects made of or containing iron (i.e., ferrous material). As such, it is *extremely* unsafe for individuals with implanted material such as ferrous aneurysm clips, pacemakers, and cochlear implants to enter the magnetic field of an MRI scanner. Torsion forces cause ferrous implants to realign so they are parallel to the magnetic field, meaning that implants shift inside a person's body. Ferrous material outside the body is also dangerous because such objects become projectiles that move toward the scanner bore if placed inside the magnetic field. Given the strength of the static magnetic field, ferrous objects of any size can move toward the scanner bore at great speeds. Metallic fibers sewn into modern exercise clothing such as yoga pants can also heat up and cause burns (Pietryga et al., 2013). Therefore, one of the key aspects of MR safety is to ensure no ferrous materials enter the scanner's magnetic field. MRI technicians in clinical and research settings conduct thorough safety screenings before a patient receives an MRI scan. For patients admitted to the emergency department whose MR safety is unknown, alternative scanning (usually CT) is performed instead. Despite such safety measures, unfortunately, fatal accidents have occurred (Chaljub et al., 2001; Chen, 2001).

However, besides the risks of ferrous material, the static magnetic field has no negative effects on people. For most people, the major risk of MRI is discomfort. Claustrophobia can be an issue, especially for brain MRI, as patients' upper bodies are placed in a relatively small bore (typically 24–28 inches in diameter), and equipment, such as a head coil (i.e., a helmet-like structure that resembles a bird cage), often surrounds the head. Loud noise is also an issue in MRI. Rapid current changes in the gradient coils cause vibrations within the coils that sound like knocking or banging. Although the nature of these sounds depends on the pulse sequence, all pulse sequences generate loud noises, and as such, hearing protection is advised. While less common than discomfort due to claustrophobia or loud noises, heating of the body can occur during a scan due to the fact that not all RF energy absorbed by hydrogen atoms is re-emitted.

Electroencephalography and Magnetoencephalography

In 1929, Hans Berger discovered that electrical activity in the brain could be measured in humans by placing sensors on the scalp (Berger, 1929). This discovery led to the advent of EEG and ultimately contributed to the invention of MEG. Like fMRI, EEG and MEG measure brain function but not brain structure.

Unlike fMRI, SPECT, and PET, EEG and MEG are direct measurements of neuronal activity. These two methods detect changes that occur as a result of synaptic activity of activated neurons. The signal generated by a single neuron is quite small; therefore, the success of EEG and MEG hinges on a sufficient population of neurons in close spatial proximity firing together. Specifically, EEG and MEG detect the activity of functional assemblies of *pyramidal neurons*. Pyramidal neurons are large and typically arranged with their dendrites perpendicular to the surface of the brain and parallel to one another (in a row, like planks in a fence), allowing for better signal detection than other types of neurons. When these neurons are excited, electrical current travels down their axons until they synapse with neighboring neurons, causing a change in the polarization of the neighboring cells. These changes, or *postsynaptic potentials*, accumulate over the population of neurons creating a **local field potential (LFP)** in the extracellular space surrounding the neuron. LFPs form the basis of EEG signal. At the same time, changes in neuronal polarization and electrical activity generate small magnetic fields, called **local magnetic fields (LMFs)**, which are the basis of the MEG signal.

Because EEG and MEG detect different types of signals, electrical and magnetic, respectively, they require different types of equipment. In EEG, electricity sensors, or **electrodes**, are placed either directly on the scalp or are affixed to a cap worn by the patient or participant (Figure 9–17). External environmental factors do not impact EEG data collection, and as such, EEG can be performed in many different settings. On the other hand, MEG is very sensitive to external influences in the environment that cause even small fluctuations in the magnetic field (e.g., iron tooth fillings or ferrous objects in the vicinity). Therefore, MEG data are collected by a scanner that must be contained in a magnetically shielded room (Figure 9–18).

Raw EEG and MEG data are recorded in the **encephalogram** and **magnetoencephalogram**, respectively, which are visualized as a series of lines (one for each measured source) that fluctuate over time (see Figure 9–17). These fluctuations, or **oscillations**, in electrical or magnetic activity are usually characterized based on frequency (measured in hertz [Hz]), but also are described in terms of amplitude, synchrony, shape, and location. Classic EEG/MEG frequency bands include delta (~0.5–3.5 Hz), theta (~4–8 Hz), alpha (~8–13.5 Hz), beta (~14–30 Hz), and gamma (~30–100 Hz) oscillations. Research regarding links between specific oscillations and sensorimotor and cognitive processes is ongoing (Canolty & Knight, 2010; Cohen, 2017; Herrmann et al., 2016; Karakaş & Barry, 2017; Singer, 2018).

While neural oscillations can be measured during sensory, motor, or cognitive tasks, they are not time-locked to specific task events or stimuli (e.g., visual cues, auditory tones, words, etc.). In contrast, **event-related potentials (ERPs)** derived from continuous EEG reflect the brain's characteristic electrophysiological response, manifesting as changes in voltage, within a given time window following a specific stimulus or event. There is good evidence to

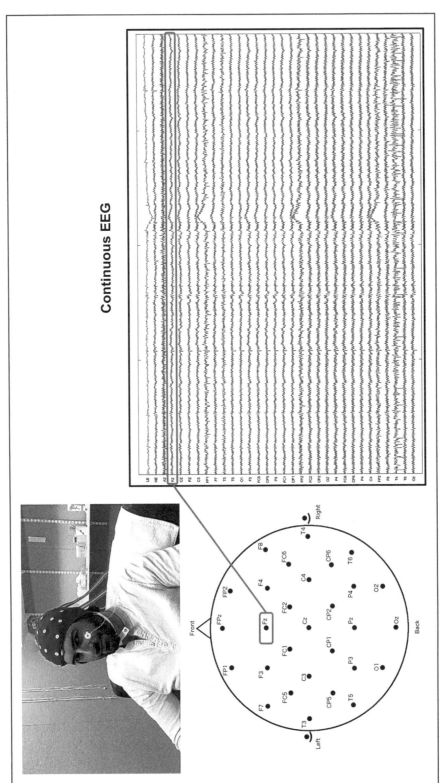

FIGURE 9–17. Setup and raw data of an example EEG experiment. At top left, a participant wears an electrode cap that is connected to a computer that collects the data. The image at bottom left shows the electrode montage, in which the top and bottom of the image correspond to the front and back of the head, respectively; the electrodes are denoted by black circles and named according to their location. A snapshot in time of the continuous EEG is shown at right, with electrode Fz highlighted. Courtesy of Shannon M. Sheppard.

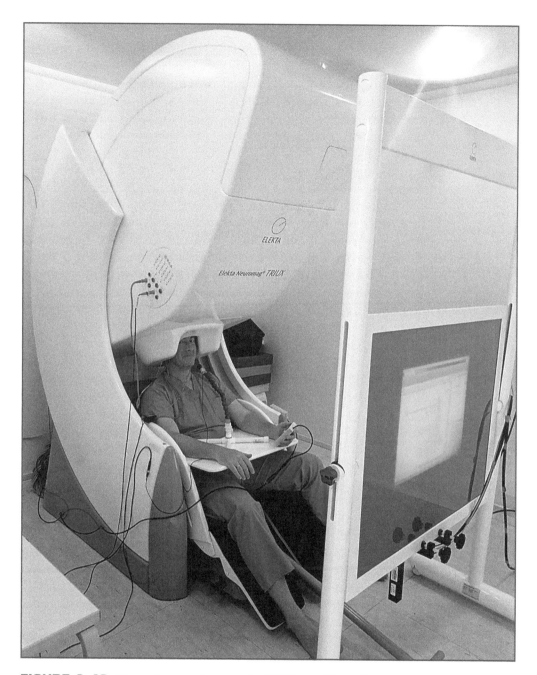

FIGURE 9–18. Magnetoencephalography (MEG) machine with an experiment presented on the screen in front of the participant. Courtesy of Carrie Niziolek.

support associations between different ERP components and specific sensory, cognitive, and language functions (Box 9–8); as such, ERPs are studied extensively in communication sciences and disorders research.

Box 9–8. Event-Related Potentials

ERPs and the equivalent measure in MEG, **event-related fields (ERFs)**, are the subject of investigation in most EEG and MEG studies in the field of communication sciences and disorders. So, what are ERPs and EMFs (hereafter, just referred to as ERPs)?

In an EEG or MEG experiment, there are many trials corresponding to different task conditions that are recorded in the ongoing encephalogram or magnetoencephalogram. EEG and MEG recordings for one experimental trial include the brain's response to that trial but also a good deal of noise. Therefore, to achieve a reliable brain response, ERPs are obtained by averaging activity for all trials within a given experimental condition over the course of an experiment. As shown in Figure 9–19, ERPs have an onset (which corresponds to a deviation in electrical activity from baseline), a peak (which corresponds to the highest amplitude and latency of the response), and an offset (which corresponds to a return to baseline activity). Several different ERP components exist and often are named according to their polarity (i.e., negative or positive) and latency (i.e., time between stimulus offset and the ERP onset). Earlier components reflect reflexive or passive perceptual or sensory encoding, whereas later components index conscious, higher-level cognitive or language processes.

Two classic ERP waveforms studied in language research are the N400 and P600. The N400 component is a large, negative waveform mainly over centro-parietal regions that occurs, in classic paradigms, approximately 400 ms following a semantically incongruent word within a sentence (e.g., "He takes his coffee with cream and *cat*"); therefore, this component is believed to index lexical-semantic processing and integration (Beres, 2017; Kutas & Federmeier, 2011; Kutas & Hillyard, 1980, 1984; McWeeny & Norton, 2020). The P600 component is commonly observed in temporo-parietal areas approximately 600 ms after a syntactically ambiguous stimulus (e.g., "While the boy walked the dog got hot and smelly") or in response to an overt syntactic violation (e.g., "They walks to the store") and is believed to index syntactic processing in language paradigms (Ainsworth-Darnell et al., 1998; Neville et al., 1991; Osterhout & Holcomb, 1992; Osterhout & Mobley, 1995). Other components also have been the subject of

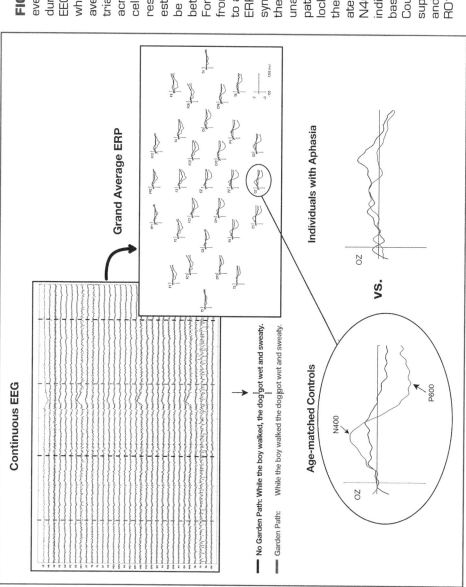

Continuous EEG

Grand Average ERP

1000 (ms)

Individuals with Aphasia

OZ

vs.

Age-matched Controls

N400

P600

OZ

— No Garden Path: **While the boy walked, the dog got wet and sweaty.**

— Garden Path: While the boy walked the dog got wet and sweaty.

FIGURE 9-19. N400 and P600 event-related potentials (ERPs) elicited during a sentence comprehension task. EEG is collected from each participant while presenting multiple trials. Grand average ERPs are made by averaging trials together from each condition across all participants, which cancels out noise and retains the brain's response to each condition of interest. Comparisons (i.e., contrasts) can be made between conditions and also between different participant groups. For example, the figure depicts ERPs from a group of controls compared to a group of individuals with aphasia. ERPs were measured in the context of syntactically ambiguous sentences (i.e., the garden path condition in red) and unambiguous sentences (i.e., no garden path condition in black), and were time-locked to the verb "got," which is when the syntactic structure was disambiguated. Age-matched controls show clear N400 and P600 effects, whereas the individuals with aphasia do not. Data based on Sheppard et al. (2017).

Courtesy of Shannon M. Sheppard, work supported by NIH/NICHD HD25889 and NIH/NIDCD RO1DC009272, RO1DC000494, and T32DC007361.

study in communication disorders research; the components examined in specific studies depend on the patient population and the specific deficits and/or cognitive processes under investigation.

Benefits, Advantages, Risks, and Disadvantages of Electroencephalography and Magnetoencephalography

One major advantage of EEG and MEG is superb temporal resolution. Unlike SPECT, PET, and fMRI, EEG and MEG can provide information about neural processing on the order of milliseconds, rather than several seconds. Unlike imaging modalities that rely on hemodynamic response (e.g., fMRI), EEG and MEG reflect direct measurement of synaptic activity, which provides a closer link to true brain activity. Additionally, EEG in particular is quite inexpensive, especially compared to fMRI and PET. Once EEG equipment has been purchased, the only cost is semi-routine maintenance (e.g., replacement electrodes or electrode caps, gel to improve electrode-to-scalp contact, etc.). EEG systems are available for purchase from many commercial vendors. In contrast, relatively few MEG systems exist compared to the prevalence of EEG, PET, and MRI. Crucially, there are no known risks of either EEG or MEG. Unlike many other modalities, EEG and MEG do not require injection of contrast and are noninvasive.

There are also several disadvantages to EEG/MEG. EEG and MEG both have poorer spatial resolution than fMRI. This stems from the fact that in EEG and MEG, the signal from a single population of neurons is detected by many adjacent sensors, making it difficult to tell where the activity originates. Furthermore, EEG signal detection is complicated by the fact that to reach the scalp, LFPs must travel through many different types of tissue (e.g., dura, skull, skin) that have their own electrical conductivity capacity, which attenuates and distorts the signal. Frontal electrodes are also susceptible to artifacts (i.e., distortions in the data) caused by contractions of the eye and jaw muscles during blinking and jaw clenching. Unlike MRI, it is not unsafe to have ferromagnetic material near a MEG machine, but such material (even something as innocuous as iron tooth fillings) easily corrupts MEG data.

As of now, EEG and MEG are used most often in research rather than clinical practice. For years, scientists believed that neural oscillations that comprise EEG/MEG constituted noise rather than meaningful data. As such, investigations into the clinical applications of frequency bands truly have emerged only in the last 10 to 15 years (Helfrich & Knight, 2019). Similarly, the clinical utility of ERPs is limited at this time, as no established ERP biomarkers of any neurologic or developmental disorder exist (Helfrich & Knight, 2019). Nevertheless, there are some exceptions to these general statements. For example, the **auditory brain stem response (ABR)** —which, like ERPs, is an evoked EEG response to external stimuli—is critical for newborn hearing screenings and is used in most American hospitals. Other clinical applications are addressed in the Clinical Applications of Neuroimaging Modalities section.

Of note, EEG and MEG are suitable, and even optimal, modalities for eventually identifying neural biomarkers of different neurologic and developmental disorders. For example, ERPs provide information about processing even before a behavioral response is given, provide time course information that can also be used to identify locus of impairment, and can be elicited in individuals who are nonverbal (e.g., infants, patients with severe aphasia, or individuals in a coma) (McWeeny & Norton, 2020). Nonetheless, for most clinicians, it is not necessary to have more in-depth knowledge about specific frequency bands or ERP components at this time. Rather, it is useful to have a general grasp on what ERPs/EMFs and neural oscillations are and what information they can provide in order to understand EEG- and MEG-based research findings.

Other Brain Mapping Techniques

While some of the tools described in this chapter are used to generate neuroanatomic images (e.g., CT and various MRI techniques), it should be clear by now that neuroimaging also encompasses techniques that are used to measure neural functions and localize them to specific areas in the brain (i.e., "brain mapping" techniques), such as fMRI, EEG, and MEG. Thus far, we have described the modalities that are most commonly used in medical settings with patients whose illnesses have implications for speech and language or those that are most widely used in research on speech, language, and communication disorders. However, in this section, we describe several additional brain mapping techniques with which SLPs should be familiar, given their application to certain relevant clinical conditions and/or their utilization in research on the neural bases of speech, language, and cognition.

The Wada Test

The Wada test, named for its creator, Juhn Wada, is a procedure for determining hemispheric language and memory dominance in the brain. Its primary clinical application is in assessing the risk of language or memory impairment as a side effect of surgical intervention for epilepsy. If the site targeted for surgical resection is in the language- or memory-dominant hemisphere, there is a greater likelihood of such side effects. It is important to recognize that Wada testing may reveal which hemisphere is predominantly associated with the cognitive function of interest, but it generally does not provide more focal information (i.e., it does not localize language or memory functions to precise areas *within* the dominant hemisphere). Nonetheless, the information provided by the Wada test can assist the patient and their medical team in making decisions as to whether and how to proceed with surgery; it may also justify more invasive but finer-grained functional mapping techniques (Binder, 2011).

The Wada testing procedure begins with an angiogram, which is conducted to ensure that the subsequent test will proceed as expected and will not be disrupted by vascular abnormalities. During the angiogram, a catheter is guided to the internal carotid artery. A contrast agent is injected, and its flow through the cerebral vasculature is monitored under x-ray. After the angiogram is complete, a sedative is administered via the catheter to temporarily anesthetize one hemisphere of the brain. Once changes in brain activity, as indicated by EEG recordings, and a loss of motor function indicate the targeted hemisphere is sedated, formal language and memory tests are administered (Bi et al., 2016). Speech-language tests may include reading, counting, naming objects, and following commands (Abou-Khalil, 2007). Memory may be assessed by waiting until the sedative wears off and asking the patient to recall various items or pictures they were shown while they were "under." Impaired test performance indicates that the sedated hemisphere underlies or contributes to the relevant behavior. After the sedative wears off, usually within about 15 min or less, the catheter is repositioned, and the procedure (i.e., angiogram, sedation, testing) is repeated to examine the other hemisphere.

Wada testing has several notable limitations. As indicated, it reveals hemispheric lateralization of cognitive functions but does not support more granular functional localization. This is fairly limiting, given that language is complex and involves the integration of a variety of regions and networks throughout the brain. Furthermore, people rarely use just one cerebral hemisphere to accomplish complex cognitive or linguistic tasks. As such, complementary or alternative techniques may be warranted when more precise localization is desired. Wada testing is also limited by its duration (Bi et al., 2016); that is, because each hemisphere is only anesthetized for a brief period of time, extensive, comprehensive, and highly nuanced evaluations are not possible. Given its invasive nature, the Wada test carries risks such as seizure, stroke, allergic reaction to the contrast agent, and infection, among others, with studies indicating overall complication rates as low as 1.09% (Haag et al., 2008) and as high as 10.9% (Loddenkemper et al., 2008).

Electrical Stimulation Mapping

Electrical stimulation mapping (ESM), also known as direct electrical stimulation or cortical stimulation mapping, is an invasive procedure for identifying areas of cortex involved in motor, sensory, and cognitive functions, including speech and language. Like the Wada test, it is predominantly used to guide neurosurgery for epilepsy or tumor management so that surgeons can avoid removing or damaging functionally critical tissue (Duffau, 2013; Ritaccio et al., 2018). ESM is invasive because it requires that a craniotomy be performed to allow the surgical team access to the patient's brain; however, this allows brain–behavior relationships to be mapped at the level of actual cortical tissue. The mapping procedure itself can be performed either intraoperatively or extraoperatively. For intraoperative mapping, the patient may be given local anesthesia so that they remain awake and conscious for the entire procedure. In other cases, the patient receives general anesthesia during the craniotomy and is then awakened for the mapping procedure. In either case, an electrode array or handheld stimulator is used to administer electrical current to various cortical and subcortical sites while behavioral responses from the patient are monitored. During speech or language mapping, the patient may be asked to count, read aloud, name pictures, form sentences, or actively perform other relevant tasks. If the delivery of electrical current inhibits or interferes with the patient's performance (e.g., if they are briefly unable to name a picture they could otherwise name without difficulty), the underlying tissue is deemed "eloquent" (i.e., it supports the behavior of interest). The procedure is repeated in the area of the intended surgical intervention, and the locations of eloquent and noneloquent cortical tissue are tracked, allowing for the creation of a functional map of the patient's brain. This map is then used to guide the subsequent tissue/tumor resection so that eloquent tissue can be spared whenever possible, thereby preserving the associated behavioral functions. As discussed by So and Alwaki (2018), in the case of language mapping, it is critical for the surgical team to have a thorough understanding of the patient's baseline language skills so that ESM tasks can be customized to the patient's ability level, and stimulation-related errors can be readily distinguished from errors the patient might be prone to make anyway.

ESM can also be performed extraoperatively. In this case, a craniotomy is performed, and an electrode array is placed on the cortex; the patient's skull is then closed, and the patient is monitored in the hospital. As in the intraoperative procedure, electrical stimulation is delivered via the electrodes, and the effects of this stimulation on motor, sensory, or cognitive functions are mapped accordingly. Once monitoring and behavioral testing are complete and a viable cortical map has been generated, a second surgery is performed to remove the electrodes and, if necessary and appropriate, resect the pathological tissue. Since extraoperative ESM does not occur in the midst of surgery, mapping can be conducted at several different points in time, a more comprehensive evaluation may be conducted, and the consequences of a stimulation-induced seizure (one of the risks associated with ESM) may be less severe than in the intraoperative approach (Marks & Laxer, 209; Vakani & Nair, 2019). However, the surgical risks of extraoperative ESM may be greater than those of intraoperative ESM, given that the former involves two separate surgeries (Vakani & Nair, 2019). In either case, Ritaccio et al. (2018) note that ESM should be paired with electrocorticography (ECoG, described in detail later) in order to monitor for stimulus-related after-discharges (i.e., abnormal spikes in brain activity that follow administration of electrical stimulation and may presage the onset of a seizure). In addition to its clinical uses, ESM is utilized for research on the brain bases of cognitive-linguistic functions, often in patients who are already undergoing presurgical mapping to treat a medical condition (e.g., Mandonnet et al., 2007; Moritz-Gasser & Duffau, 2009).

Electrocorticography

Another technique for monitoring and localizing brain activity is electrocorticography (ECoG). ECoG is similar to EEG in that it involves the use of electrodes to monitor and measure electrical signals related to neural activity in the brain. However, in contrast to conventional EEG, the electrodes for ECoG are placed directly on the cortex, giving ECoG far better spatial resolution than EEG. Note that ECoG specifically refers to recording electrophysiological signals at the level of the cortex and is distinct from ESM. It is, however, often performed *during* ESM in order to monitor post-stimulation brain activity (Figure 9–20). ECoG can be performed intraoperatively or extraoperatively and is most commonly used to aid in planning epilepsy surgery by revealing regions of cortical tissue associated with seizures based on abnormal electrical signals (Yang et al., 2014). It may also be used to track brain activity during the performance of motor, cognitive, or language tasks.

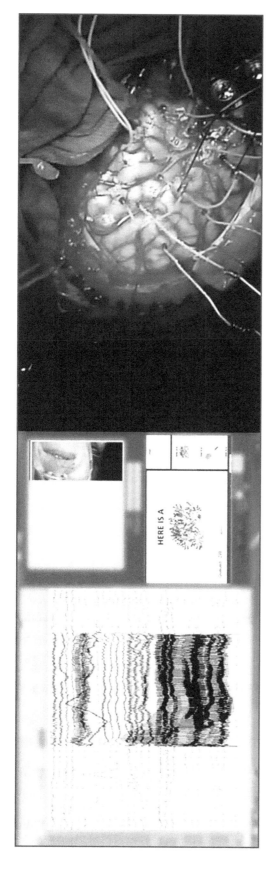

FIGURE 9-20. Intraoperative electrical stimulation mapping (ESM) and electrocorticography (ECoG), from Mahon et al. (2019). As the anesthetized but awake patient looks on, pictures, such as the tree in the center of the figure, are presented on a computer screen. The patient attempts to name the picture (e.g., "Here is a tree") as electrical pulses are delivered to her cortex with a handheld stimulator (not shown). When stimulation at a given site interferes with her naming performance, the site is flagged as eloquent tissue (i.e., it is pertinent to naming). The small, numbered tags on the cortex denote sites of interest to the surgical team—often, these sites represent eloquent tissue identified via ESM. The white leads with black tips positioned around the cortex are ECoG electrodes, which monitor electrophysiologic activity in the underlying tissue. On the far left, the ECoG readout is shown, with each line on the plot corresponding to an electrode. The dark black lines indicate changes in brain activity during and immediately following a pulse from the stimulator. Images courtesy of *JoVE*, with thanks to Bradford Z. Mahon and Benjamin L. Chernoff. (Mahon, B. Z., Mead, J. A., Chernoff, B. L., Sims, M. H., Garcea, F. E., Prentiss, E., . . . Pilcher, W. H. [2019]. Translational brain mapping at the University of Rochester Medical Center: Preserving the mind through personalized brain mapping. *Journal of Visualized Experiments*, 150. https://doi.org/10.3791/59592]

In fact, recent research suggests the precision of passive ECoG-based language mapping may be similar to that of ESM-based mapping, with the added benefit of a lower risk of seizure since ECoG does not require the application of electrical current to the cortex (Taplin et al., 2016). Like ESM, ECoG is not strictly limited to clinical applications; it is also used for research on speech, language, and other cognitive domains (e.g., Fedorenko et al., 2016).

Transcortical Magnetic Stimulation

TMS is another tool that supports functional brain mapping, and, in contrast to other techniques described in this section, it is noninvasive. Modern TMS was introduced in the 1980s as a more accessible, comfortable alternative to external electrical cortical stimulation (Barker et al., 1985). A TMS machine or stimulator produces an electrical current that passes through a coil, creating a brief but powerful and focal magnetic field beneath the coil. The coil is positioned over the scalp and the magnetic field from the coil induces a stimulating current in the underlying cortical tissue (Chervyakov et al., 2015; Peterchev et al., 209). If the stimulation is sufficiently strong, the current results in an action potential that propagates along stimulated neurons and may ultimately evoke an observable behavioral response. For example, when the coil is positioned over motor cortex, a single TMS pulse can cause twitches or movement in the muscles innervated by the stimulated neurons. By methodically administering pulses and logging the location of the coil over the skull and the evoked behavioral response, TMS can be used to map brain–behavior relationships in a similar fashion as ESM, albeit with poorer spatial resolution. The precision of TMS-based mapping can be enhanced via complementary neuronavigation systems that use ultrasound or other methods to track the location of the TMS coil in space and record the strength and position of the pulses relative to a computer model of the patient or subject's brain.

Whereas single TMS pulses can produce a visible motor response, repetitive TMS (rTMS), the administration of a series of pulses in rapid succession, has been found to interfere with various behaviors, including speech production and language functions (Devlin & Watkins, 2007). In other words, rTMS applied to certain brain regions, but not others, can cause transient disruptions in the performance of tasks like counting aloud or naming pictures, which helps researchers localize these functions in the brain. Thus, of interest to the SLP, TMS and rTMS have become increasingly popular tools for research on the neural bases of communicative functions like speech perception (Murakami et al., 2013) and picture naming (Naeser et al., 2011), as well as swallowing (Li et al.,

2020; Plowman-Prine et al., 2008). Given the capabilities and non-invasive nature of TMS, it plays a role in presurgical brain mapping for tumor and epilepsy management (see Clinical Applications of Neuroimaging Modalities), but its current utilization in the communication sciences and disorders is primarily in research, where it is used to map brain functions and as a potential neuromodulatory rehabilitation tool, as described in Box 9–9.

Box 9–9. Neuromodulation in Speech, Language, and Swallowing Disorders

Neuromodulation refers to the application of an external stimulus intended to alter neural function, often with the goal of evoking a positive and lasting change in behavior. rTMS and a related tool called transcranial direct current stimulation (tDCS) are two examples of neuromodulatory techniques that are the subject of much interest in speech-language pathology research today. The basic idea is that these techniques may be utilized instead of or in conjunction with traditional speech-language therapy to boost rehabilitation outcomes for patients with neurologic damage or disease. Indeed, there is a growing body of research suggesting that rTMS and tDCS may aid in recovery from disorders of speech, language, cognition, and swallowing (Coslett, 2016; Dionísio et al., 2018; Fridriksson et al., 2018; Murdoch & Barwood, 2013; Shigematsu et al., 2013). While these neuromodulatory approaches are mostly confined to the realm of research at present, they are on the cusp of entering the clinical arena, and it is likely that many SLPs working in health care settings will encounter them in practice in the future.

Like ESM, an important benefit of TMS is that it allows for causal evaluation of brain–behavior dynamics. That is, stimulation applied over a particular region of the brain can evoke an observable behavioral response in real time, thereby demonstrating or confirming a direct link between the two. TMS has the important added benefit of being noninvasive, making it safer and more appropriate for research purposes than ESM. However, TMS has lower spatial resolution than ESM, as well as several risks of its own. These include seizure (rare in standard TMS, slightly less so in rTMS), the potential to cause heating or displacement of metal implants in the head or eyes, transient headache, discomfort or pain at the stimulation site, and the possibility of transient hearing changes (Rossi et al., 2009). As such, patients are typically screened for a recent history of seizures, cochlear and other implants, and the presence of metal in the head or eyes prior to undergoing TMS; hearing protection is provided during the procedure.

Clinical Applications of Neuroimaging Modalities

The type of imaging that is done in clinical settings depends on the equipment that is available and the pathology that is suspected to underlie the patient's symptoms. You may have noticed when reading this chapter that certain neuroimaging modalities can provide similar information regarding brain structure or function. For example, CTA and MRA both provide information about the gross structure of blood vessels. Perfusion imaging of the microvasculature can be performed with CT perfusion, MR-based ASL and contrast-enhanced PWI, and PET and SPECT with specific radiotracers. The use of one modality over another depends on the specific information clinicians or researchers aim to gather, what types of neuroimaging devices are accessible, and contraindications for certain scans patients may have.

Overall, the goal of clinical neuroimaging is to identify brain abnormalities, determine the etiology of those abnormalities, and use that information to establish a treatment plan for the patient. As such, all neuroimaging modalities can be thought of as diagnostic tools, where clinicians aim to determine *how*, *where*, and *why* brain structure or function has changed in patients with specific behavioral symptoms. To further illustrate these concepts, let's use dementia as an example. There are many forms of dementia (see the Neurodegenerative Diseases section later). All dementias are characterized by similar changes in brain structure (i.e., the *how*) but in different parts of the brain (i.e., the *where*) and for different underlying reasons (i.e., the *why*). For example, in dementia associated with Alzheimer's disease, there is neuronal cell loss in bilateral temporoparietal areas, especially the medial temporal lobes, due to beta-amyloid plaques and neurofibrillary tau protein tangle aggregation. In contrast, in dementia associated with Huntington's disease, neuronal cell loss occurs in the head of the caudate and other striatal structures due to an autosomal dominant gene mutation that causes toxicities in the protein huntingtin. This example oversimplifies the intricacies of differential diagnosis, especially for disorders with closer underlying pathology, but it still illustrates the general uses of neuroimaging.

Although SLPs do not diagnose medical diseases, it is important that they understand how other medical professionals (e.g., neurologists, oncologists) do and how neuroimaging factors into diagnoses. For many CNS disorders, clinical diagnosis involves combining information gleaned from multiple sources (e.g., the medical history, neurologic exam, behavioral tests, genetic tests, body fluid tests, neuroimaging examinations) to narrow down many potential conditions to one likely candidate disorder. The type of information used to determine a differential diagnosis varies by disorder. Currently, neuroimaging biological markers (i.e., **biomarkers**) are critical for differential diagnosis of certain disorders included within the scope of medical SLP (e.g., ischemic and hemorrhagic stroke, moderate to severe traumatic brain injury, hydrocephalus, brain and head and neck cancer). For other disorders (e.g., concussion, different types of dementia, Parkinson's disease, multiple sclerosis), neuroimaging can be used to support a clinical diagnosis, but as of now, neuroimaging techniques are not advanced enough to provide a definitive imaging biomarker for differential diagnosis.

To avoid misdiagnosis, clinical imaging is often used to differentiate a specific disorder from other disorders with similar symptoms (i.e., *mimics*). For example, stroke mimics include transient ischemic attack, conversion disorder, seizure, brain tumor, infection, low blood sugar, and migraine (Barthel et al., 2015; Moulin & Leys, 2019; Vilela, 2017). Clinical imaging can be important even for disorders for which imaging cannot solely provide a differential diagnosis; for example, for individuals with suspected multiple sclerosis, MRI is often used to exclude stroke, tumor, small vessel disease, cerebral amyloid angiopathy, and other conditions (Aliaga & Barkhof, 2014; Chen et al., 2016).

In the remainder of this section, we describe neuroimaging modalities commonly used to assess brain structure or function abnormalities in disorders with speech, language, cognitive, or swallowing symptoms. We mainly focus on imaging used in routine clinical testing, but we also highlight advances in research that show promise for entering the clinical arena in the near future.

Stroke

When a patient is admitted to the emergency department with a suspected stroke, noncontrast CT or MRI is used to quickly confirm that the patient had a stroke, to establish whether the stroke was due to *ischemia* (i.e., blocked artery) or *hemorrhage* (i.e., brain bleed), and to determine what brain tissue is at risk. In most hospitals, patients often first undergo CT, since CT scanning is faster than MRI sequences and, despite radiation exposure, is safe for most people (with the exception of young children or women who are pregnant) (Domingues et al., 2015; Hakimi & Garg, 2016; Macdonald & Schweizer, 2017). For individuals who are MR-safe, follow-up MRI scans including multiple pulse sequences (T1-weighted, T2-weighted, FLAIR, DWI, PWI, and sometimes SWI) are often performed.

CT and MRI have similar sensitivity and specificity for identifying acute hemorrhage (Figure 9–21A and B) (Domingues et al., 2015; Fiebach et al., 2004). However, after about a week post-hemorrhage, the stroke lesion has the same density as surrounding

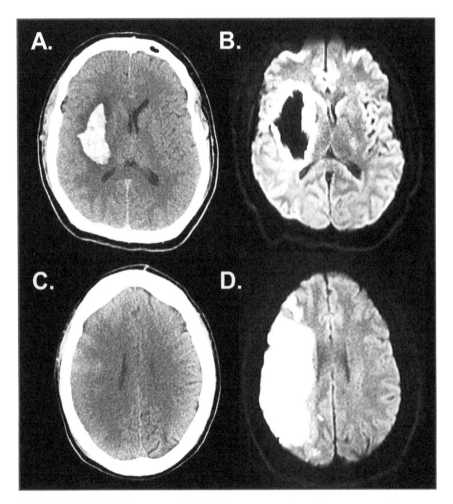

FIGURE 9–21. CT versus MR-DWI for acute stroke. A large, acute intracranial hemorrhage within the left hemisphere is visible on both CT (**A**) and DWI (**B**) trace images, whereas a large, acute ischemic stroke in another patient is difficult to see on CT (**C**) but very visible on DWI (**D**). Author-created image constructed using data from NIH/NIDCD R01DC005375, R01DC015466, and P50DC014664 (PI: Argye E. Hillis).

functional tissue and is therefore much more difficult to identify using CT than MRI (Hakimi & Garg, 2016). In the case of hemorrhage due to a ruptured aneurysm, CTA or MRA is often done to visualize the structure of the vessels. In cases where an unruptured aneurysm was found on CT or other MRI sequences, CTA or MRA can be used as a follow-up to assist with surgical planning (Ajiboye et al., 2015). For example, Figure 9–22 shows snapshots of a head MRA performed in a patient with an aneurysm within the left inferior frontal lobe. Besides ruptured aneurysms, other

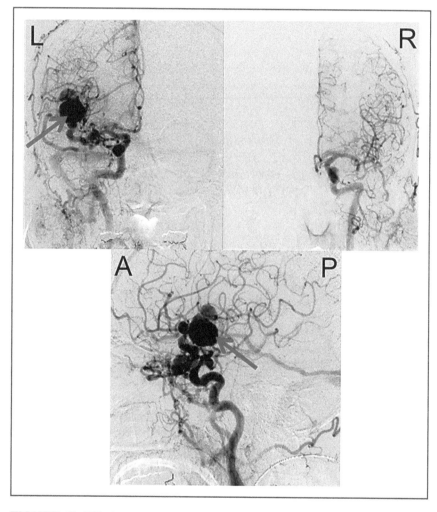

FIGURE 9–22. Images obtained from magnetic resonance angiography (MRA) performed in a patient with a large, left frontal aneurysm. The aneurysm, denoted by the red arrows, is visible in the coronal (*top left*) and sagittal (*bottom*) MRA images showing the left hemisphere vasculature. The MRA image at the top right shows normal right-sided vasculature. L = left, R = right, A = anterior, P = posterior. Author-created image constructed using data from NIH/NIDCD R01DC005375, R01DC015466, and P50DC014664 (PI: Argye E. Hillis).

common causes of nontraumatic hemorrhage are cerebral amyloid angiopathy and arterial vasculopathy due to increased blood pressure (Brody et al., 2015; Hakimi & Garg, 2016). In such cases, CT is inferior to MRI, SWI in particular, in determining the underlying cause of hemorrhage and identifying small microbleeds.

For acute ischemic stroke, MRI is superior to CT (Figure 9–21C and D). Specifically, DWI is the gold-standard sequence for detecting acute ischemic stroke and for determining candidacy for thrombolytic therapy like tissue plasminogen activator (tPA), which is used to break up blood clots (Cohen et al., 2011; Hjort et al., 2005; Ledezma et al., 2009; Merino & Warach, 2010). Acute lesions appear **hyperintense** (i.e., bright white) on trace DWI and dark black on ADC images. In addition to DWI, PWI is frequently used in acute ischemic stroke to evaluate changes in cerebral microvasculature. Specifically, low cerebral blood flow (i.e., *hypoperfusion*) and decreased blood volume in the infarction core will ultimately result in tissue death (i.e., *necrosis*), but hypoperfusion and prolonged blood flow transit times are also observed in the ischemic *penumbra* (i.e., the area surrounding the core of the infarct) in the immediate aftermath of stroke. Mismatch between the area of acute infarct visible on DWI and the area of hypoperfusion evident through PWI—**PWI/DWI mismatch**—can explain the extent of behavioral deficits seen in patients after ischemic stroke (Figure 9–23) (Beaulieu et al., 1999; Hakimelahi et al., 2012; Hillis et al., 2001, 2002, 2004, 2008; Sorensen et al., 1996).

In chronic ischemic stroke (months to years after infarct), T1-weighted, T2-weighted, and FLAIR scans are used to visualize changes in brain structure. By the chronic stage of recovery, tissue that has died has been sectioned off from intact tissue by astrocytes, and the stroke core is a CSF-filled cavity, often surrounded by gliosis. As such, chronic strokes appear black on T1-weighted images and bright white on T2-weighted images. On FLAIR, CSF-filled lesions appear dark black, and the surrounding gliosis is white. Note that the ability to visualize ischemic stroke lesions on different MRI sequences depends on stroke chronicity. Figure 9–24 shows different images for a patient with a large acute left hemisphere ischemic stroke (easily visible on the DWI trace image) and a prior, chronic right inferior frontal lobe lesion (most visible on T1-weighted, T2-weighted and FLAIR images).

Traumatic Brain Injury

In traumatic brain injuries (TBIs), the primary injury is direct structural damage due to trauma, but secondary injury mechanisms

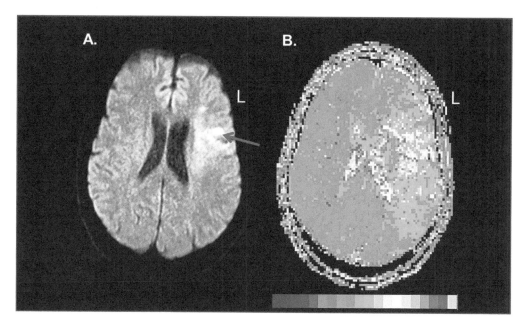

FIGURE 9–23. Mismatch in diffusion-weighted imaging (DWI) (**A**) and perfusion-weighted imaging (PWI) (**B**) in a patient with a new left hemisphere ischemic stroke. Note that the figures are shown in radiologic orientation, with the left hemisphere depicted on the right, and vice versa. Bright white hyperintense areas (*indicated by the red arrow*) in the DWI shown in **A** reflect the infarct core. In the PWI in **B**, voxels in the infarct core appear yellow, orange, or red, whereas lighter green voxels in the left hemisphere reflect hypoperfused tissue surrounding the infarct core. Normally perfused tissue in the right hemisphere is teal/dark green. L = left. Author-created image constructed using data from NIH/NIDCD R01DC005375, R01DC015466, and P50DC014664 (PI: Argye E. Hillis).

occur at a cellular level (e.g., hydrocephalus, edema, disruption of the blood brain barrier, reduced metabolism, etc.). Many different types of injuries fall within the broad umbrella of TBI, including, but not limited to, concussion; hematomas (i.e., collections of blood) and hemorrhages in different locations in the brain; and **traumatic axonal injury** (TAI; i.e., damage to white matter axons due to strain and shearing forces). When a patient is admitted to the emergency department with a suspected head injury, the first scan that is done is often noncontrast CT. As referenced previously, CT is able to quickly identify traumatic hemorrhages as well as skull fractures, contusions, and hematomas in emergency situations. In the case of moderate to severe TBI, CT can quickly reveal the need for surgical intervention (Mutch et al., 2016).

In cases of concussion or mild TBI, modern MRI structural sequences (T1, T2, FLAIR) are superior to noncontrast CT in identifying very small hemorrhages or contusions (Brody et al., 2015; Mutch et al., 2016). Nonetheless, routine clinical scans may appear

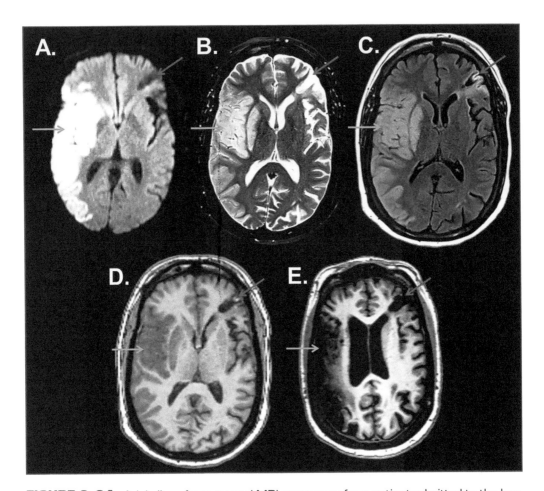

FIGURE 9–24. Axial slices from several MRI sequences for a patient admitted to the hospital with a new, large left hemisphere ischemic stroke (*denoted by blue arrows*) and a prior right inferior frontal stroke (*denoted by red arrows*). The acute MRI performed 1 day poststroke included diffusion-weighted imaging (DWI) (**A**), T2-weighted (**B**), fluid-attenuated inversion recovery (FLAIR) (**C**), and T1-weighted (**D**) sequences. In the acute images, the large left hemisphere stroke is most visible on DWI and least visible on T1-weighted imaging. In contrast, the left hemisphere stroke is very visible in **E**, an axial slice taken from a T1-weighted magnetization-prepared rapid acquisition with gradient echo (MPRAGE) sequence conducted approximately 9 months after the left hemisphere stroke occurred. The patient's prior right inferior frontal stroke occurred several years prior to the left hemisphere stroke; as such, it is visible in all images. Author-created image constructed using data from NIH/NIDCD R01DC005375, R01DC015466, and P50DC014664 (PI: Argye E. Hillis).

normal in concussion and mild TBI due to the nature of the injury (Blennow et al., 2016; Brody et al., 2015; Mutch et al., 2016). Specifically, TAI is essentially undetectable on routine clinical CT and MRI sequences. While DTI is optimal for revealing changes to the white matter microstructure due to TAI (Blennow et al., 2016; Hulkower et al., 2013; Niogi & Mukherjee, 2010; Wintermark et al., 2015), DTI sequences have not been incorporated into routine MRI scans in most hospitals. Unlike other MRI sequences, SWI can detect blood products and microhemorrhages often seen in patients with TBI, and as such, SWI is now often added to clinical imaging routines (Bonfante et al., 2018; Mutch et al., 2016; Wintermark et al., 2015). PET and SPECT are also able to identify changes in cerebral blood flow and brain metabolism, even in the event of normal structural CT or MRI scans (Blennow et al., 2016; Bonfante et al., 2018; Byrnes et al., 2014; Raji et al., 2014; Wintermark et al., 2015).

Each of the aforementioned scans and sequences are used to evaluate longitudinal changes in brain structure or function following TBI. For example, Figure 9–25 shows the evolution of an intracranial hematoma from an initial CT scan to a CT scan several hours after injury. Neuroimaging can even be used to evaluate persistent changes in brain metabolism in the months to years postinjury. In cases of severe TBI that result in coma, EEG-based neural oscillations and ERPs (especially the MMN and P300) also appear to have good prognostic value in predicting outcomes and awakening from coma (Boccagni et al., 2011; Daltrozzo et al., 2007; Fingelkurts et al., 2019; Morlet & Fischer, 2014). Brain injury can also result in seizure activity, which is often monitored in hospital settings using continuous EEG (Barkley & Baumgartner, 2003; Britton et al., 2016).

Neurodegenerative Diseases

Neurodegenerative diseases are characterized by progressive loss of neuronal tissue in areas of the brain involved in cognitive-linguistic, motor and/or sensory processing. Neurodegenerative diseases that have symptoms that fall within the SLP scope include Alzheimer's disease, Huntington's disease, Parkinson's disease, subtypes of frontotemporal dementia (FTD) (i.e., behavioral variant of FTD, nonfluent and semantic variants of primary progressive aphasia, supranuclear palsy, cortico-basal degeneration), Lewy body dementia, vascular dementia, and amyotrophic lateral sclerosis (ALS). Differential diagnosis of these disorders is challenging, particularly in early disease stages, and no single test or marker can definitively provide a diagnosis. Therefore, neuroimaging biomarkers are used in combination with clinical assessment and fluid biomarkers to differentiate these disorders (Eisenmenger et al., 2016; Gorno-Tempini et al., 2011).

As a first line of inquiry, CT scans and/or various structural MRI sequences (e.g., T1-weighted, T2-weighted, FLAIR scans) are used to assess morphologic changes in cortical structures due

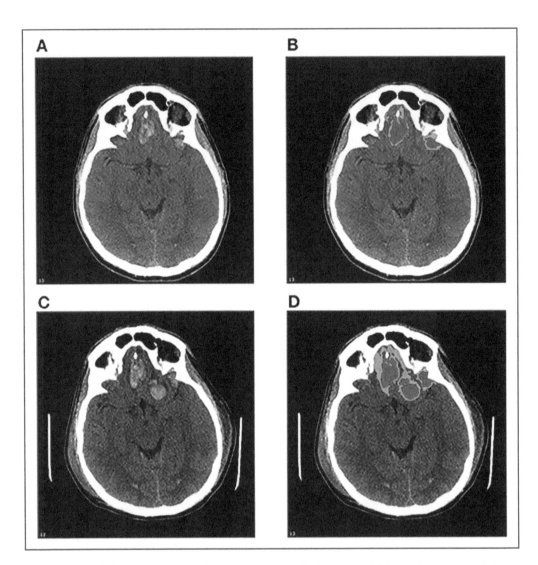

FIGURE 9–25. Change over time in a traumatic intracranial hematoma on CT, from Wilkes et al. (2018). An axial slice from an initial CT scan post-injury is shown without annotation (**A**) and with the lesion annotated (**B**). At a few (9–36) hours post-injury, the hematoma has evolved, as shown in unannotated (**C**) and annotated (**D**) axial images. In **B** and **D**, high-density areas that reflect blood are annotated in red and low-density areas that reflect edema surrounding the hematoma are annotated in green. (Wilkes, S., McCormack, E., Kenney, K., Stephens, B., Passo, R., Harburg, L., . . . Diaz-Arrastia, R. [2018]. Evolution of traumatic parenchymal intracranial hematomas (ICHs): Comparison of hematoma and edema components. *Frontiers in Neurology, 9.* https://doi.org/10.3389/fneur.2018.00527)

to neuronal loss (Barthel et al., 2015; Zukotynski et al., 2018). However, cortical atrophy and ventricular enlargement visible on structural scans occur at later stages of neurodegenerative disease (Figure 9–26). On the other hand, pathologic changes in brain

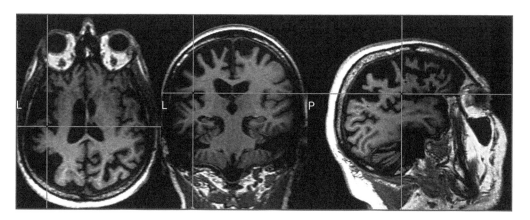

FIGURE 9–26. A T1-weighted MPRAGE image in an individual with primary progressive aphasia. Pronounced atrophy is visible in the left hemisphere compared to the relatively intact structure of the right hemisphere. L = left, P = posterior. Author-created image constructed using data from NIH/NIDCD RO1DCO11317 and RO1DCO15466 (PI: Argye E. Hillis).

metabolism and biochemistry precede changes in brain structure (Barthel et al., 2015; Eisenmenger et al., 2016; Goffin & van Laere, 2016). Therefore, nuclear imaging techniques—and PET in particular for most forms of dementia—are important for early detection and diagnosis (Barthel et al., 2015).

Breakthroughs in Alzheimer's disease research show that PET imaging can be used to identify beta-amyloid and neurofibrillary tau protein tangles—biomarkers of AD—even before clinical symptoms manifest and changes in brain structure occur (Agosta et al., 2017; Bao et al., 2017; Barthel et al., 2015; Betthauser, 2019; Eisenmenger et al., 2016; Hall et al., 2017; Jack et al., 2018; Meyer et al., 2019; Scheltens et al., 2016; Syed & Deeks, 2015; Valkanova & Ebmeier, 2014; Valotassiou et al., 2018; Zhang et al., 2017). Negative beta-amyloid findings and the additional presence of alpha-synuclein protein in PET imaging are suggestive of FTD pathology instead of Alzheimer's disease (Agosta et al., 2017; Barthel et al., 2015; Diehl-Schmid et al., 2014; Eisenmenger et al., 2016; Gordon et al., 2016; Whitwell, 2019). As another example, PET and SPECT imaging with radiotracers that target dopamine synthesis can be used to differentiate Parkinson's disease from other parkinsonian syndromes (Barthel et al., 2015; Eisenmenger et al., 2016; Pagano et al., 2016). PET imaging is also an emerging tool for the detection of tau protein buildup in patients with chronic traumatic encephalopathy (Barrio et al., 2015; Blennow et al., 2016; Dallmeier et al., 2019; Eisenmenger et al., 2016). As shown in Figure 9–27, PET imaging with radiotracers sensitive to tau deposition have been used to differentiate healthy individuals and patients with different

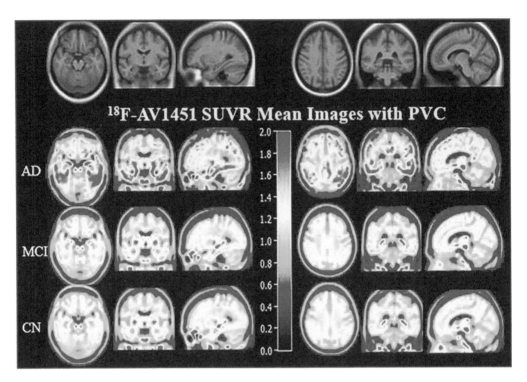

FIGURE 9–27. Differences in brain metabolism per PET imaging between different patient and control groups, modified from Zhao et al. (2019). Greater accumulation of the radiotracer ([18F-AV1451) according to the standardized uptake value ratio (SUVR)—indicative of greater pathologic tau—is evident in patients with Alzheimer's disease (AD) compared to patients with mild cognitive impairment (MCI) and healthy controls (CN). Note that because of the low spatial resolution of PET, the authors implemented a partial volume correction (PVC). (Zhao, Q., Liu, M., Ha, L., Zhou, Y., & Alzheimer's Disease Neuroimaging Initiative. [2019]. Quantitative 18F-AV1451 brain tau PET imaging in cognitively normal older adults, mild cognitive impairment, and Alzheimer's disease patients. *Frontiers in Neurology*, 10. https://doi.org/10.3389/fneur.2019.00486)

neurodegenerative disorders from each other and to track disease progression. While these research advances show promise, SPECT and PET findings are not yet part of consensus criteria in clinical diagnosis of any neurodegenerative disease.

While most of the aforementioned neurodegenerative disorders involve neuronal cell loss within cerebral cortex structures, ALS is characterized by progressive loss of motor neurons in the spinal cord or brainstem. Differential diagnosis of ALS requires evidence of lower-motor neuron symptoms according to clinical, neurologic, and/or electrophysiologic testing (Brooks et al., 2000). While patients with suspected ALS often undergo structural MRI scanning, brain imaging findings are not included in the current consensus criteria for ALS diagnosis. Instead, recent diagnostic criteria emphasize the role of **electromyography (EMG)**, which measures electrical muscle activity, in providing critical information regarding muscle function (Bashford et al., 2020; de Carvalho et al., 2008; Geevasinga et al., 2016). Although not part of routine clinical imaging, advanced MR-based techniques such as DTI and MR spectroscopy show promise in aiding diagnosis and monitoring disease progression in ALS (Cardenas-Blanco et al., 2016; El Mendili et al., 2019; Kassubek & Pagani, 2019; Li et al., 2019).

Autoimmune Disorders

Autoimmune disorders are diseases in which the immune system attacks tissues within a person's body. One common autoimmune disorder is multiple sclerosis (MS), which is characterized by inflammation, demyelination, and loss of axons. In patients with MS, damaged white matter (often called *plaques* or *lesions*) show up as hyperintensities on MRI-based T2-weighted and FLAIR sequences. Chronic plaques appear as black areas on T1-weighted images (Chen et al., 2016). Because timing is crucial for the different subtypes of MS (i.e., clinically isolated, relapsing–remitting, primary progressive, and secondary progressive MS), lesion distribution throughout the brain and when lesions appear on the aforementioned MRI scans are important factors to consider. However, T2 hyperintensities and T1 "black holes" also occur in other disorders, so these imaging abnormalities cannot be used for differential MS diagnosis (Chen et al., 2016; Filippi et al., 2016; Giorgio & De Stefano, 2018; Enzinger et al., 2015; Thompson et al., 2018). Although MRI findings in MS are nonspecific, MRI is still recommended in all patients with suspected MS (Thompson et al., 2018). Nonconventional, advanced imaging methods like SWI and DTI (Figure 9–28), among others, show promise for identifying microstructural white matter changes that are specific to MS (Filippi et al., 2018; Enzinger et al., 2015), yet most of these methods currently are not ready for routine clinical implementation.

Two other autoimmune disorders medical SLPs may encounter are Guillain-Barré syndrome, characterized by acute neuropathy that causes muscle weakness and sometimes paralysis, and myasthenia gravis, a disorder in which the immune system attacks the *neuromuscular junction* (i.e., the connection between nerves and muscles). Routine clinical neuroimaging plays little to no role in differential diagnosis of either disorder. Nonetheless, in Guillain-Barré syndrome, nerve conduction studies or structural MRI of the spinal cord can support disease diagnosis and monitoring (van den Berg et al., 2014; Willison et al., 2016). Similarly, repetitive nerve

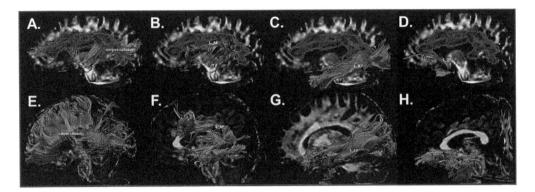

FIGURE 9–28. Major white matter pathways that play a crucial role in speech and language functions, including the corpus callosum, left arcuate fasciculus (L_AF), left inferior longitudinal fasciculus (L_ILF), and left uncinate fasciculus (L_UF). **A–D.** The afore-listed tracts are shown in a patient with multiple sclerosis (MS) who has extensive periventricular white matter lesions (shown in red) and advanced cognitive and verbal fluency impairments. Although some fibers still travel across white matter lesions, most lesions lead to white matter fiber loss and disconnection between the regions critical for language. **E–H.** The same white matter tracts are shown in a healthy subject who does not have MS. Courtesy of Zafer Keser, work supported by NIH/NINDS K23NS072134 to Flavia M. Nelson and DUNN research foundation funding to Khader M. Hasan.

stimulation testing and/or EMG can assist with diagnosis of myasthenia gravis (Gilhus et al., 2019; Mantegazza & Cavalcante, 2019; Pasnoor et al., 2018).

Tumors

Neuroimaging plays a critical role in initial cancer diagnosis, tumor monitoring, and evaluation of treatment response in oncology (Henriksen et al., 2016). CT and structural MRI sequences (T1-weighted, T2-weighted, FLAIR) can be used to assess the anatomic features (location, size) of brain, head, or neck tumors, although MRI is generally superior to CT for detection of brain tumors (Fink et al., 2015). However, current MRI sequences lack the sensitivity and specificity for detecting very small tumors and for distinguishing tumor recurrence from tumor mimics (e.g., inflammation) (Ehman et al., 2017).

PET and SPECT imaging—particularly combined PET/CT or most recently, PET/MRI—are routinely used in diagnosis and treatment evaluation for oncology patients. Besides detection, combined MRI/PET and CT/PET are used to determine if a tumor can be removed (i.e., *resected*) and what approach is best (Queiroz & Huellner, 2015). There are some advantages of PET/MRI over PET/CT for certain primary head and neck tumors (e.g., oral and pharyngeal) (Ehman et al., 2017; Fink et al., 2015; Queiroz & Huellner,

2015). However, future studies must prove the utility of PET/MRI for different types of cancers, and PET/MRI scanners must become more widely available before PET/MRI overtakes PET/CT. As Figure 9–29 shows, though, combined MRI and PET imaging can provide important complementary information for tumor diagnosis and monitoring response to treatment and future recurrence.

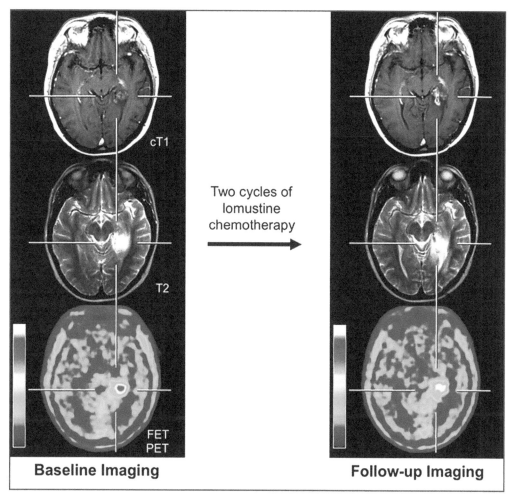

FIGURE 9–29. Monitoring treatment response in brain tumor using MRI and PET, from Galldiks and Langen (2016). This figure compares MRI (*top and middle images*) and amino acid PET (*bottom images*) scans taken before (*left*) and after (*right*) several months of chemotherapy for a tumor in the left parahippocampal region in a 31-year-old patient. While the MRI images appear to indicate that the tumor has progressed, the PET scans reveal a reduction in metabolic activity in the area of the tumor after treatment. The latter finding suggests the patient is experiencing a treatment-related phenomenon known as "pseudoprogression" rather than actual progression of the tumor. Note that the images are presented in radiologic orientation, such that the left hemisphere is shown on the right and vice versa. (Galldiks, N., & Langen, K.-J. [2016]. Amino acid PET—An imaging option to identify treatment response, posttherapeutic effects, and tumor recurrence? *Frontiers in Neurology, 7.* https://doi.org/10.3389/fneur.2016.00120)

Finally, surgical planning for tumor resection is often guided by brain mapping techniques like fMRI, ESM, and TMS (Frey et al., 2014; Nadkarni et al., 2015; Szelényi et al., 2010), which help the surgical team identify brain areas that are critical to motor, cognitive, or language functions and should be spared if possible.

Seizure Disorders

For many individuals with epilepsy or other seizure disorders, surgical intervention is the best treatment option available for stopping or reducing the frequency of seizures. Often, the goal of such intervention is to remove or destroy the brain tissue believed to be responsible for seizure activity, so it is crucial for the medical team to locate the area from which the seizures arise. Thus, patients typically undergo an extensive presurgical evaluation that includes, among other things, inpatient and/or outpatient monitoring via EEG to localize seizure or pre-seizure activity, and structural (T1, T2, and FLAIR) MRI to identify lesions or other abnormalities that may underlie the patient's disorder (Baumgartner et al., 2019; Ryvlin & Rheims, 2008). Importantly, and perhaps more relevant to the SLP, a second goal of the presurgical evaluation is to identify language- and memory-eloquent tissue in the brain to help the surgical team avoid, as much as possible, damaging areas that will result in a functional deficit (Baumgartner et al., 2019; Ryvlin & Rheims, 2008). Thus, patients may undergo Wada testing to determine if their language and/or memory functions are predominantly lateralized to the same hemisphere as the source of their seizures. More focal evaluations may also be performed via fMRI, TMS, MEG, or intra- or extraoperative ESM or ECoG (Ritaccio et al., 2018) in order to derive precise functional maps of brain–behavior relationships that can be used to guide surgery.

Practical Tips for Clinical Practice

Before we conclude this chapter, there are several practical considerations regarding the role of neuroimaging in clinical speech-language pathology that practitioners would do well to keep in mind:

■ Despite the many factors that impact the selection of one neuroimaging modality over another (see Clinical Applications of Neuroimaging Modalities), many hospitals typically adhere to certain routine protocols in emergency situations. For instance, a patient admitted to the emergency department with a suspected acute stroke is likely to undergo an initial CT scan, especially if their suitability for MRI from a safety perspective is unknown. A multisequence structural MRI may be performed as a follow-up, depending on the results of the CT scan and assuming the patient's MR safety can be confirmed. If the patient is admitted to the hospital, subsequent MRI or CT scans would likely be repeated in the first few days to monitor the evolution of the stroke and verify findings from the initial scans. In a case of intracerebral hemorrhage, the patient would undergo further evaluation via CTA or MRA to assess the cerebral vasculature.

Not all scans, even those that are ostensibly the same, are created equal. For example, the quality of two T1 MRI images obtained from different machines may be visibly different, depending on the types and ages of the scanners and the specific scan parameters used.

After a scan, a radiologist reviews the images and typically documents their main findings in a report that is available in a patient's medical record. These reports can be as valuable as the images themselves (and in some cases, even more so), as they provide an expert's interpretation of the pathology they observed.

For many neuroimaging modalities, patient motion during scanning degrades image quality and limits the amount or value of information that can be gleaned from the images (Figure 9–30A). In some cases, it can be challenging to distinguish motion from pathology, so check the imaging report for any reference to the impact patient motion had on image quality.

In MRI, susceptibility artifacts (i.e., distortions in the magnetic field that appear as blurring or loss of signal on an image) can be caused by magnetic field inhomogeneities in tissues near air-filled sinuses. These artifacts are often found in the frontal and temporal lobes and should not be confused with brain pathology (Figure 9–30B).

SLPs may encounter nonspecific brain abnormalities such as *white matter hyperintensities* on T2 and FLAIR MRI images or references to such abnormalities in imaging reports (Figure 9–30C). While these abnormalities may reflect underlying pathology, they are not specific to any one disorder.

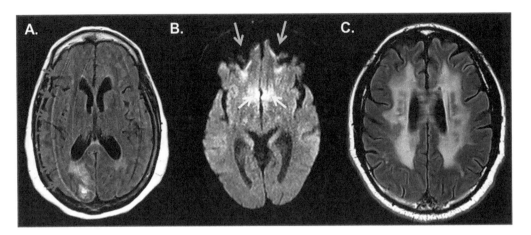

FIGURE 9–30. Artifacts and nonspecific findings visible on MRI, including motion arti-fact (*denoted by red arrows*) visible on a FLAIR axial slice (**A**), distortions (*denoted by blue arrows*) and artifacts due to scan parameters (*denoted by yellow arrows*) visible on DWI (**B**), and extensive white matter hyperintensities visible on a FLAIR axial slice in another partici-pant (**C**). Author-created image constructed using data from NIH/NIDCD RO1DC005375, RO1DC015466, and P50DC014664 (PI: Argye E. Hillis).

> ▪ In most medical settings, SLPs are part of a larger team. Other team members may have extensive experience reading imaging reports and viewing neuroimages, so ask questions and take advantage of your colleagues' expertise.

Conclusion

Although most SLPs are not directly involved in acquiring, pro-cessing, or reading neuroimages, the domain of neuroimaging is immensely relevant to the field of speech-language pathology. The various modalities described in this chapter are crucial to the diag-nosis and management of many neurogenic disorders that affect communication and swallowing and are instrumental to modern research on normal and dysfunctional speech, language, hearing, and cognitive processes. For the medical SLP, neuroimages and neuroimaging reports are no substitute for a thorough behavioral evaluation, but they can be an excellent source of supplementary information. Moreover, as our understanding of the relationships between speech, language, and swallowing therapy and brain func-tion and structure continues to evolve, neuroimaging data, includ-ing that obtained via routine clinical scans, will likely become more directly relevant to prognostication and treatment planning in medical speech-language pathology settings.

Questions for Discussion

1. What is the scientific basis for CT? What about MRI? How do the scientific bases of each of these modalities relate to their chief health/safety risks?

2. A patient with a recent history of headaches and cognitive changes presents at the emergency department at his local hospital. His son mentions that he has a pacemaker. What type(s) of neuroimaging is he likely to undergo, and why?

3. How do structural and functional neuroimaging modalities differ? What are some of the primary applications of each?

4. In what ways might knowledge of neuroimaging inform or impact your clinical practice?

References

Abou-Khalil, B. (2007). An update on determination of language dominance in screening for epilepsy surgery: The Wada test and newer noninvasive alternatives. *Epilepsia*, *48*(3), 442–455. https://doi.org/10.1111/j.1528-1167.2007.01012.x

Agosta, F., Galantucci, S., & Filippi, M. (2017). Advanced magnetic resonance imaging of neurodegenerative diseases. *Neurological Sciences*, *38*(1), 41–51. https://doi.org/10.1007/s10072-016-2764-x

Ainsworth-Darnell, K., Shulman, H. G., & Boland, J. E. (1998). Dissociating brain responses to syntactic and semantic anomalies: Evidence from event-related potentials. *Journal of Memory and Language*, *38*(1), 19–130. https://doi.org/10.1006/jmla.1997.2537

Ajiboye, N., Chalouhi, N., Starke, R. M., Zanaty, M., & Bell, R. (2015). Unruptured cerebral aneurysms: Evaluation and management. *Scientific World Journal*, *2015*, 1–10. https://doi.org/10.1155/2015/954954

Aliaga, E. S., & Barkhof, F. (2014). MRI mimics of multiple sclerosis. In D. S. Goodin (Ed.), *Handbook of clinical neurology* (Vol. 122, pp. 291–316). Elsevier. https://doi.org/10.1016/B978-0-444-52001-2.00012-1

Almandoz, J. E. D., Kamalian, S., González, R. G., Lev, M. H., & Romero, J. M. (2011). Imaging of acute ischemic stroke: Stroke CT angiography (CTA). In R. G. González, J. A. Hirsch, M. H. Lev, P. W. Schaefer, & L. H. Schwamm (Eds.), *Acute ischemic stroke* (pp. 57–82). Springer Berlin Heidelberg. https://doi.org/10.1007/978-3-642-12751-9_4

Bao, W., Jia, H., Finnema, S., Cai, Z., Carson, R. E., & Huang, Y. H. (2017). PET imaging for early detection of Alzheimer's disease. *PET Clinics*, *9*(3), 329–350. https://doi.org/10.1016/j.cpet.2017.03.001

Barker, A. T., Jalinous, R., & Freeston, I. L. (1985). Non-invasive magnetic stimulation of human motor cortex. *The Lancet*, *325* (8437), 1106–1107. https://doi.org/10.1016/S0140-6736(85)92413-4

Barkley, G. L., & Baumgartner, C. (2003). MEG and EEG in epilepsy. *Journal of Clinical Neurophysiology, 20*(3), 163–178. https://doi.org/10.1097/00004691-200305000-00002

Barrio, J. R., Small, G. W., Wong, K.P., Huang, S.C., Liu, J., Merrill, D. A., . . . Kepe, V. (2015). In vivo characterization of chronic traumatic encephalopathy using [F-18] FDDNP PET brain imaging. *Proceedings of the National Academy of Sciences, 19*(16), E2039–E2047. https://doi.org/10.1073/pnas.1409952112

Barthel, H., Schroeter, M. L., Hoffmann, K. T., & Sabri, O. (2015). PET/MR in dementia and other neurodegenerative diseases. *Seminars in Nuclear Medicine, 45*(3), 224–233. https://doi.org/10.1053/j.semnuclmed.2014.12.003

Bashford, J., Mills, K., & Shaw, C. (2020). The evolving role of surface electromyography in amyotrophic lateral sclerosis: A systematic review. *Clinical Neurophysiology, 131*(4), 942–950. https://doi.org/10.1016/j.clinph.2019.12.007

Bates, E., Wilson, S. M., Saygin, A. P., Dick, F., Sereno, M. I., Knight, R. T., & Dronkers, N. F. (2003). Voxel-based lesion–symptom mapping. *Nature Neuroscience, 6*(5), 448–450. https://doi.org/10.1038/nn1050

Baumgartner, C., Koren, J. P., Britto-Arias, M., Zoche, L., & Pirker, S. (2019). Presurgical epilepsy evaluation and epilepsy surgery. *F1000Research, 8*, 1818. https://doi.org/10.12688/f1000research.17714.1

Beaulieu, C., De Crespigny, A., Tong, D. C., Moseley, M. E., Albers, G. W., & Marks, M. P. (1999). Longitudinal magnetic resonance imaging study of perfusion and diffusion in stroke: Evolution of lesion volume and correlation with clinical outcome. *Annals of Neurology, 46*(4), 568–578. https://doi.org/10.1002/1531-8249(199910)46:4<568::AID-ANA4>3.0.CO;2-R

Beres, A. M. (2017). Time is of the essence: A review of electroencephalography (EEG) and event-related brain potentials (ERPs) in language research. *Applied Psychophysiology and Biofeedback, 42*(4), 247–255. https://doi.org/10.1007/s10484-017-9371-3

Berger, H. (1929). Über das Elektrenkephalogramm des Menschen. *Archiv für Psychiatrie und Nervenkrankheiten, 87*(1), 527–570. https://doi.org/10.1007/BF01797193

Betthauser, T. J. (2019). AD molecular: Imaging tau aggregates with positron emissions tomography. *Progress in Molecular Biology and Translational Science, 165*, 107–138. https://doi.org/10.1016/bs.pmbts.2019.07.007

Bi, W. L., Olubiyi, O., Tharin, S., & Golby, A. J. (2016). Neurosurgical treatment planning. In H. B. Newton (Ed.), *Handbook of neuro-oncology neuroimaging* (2nd ed., pp. 217–229). Elsevier. https://doi.org/10.1016/B978-0-12-800945-1.00023-9

Binder, J. R. (2011). Functional MRI is a valid noninvasive alternative to Wada testing. *Epilepsy & Behavior, 20*(2), 214–222. https://doi.org/10.1016/j.yebeh.2010.08.004

Blennow, K., Brody, D. L., Kochanek, P. M., Levin, H., McKee, A., Ribbers, G. M., . . . Zetterberg, H. (2016). Traumatic brain injuries. *Nature Reviews Disease Primers, 2*(1). https://doi.org/10.1038/nrdp.2016.84

Boccagni, C., Bagnato, S., Sant'Angelo, A., Prestandrea, C., & Galardi, G. (2011). Usefulness of standard EEG in predicting the outcome of patients with disorders of consciousness after anoxic coma. *Journal of Clinical Neurophysiology*, 1. https://doi.org/10.1097/WNP.0b013e318231c8c8

Bonfante, E., Riascos, R., & Arevalo, O. (2018). Imaging of chronic concussion. *Neuroimaging Clinics of North America*, *28*(1), 97–135. https://doi.org/10.1016/j.nic.2017.09.011

Boyle, M. (2010). Semantic feature analysis treatment for aphasic word retrieval impairments: What's in a name? *Topics in Stroke Rehabilitation*, *17*(6), 411–422. https://doi.org/10.1310/tsr1706-411

Britton, J. W., Frey, L. C., Hopp, J. L., Korb, P., Koubeissi, M. Z., Lievens, W. E., . . . St. Louis, E. K. (2016). *Electroencephalography (EEG): An introductory text and atlas of normal and abnormal findings in adults, children, and infants* [Internet]. (E. K. St. Louis & L. C. Frey, Eds.). American Epilepsy Society. http://www.ncbi.nlm.nih.gov/books/NBK390354/

Brody, D. L., Mac Donald, C. L., & Shimony, J. S. (2015). Current and future diagnostic tools for traumatic brain injury: CT, conventional MRI, and diffusion tensor imaging. In D, S, Goodin (Ed.), *Handbook of clinical neurology* (Vol. 127, pp. 267–275). Elsevier. https://doi.org/10.1016/B978-0-444-52892-6.00017-9

Brooks, B. R., Miller, R. G., Swash, M., & Munsat, T. L. (2000). El Escorial revisited: Revised criteria for the diagnosis of amyotrophic lateral sclerosis. *Amyotrophic Lateral Sclerosis and Other Motor Neuron Disorders*, *1*(5), 293–299. https://doi.org/10.1080/146608200300079536

Byrnes, K. R., Wilson, C. M., Brabazon, F., von Leden, R., Jurgens, J. S., Oakes, T. R., & Selwyn, R. G. (2014). FDG-PET imaging in mild traumatic brain injury: A critical review. *Frontiers in Neuroenergetics*, *5*. https://doi.org/10.3389/fnene.2013.00013

Canolty, R. T., & Knight, R. T. (2010). The functional role of cross-frequency coupling. *Trends in Cognitive Sciences*, *14*(11), 506–515. https://doi.org/10.1016/j.tics.2010.09.001

Cardenas-Blanco, A., Machts, J., Acosta-Cabronero, J., Kaufmann, J., Abdulla, S., Kollewe, K., . . . Nestor, P. J. (2016). Structural and diffusion imaging versus clinical assessment to monitor amyotrophic lateral sclerosis. *NeuroImage: Clinical*, *11*, 408–414. https://doi.org/10.1016/j.nicl.2016.03.011

Center for Devices and Radiological Health. (2019). *Computed tomography (CT)*. FDA. https://www.fda.gov/radiation-emitting-products/medical-x-ray-imaging/computed-tomography-ct

Chaljub, G., Kramer, L. A., Johnson, R. F., Johnson, R. F., Singh, H., & Crow, W. N. (2001). Projectile cylinder accidents resulting from the presence of ferromagnetic nitrous oxide or oxygen tanks in the MR suite. *American Journal of Roentgenology*, *177*(1), 27–30. https://doi.org/10.2214/ajr.177.1.1770027

Chen, D. W. (2001). Boy, 6, dies of skull injury during MRI. *New York Times*.

Chen, J. J., Carletti, F., Young, V., Mckean, D., & Quaghebeur, G. (2016). MRI differential diagnosis of suspected multiple sclerosis. *Clinical Radiology, 71*(9), 815–827. https://doi.org/10.1016/j.crad.2016.05.010

Cherry, S. R., Sorenson, J. A., & Phelps, M. E. (2019). Positron emission tomography. In S. R. Cherry, J. A. Sorenson, & M. E. Phelps (Eds.), *Physics in Nuclear Medicine* (4th ed., pp. 307–343). Elsevier. https://doi.org/10.1016/B978-1-4160-5198-5.00018-6

Chervyakov, A. V., Chernyavsky, A. Yu., Sinitsyn, D. O., & Piradov, M. A. (2015). Possible mechanisms underlying the therapeutic effects of transcranial magnetic stimulation. *Frontiers in Human Neuroscience, 9.* https://doi.org/10.3389/fnhum.2015.00303

Choi, J. W., & Moon, W.-J. (2019). Gadolinium deposition in the brain: Current updates. *Korean Journal of Radiology, 20*(1), 134. https://doi.org/10.3348/kjr.2018.0356

Cohen, J. E., Itshayek, E., Moskovici, S., Gomori, J. M., Fraifeld, S., Eichel, R., & Leker, R. R. (2011). State-of-the-art reperfusion strategies for acute ischemic stroke. *Journal of Clinical Neuroscience, 18*(3), 319–323. https://doi.org/10.1016/j.jocn.2010.10.008

Cohen, M. X. (2017). Where does EEG come from and what does it mean? *Trends in Neurosciences, 40*(4), 208–218. https://doi.org/10.1016/j.tins.2017.02.004

Coslett, H. B. (2016). Noninvasive brain stimulation in aphasia therapy. In G. Hickok & S. L. Small (Eds.), *Neurobiology of language* (pp. 1035–1054). Elsevier. https://doi.org/10.1016/B978-0-12-407794-2.00083-3

Dallmeier, J. D., Meysami, S., Merrill, D. A., & Raji, C. A. (2019). Emerging advances of in vivo detection of chronic traumatic encephalopathy and traumatic brain injury. *British Journal of Radiology, 92*(1101), 20180925. https://doi.org/10.1259/bjr.20180925

Daltrozzo, J., Wioland, N., Mutschler, V., & Kotchoubey, B. (2007). Predicting coma and other low responsive patients' outcome using event-related brain potentials: A meta-analysis. *Clinical Neurophysiology, 118*(3), 606–614. https://doi.org/10.1016/j.clinph.2006.11.019

de Carvalho, M., Dengler, R., Eisen, A., England, J. D., Kaji, R., Kimura, J., . . . Swash, M. (2008). Electrodiagnostic criteria for diagnosis of ALS. *Clinical Neurophysiology, 119*(3), 497–503. https://doi.org/10.1016/j.clinph.2007.09.143

Devlin, J. T., & Watkins, K. E. (2007). Stimulating language: Insights from TMS. *Brain, 130*(3), 610–622. https://doi.org/10.1093/brain/awl331

Diehl-Schmid, J., Onur, O. A., Kuhn, J., Gruppe, T., & Drzezga, A. (2014). Imaging frontotemporal lobar degeneration. *Current Neurology and Neuroscience Reports, 14*(10). https://doi.org/10.1007/s11910-014-0489-x

Dionísio, A., Duarte, I. C., Patrício, M., & Castelo-Branco, M. (2018). Transcranial magnetic stimulation as an intervention tool to recover from language, swallowing and attentional deficits after stroke: A systematic review. *Cerebrovascular Diseases, 46*(3–4), 178–185. https://doi.org/10.1159/000494213

Domingues, R., Rossi, C., & Cordonnier, C. (2015). Diagnostic evaluation for nontraumatic intracerebral hemorrhage. *Neurologic Clinics, 33*(2), 315–328. https://doi.org/10.1016/j.ncl.2014.12.001

Duffau, H. (2013). Brain mapping in tumors: Intraoperative or extraoperative? *Epilepsia, 54*, 79–83. https://doi.org/10.1111/epi.12449

Ehman, E. C., Johnson, G. B., Villanueva-Meyer, J. E., Cha, S., Leynes, A. P., Larson, P. E. Z., & Hope, T. A. (2017). PET/MRI: Where might it replace PET/CT? *Journal of Magnetic Resonance Imaging, 46*(5), 947–962. https://doi.org/10.1002/jmri.25711

Eisenmenger, L. B., Huo, E. J., Hoffman, J. M., Minoshima, S., Matesan, M. C., Lewis, D. H., . . . Mountz, J. M. (2016). Advances in PET imaging of degenerative, cerebrovascular, and traumatic causes of dementia. *Seminars in Nuclear Medicine, 46*(1), 57–87. https://doi.org/10.1053/j.semnuclmed.2015.09.003

El Mendili, M. M., Querin, G., Bede, P., & Pradat, P.F. (2019). Spinal cord imaging in amyotrophic lateral sclerosis: Historical concepts—novel techniques. *Frontiers in Neurology, 10*. https://doi.org/10.3389/fneur.2019.00350

Enzinger, C., Barkhof, F., Ciccarelli, O., Filippi, M., Kappos, L., Rocca, M. A., . . . Fazekas, F.; on behalf of the MAGNIMS study group. (2015). Nonconventional MRI and microstructural cerebral changes in multiple sclerosis. *Nature Reviews Neurology, 11*(9), 676–686. https://doi.org/10.1038/nrneurol.2015.194

Fedorenko, E., Scott, T. L., Brunner, P., Coon, W. G., Pritchett, B., Schalk, G., & Kanwisher, N. (2016). Neural correlate of the construction of sentence meaning. *Proceedings of the National Academy of Sciences, 113*(41), E6256–E6262. https://doi.org/10.1073/pnas.1612132113

Fiebach, J. B., Schellinger, P. D., Gass, A., Kucinski, T., Siebler, M., Villringer, A., . . . Sartor, K. (2004). Stroke magnetic resonance imaging is accurate in hyperacute intracerebral hemorrhage: A multicenter study on the validity of stroke imaging. *Stroke, 35*(2), 502–506. https://doi.org/10.1161/01.STR.0000114203.75678.88

Filippi, M., Preziosa, P., & Rocca, M. A. (2018). MRI in multiple sclerosis: What is changing? *Current Opinion in Neurology, 31*(4), 386–395. https://doi.org/10.1097/WCO.0000000000000572

Filippi, M., Rocca, M. A., Ciccarelli, O., De Stefano, N., Evangelou, N., Kappos, L., . . . Barkhof, F. (2016). MRI criteria for the diagnosis of multiple sclerosis: MAGNIMS consensus guidelines. *The Lancet Neurology, 15*(3), 292–303. https://doi.org/10.1016/S1474-4422(15)00393-2

Fingelkurts, A. A., Fingelkurts, A. A., Bagnato, S., Boccagni, C., & Galardi, G. (2019). EEG oscillatory states as neuro-phenomenology of consciousness as revealed from patients in vegetative and minimally conscious states. *Consciousness and Cognition, 21*(1), 149–169. https://doi.org/10.1016/j.concog.2011.10.004

Fink, J. R., Muzi, M., Peck, M., & Krohn, K. A. (2015). Multimodality brain tumor imaging: MR imaging, PET, and PET/MR imaging. *Journal of Nuclear Medicine, 56*(10), 1554–1561. https://doi.org/10.2967/jnumed.113.131516

Fox, M. D., & Raichle, M. E. (2007). Spontaneous fluctuations in brain activity observed with functional magnetic resonance imaging. *Nature Reviews Neuroscience, 8*(9), 700–711. https://doi.org/10.1038/nrn2201

Fox, M. D., Snyder, A. Z., Vincent, J. L., Corbetta, M., Van Essen, D. C., & Raichle, M. E. (2005). The human brain is intrinsically organized into dynamic, anticorrelated functional networks. *Proceedings of the National Academy of Sciences of the United States of America*, *102*(27), 9673–9678.

Frey, D., Schilt, S., Strack, V., Zdunczyk, A., Rosler, J., Niraula, B., . . . Picht, T. (2014). Navigated transcranial magnetic stimulation improves the treatment outcome in patients with brain tumors in motor eloquent locations. *Neuro-Oncology*, *16*(10), 1365–1372. https://doi.org/10.1093/neuonc/nou110

Fridriksson, J., Rorden, C., Elm, J., Sen, S., George, M. S., & Bonilha, L. (2018). Transcranial direct current stimulation vs. sham stimulation to treat aphasia after stroke: A randomized clinical trial. *JAMA Neurology*, *75*(9), 1470. https://doi.org/10.1001/jamaneurol.2018.2287

Galldiks, N., & Langen, K.J. (2016). Amino acid PET—An imaging option to identify treatment response, post-therapeutic effects, and tumor recurrence? *Frontiers in Neurology*, *7*. https://doi.org/10.3389/fneur.2016.0090

Geevasinga, N., Loy, C. T., Menon, P., de Carvalho, M., Swash, M., Schrooten, M., . . . Vucic, S. (2016). Awaji criteria improves the diagnostic sensitivity in amyotrophic lateral sclerosis: A systematic review using individual patient data. *Clinical Neurophysiology*, *97*(7), 2684–2691. https://doi.org/10.1016/j.clinph.2016.04.005

Gilhus, N. E., Tzartos, S., Evoli, A., Palace, J., Burns, T. M., & Verschuuren, J. J. G. M. (2019). Myasthenia gravis. *Nature Reviews Disease Primers*, *5*(1). https://doi.org/10.1038/s41572-019-0079-y

Gilmore, N., Meier, E. L., Johnson, J. P., & Kiran, S. (2020). Typicality-based semantic treatment for anomia results in multiple levels of generalisation. *Neuropsychological Rehabilitation*, *30*(5), 802–828. https://doi.org/10.1080/09602011.2018.1499533

Giorgio, A., & De Stefano, N. (2018). Effective utilization of MRI in the diagnosis and management of multiple sclerosis. *Neurologic Clinics*, *36*(1), 27–34. https://doi.org/10.1016/j.ncl.2017.08.013

Goffin, K., & van Laere, K. (2016). Single-photon emission tomography. In J. C. Masdeu & R. Gilberto González (Eds.), *Handbook of clinical neurology* (Vol. 135, pp. 241–250). Elsevier. https://doi.org/10.1016/B978-0-444-53485-9.00013-1

Gordon, E., Rohrer, J. D., & Fox, N. C. (2016). Advances in neuroimaging in frontotemporal dementia. *Journal of Neurochemistry*, *138*, 193–210. https://doi.org/10.1111/jnc.13656

Gorno-Tempini, M. L., Hillis, A. E., Weintraub, S., Kertesz, A., Mendez, M., Cappa, S. F., . . . Grossman, M. (2011). Classification of primary progressive aphasia and its variants. *Neurology*, *76*(11), 1006–1014. https://doi.org/10.1212/WNL.0b013e31821103e6

Haacke, E. M., Xu, Y., Cheng, Y. C. N., & Reichenbach, J. R. (2004). Susceptibility weighted imaging (SWI). *Magnetic Resonance in Medicine*, *52*(3), 69–618. https://doi.org/10.1002/mrm.20198

Haag, A., Knake, S., Hamer, H. M., Boesebeck, F., Freitag, H., Schulz, R., . . . Rosenow, F. (2008). The Wada test in Austrian, Dutch, German, and Swiss epilepsy centers from 2000 to 2005: A review of 1421 procedures. *Epilepsy & Behavior, 13*(1), 83–89. https://doi.org/10.1016/j.yebeh.2008.02.012

Hakimelahi, R., Yoo, A. J., He, J., Schwamm, L. H., Lev, M. H., Schaefer, P. W., & González, R. G. (2012). Rapid identification of a major diffusion/perfusion mismatch in distal internal carotid artery or middle cerebral artery ischemic stroke. *BMC Neurology, 9*(1). https://doi.org/10.1186/1471-2377-12-132

Hakimi, R., & Garg, A. (2016). Imaging of hemorrhagic stroke. *CONTINUUM: Lifelong Learning in Neurology, 22*(5), 1424–1450. https://doi.org/10.1212/CON.0000000000000377

Hall, B., Mak, E., Cervenka, S., Aigbirhio, F. I., Rowe, J. B., & O'Brien, J. T. (2017). In vivo tau PET imaging in dementia: Pathophysiology, radiotracer quantification, and a systematic review of clinical findings. *Ageing Research Reviews, 36*, 50–63. https://doi.org/10.1016/j.arr.2017.03.002

Harrigan, M. R., & Deveikis, J. P. (2013). *Handbook of cerebrovascular disease and neurointerventional technique*. Humana Press. https://doi.org/10.1007/978-1-61779-946-4

Haussen, D. C., & Nogueira, R. G. (2017). Conventional cerebral arteriography. In L. R. Caplan, J. Biller, M. C. Leary, E. H. Lo, A. J. Thomas, M. Yenari, & J. H. Zhang (Eds.), *Primer on cerebrovascular diseases* (2nd ed., pp. 707–712). Elsevier. https://doi.org/10.1016/B978-0-12-803058-5.00134-X

Helfrich, R. F., & Knight, R. T. (2019). Cognitive neurophysiology: Event-related potentials. In K. H. Levin & P. Chauvel (Eds.), *Handbook of clinical neurology* (Vol. 160, pp. 543–558). Elsevier. https://doi.org/10.1016/B978-0-444-64032-1.00036-9

Henriksen, O. M., Marner, L., & Law, I. (2016). Clinical PET/MR imaging in dementia and neuro-oncology. *PET Clinics, 11*(4), 441–452. https://doi.org/10.1016/j.cpet.2016.05.003

Herrmann, C. S., Strüber, D., Helfrich, R. F., & Engel, A. K. (2016). EEG oscillations: From correlation to causality. *International Journal of Psychophysiology, 103*, 9–21. https://doi.org/10.1016/j.ijpsycho.2015.02.003

Hillis, A. E., Barker, P. B., Wityk, R. J., Aldrich, E. M., Restrepo, L., Breese, E. L., & Work, M. (2004). Variability in subcortical aphasia is due to variable sites of cortical hypoperfusion. *Brain and Language, 89*(3), 524–530. https://doi.org/10.1016/j.bandl.2004.01.007

Hillis, A. E., Gold, L., Kannan, V., Cloutman, L., Kleinman, J. T., Newhart, M., . . . Gottesman, R. F. (2008). Site of the ischemic penumbra as a predictor of potential for recovery of functions. *Neurology, 71*(3), 184–189. https://doi.org/10.1212/01.wnl.0000317091.17339.98

Hillis, A. E., Wityk, R. J., Barker, P. B., Beauchamp, N. J., Gailloud, P., Murphy, K., . . . Metter, E. J. (2002). Subcortical aphasia and neglect in acute stroke: The role of cortical hypoperfusion. *Brain, 95*(5), 1094–1104. https://doi.org/10.1093/brain/awf113

Hillis, A. E., Wityk, R. J., Tuffiash, E., Beauchamp, N. J., Jacobs, M. A., Barker, P. B., & Selnes, O. A. (2001). Hypoperfusion of Wernicke's area predicts severity of semantic deficit in acute stroke. *Annals of Neurology, 50*(5), 561–566. https://doi.org/10.1002/ana.1265

Hjort, N., Christensen, S., Sølling, C., Ashkanian, M., Wu, O., Røhl, L., . . . Østergaard, L. (2005). Ischemic injury detected by diffusion imaging 11 minutes after stroke. *Annals of Neurology, 58*(3), 462–465. https://doi.org/10.1002/ana.20595

Hulkower, M. B., Poliak, D. B., Rosenbaum, S. B., Zimmerman, M. E., & Lipton, M. L. (2013). A decade of DTI in traumatic brain injury: 10 years and 100 articles later. *American Journal of Neuroradiology, 34*(11), 2064–2074. https://doi.org/10.3174/ajnr.A3395

Jack, C. R., Bennett, D. A., Blennow, K., Carrillo, M. C., Dunn, B., Haeberlein, S. B., . . . Silverberg, N. (2018). NIA-AA research framework: Toward a biological definition of Alzheimer's disease. *Alzheimer's & Dementia, 14*(4), 535–562. https://doi.org/10.1016/j.jalz.2018.02.018

Kanda, T., Ishii, K., Kawaguchi, H., Kitajima, K., & Takenaka, D. (2014). High signal intensity in the dentate nucleus and globus pallidus on unenhanced T1-weighted MR images: Relationship with increasing cumulative dose of a gadolinium-based contrast material. *Radiology, 270*(3), 834–841. https://doi.org/10.1148/radiol.13131669

Karakaş, S., & Barry, R. J. (2017). A brief historical perspective on the advent of brain oscillations in the biological and psychological disciplines. *Neuroscience & Biobehavioral Reviews, 75*, 335–347. https://doi.org/10.1016/j.neubiorev.2016.12.009

Kassubek, J., & Pagani, M. (2019). Imaging in amyotrophic lateral sclerosis: MRI and PET. *Current Opinion in Neurology, 32*(5), 740–746. https://doi.org/10.1097/WCO.0000000000000728

Kidwell, C. S., & Hsia, A. W. (2006). Imaging of the brain and cerebral vasculature in patients with suspected stroke: Advantages and disadvantages of CT and MRI. *Current Neurology and Neuroscience Reports, 6*(1), 9–16. https://doi.org/10.1007/s11910-996-0003-1

Kutas, M., & Federmeier, K. D. (2011). Thirty years and counting: Finding meaning in the N400 component of the event-related brain potential (ERP). *Annual Review of Psychology, 62*(1), 621–647. https://doi.org/10.1146/annurev.psych.093008.131123

Kutas, M, & Hillyard, S. (1980). Reading senseless sentences: Brain potentials reflect semantic incongruity. *Science, 207*(4427), 203–205. https://doi.org/10.1126/science.7350657

Kutas, M., & Hillyard, S. A. (1984). Brain potentials during reading reflect word expectancy and semantic association. *Nature, 307*(5947), 161–163. https://doi.org/10.1038/307161a0

Ledezma, C. J., Fiebach, J. B., & Wintermark, M. (2009). Modern imaging of the infarct core and the ischemic penumbra in acute stroke patients: CT versus MRI. *Expert Review of Cardiovascular Therapy, 7*(4), 395–403. https://doi.org/10.1586/erc.09.7

Li, J., Pan, P., Song, W., Huang, R., Chen, K., & Shang, H. (2019). A meta-analysis of diffusion tensor imaging studies in amyotrophic lateral sclerosis. *Neurobiology of Aging, 33*(8), 1833–1838. https://doi.org/10.1016/j.neurobiolaging.2011.04.007

Li, W., Lin, T., Li, X., Jing, Y., Wu, C., Li, M., . . . Xu, G. (2020). TMS brain mapping of the pharyngeal cortical representation in healthy subjects. *Brain Stimulation, 13*(3), 891–899. https://doi.org/10.1016/j.brs.2020.02.031

Loddenkemper, T., Morris, H. H., & Möddel, G. (2008). Complications during the Wada test. *Epilepsy & Behavior, 13*(3), 551–553. https://doi.org/10.1016/j.yebeh.2008.05.014

Macdonald, R. L., & Schweizer, T. A. (2017). Spontaneous subarachnoid haemorrhage. *The Lancet, 389*(10069), 655–666. https://doi.org/10.1016/S0140-6736(16)30668-7

Mahon, B. Z., Mead, J. A., Chernoff, B. L., Sims, M. H., Garcea, F. E., Prentiss, E., . . . Pilcher, W. H. (2019). Translational brain mapping at the University of Rochester Medical Center: Preserving the mind through personalized brain mapping. *Journal of Visualized Experiments, 150.* https://doi.org/10.3791/59592

Mandonnet, E., Nouet, A., Gatignol, P., Capelle, L., & Duffau, H. (2007). Does the left inferior longitudinal fasciculus play a role in language? A brain stimulation study. *Brain, 130*(3), 623–629. https://doi.org/10.1093/brain/awl361

Manias, K. A., & Peet, A. (2018). What is MR spectroscopy? *Archives of Disease in Childhood—Education & Practice Edition, 103*(4), 213–216. https://doi.org/10.1136/archdischild-2017-312839

Mantegazza, R., & Cavalcante, P. (2019). Diagnosis and treatment of myasthenia gravis. *Current Opinion in Rheumatology, 31*(6), 623–633. https://doi.org/10.1097/BOR.0000000000000647

Marks, W. J., & Laxer, K. D. (2019). Invasive clinical neurophysiology in epilepsy and movement disorders. In M. J. Aminoff (Ed.), *Aminoff's electrodiagnosis in clinical neurology* (6th ed., pp. 165–185). Elsevier. https://doi.org/10.1016/B978-1-4557-0308-1.00007-8

McWeeny, S., & Norton, E. S. (2020). Understanding event-related potentials (ERPs) in clinical and basic language and communication disorders research: A tutorial. *International Journal of Language & Communication Disorders, 55*(4), 445–457. https://doi.org/10.1111/1460-6984.12535

Merino, J. G., & Warach, S. (2010). Imaging of acute stroke. *Nature Reviews. Neurology, 6*(10), 560–571. https://doi.org/10.1038/nrneurol.2010.129

Meyer, P. F., McSweeney, M., Gonneaud, J., & Villeneuve, S. (2019). AD molecular: PET amyloid imaging across the Alzheimer's disease spectrum: From disease mechanisms to prevention. In J. T. Becker & A. D. Cohen (Eds.), *Progress in Molecular Biology and Translational Science* (Vol. 165, pp. 63–106). Elsevier. https://doi.org/10.1016/bs.pmbts.2019.05.001

Moritz-Gasser, S., & Duffau, H. (2009). Evidence of a large-scale network underlying language switching: A brain stimulation study: Case report. *Journal of Neurosurgery, 111*(4), 729–732. https://doi.org/10.3171/2009.4.JNS081587

Morlet, D., & Fischer, C. (2014). MMN and novelty P3 in coma and other altered states of consciousness: A review. *Brain Topography, 27*(4), 467–479. https://doi.org/10.1007/s10548-013-0335-5

Moulin, S., & Leys, D. (2019). Stroke mimics and chameleons. *Current Opinion in Neurology*, *32*(1), 54–59. https://doi.org/10.1097/WCO.0000000000000620

Murakami, T., Ugawa, Y., & Ziemann, U. (2013). Utility of TMS to understand the neurobiology of speech. *Frontiers in Psychology*, *4*. https://doi.org/10.3389/fpsyg.2013.00446

Murdoch, B. E., & Barwood, C. H. S. (2013). Non-invasive brain stimulation: A new frontier in the treatment of neurogenic speech-language disorders. *International Journal of Speech-Language Pathology*, *15*(3), 234–244. https://doi.org/10.3109/17549507.2012.745605

Mutch, C. A., Talbott, J. F., & Gean, A. (2016). Imaging evaluation of acute traumatic brain injury. *Neurosurgery Clinics of North America*, *27*(4), 409–439. https://doi.org/10.1016/j.nec.2016.05.011

Nadkarni, T. N., Andreoli, M. J., Nair, V. A., Yin, P., Young, B. M., Kundu, B., . . . Prabhakaran, V. (2015). Usage of fMRI for pre-surgical planning in brain tumor and vascular lesion patients: Task and statistical threshold effects on language lateralization. *NeuroImage: Clinical*, *7*, 415–423. https://doi.org/10.1016/j.nicl.2014.12.014

Naeser, M. A., Martin, P. I., Theoret, H., Kobayashi, M., Fregni, F., Nicholas, M., . . . Pascual-Leone, A. (2011). TMS suppression of right pars triangularis, but not pars opercularis, improves naming in aphasia. *Brain and Language*, *119*(3), 206–213. https://doi.org/10.1016/j.bandl.2011.07.005

Neville, H., Nicol, J. L., Barss, A., Forster, K. I., & Garrett, M. F. (1991). Syntactically based sentence processing classes: Evidence from event-related brain potentials. *Journal of Cognitive Neuroscience*, *3*(2), 151–165. https://doi.org/10.1162/jocn.1991.3.2.151

Niogi, S. N., & Mukherjee, P. (2010). Diffusion tensor imaging of mild traumatic brain injury. *Journal of Head Trauma Rehabilitation*, *25*(4), 241–255. https://doi.org/10.1097/HTR.0b013e3181e52c2a

O'Donnell, L. J., & Westin, C.F. (2011). An introduction to diffusion tensor image analysis. *Neurosurgery Clinics of North America*, *22*(2), 185–196. https://doi.org/10.1016/j.nec.2010.12.004

Osterhout, L., & Holcomb, P. J. (1992). Event-related brain potentials elicited by syntactic anomaly. *Journal of Memory and Language*, *31*(6), 785–806. https://doi.org/10.1016/0749-596X(92)90039-Z

Osterhout, L., & Mobley, L. A. (1995). Event-related brain potentials elicited by failure to agree. *Journal of Memory and Language*, *34*(6), 739–773. https://doi.org/10.1006/jmla.1995.1033

Öz, G., Alger, J. R., Barker, P. B., Bartha, R., Bizzi, A., Boesch, C., . . . Kauppinen, R. A.; for the MRS Consensus Group. (2014). Clinical proton MR spectroscopy in central nervous system disorders. *Radiology*, *270*(3), 658–679. https://doi.org/10.1148/radiol.13130531

Pagano, G., Niccolini, F., & Politis, M. (2016). Imaging in Parkinson's disease. *Clinical Medicine*, *16*(4), 371–375. https://doi.org/10.7861/clinmedicine.16-4-371

Pasnoor, M., Dimachkie, M. M., Farmakidis, C., & Barohn, R. J. (2018). Diagnosis of myasthenia gravis. *Neurologic Clinics*, *36*(2), 261–274. https://doi.org/10.1016/j.ncl.2018.01.010

Peterchev, A. V., Wagner, T. A., Miranda, P. C., Nitsche, M. A., Paulus, W., Lisanby, S. H., . . . Bikson, M. (2019). Fundamentals of transcranial electric and magnetic stimulation dose: Definition, selection, and reporting practices. *Brain Stimulation, 5*(4), 435–453. https://doi .org/10.1016/j.brs.2011.10.001

Pietryga, J. A., Fonder, M. A., Rogg, J. M., North, D. L., & Bercovitch, L. G. (2013). Invisible metallic microfiber in clothing presents unrecognized MRI risk for cutaneous burn. *American Journal of Neuroradiology, 34*(5), E47–E50. https://doi.org/10.3174/ajnr.A2827

Pinter, N. K., Klein, J. P., & Mechtler, L. L. (2016). Potential safety issues related to the use of gadolinium-based contrast agents. *Continuum, 22*(5), 1678–1684. https://doi.org/10.1212/CON.0000000000000378

Plowman-Prine, E. K., Triggs, W. J., Malcolm, M. P., & Rosenbek, J. C. (2008). Reliability of transcranial magnetic stimulation for mapping swallowing musculature in the human motor cortex. *Clinical Neurophysiology, 119*(10), 2298–2303. https://doi.org/10.1016/j.clinph .2008.06.006

Poldrack, R. A. (2019). The future of fMRI in cognitive neuroscience. *NeuroImage, 62*(2), 916–920. https://doi.org/10.1016/j.neuroimage .2011.08.007

Queiroz, M. A., & Huellner, M. W. (2015). PET/MR in cancers of the head and neck. *Seminars in Nuclear Medicine, 45*(3), 248–265. https://doi .org/10.1053/j.semnuclmed.2014.12.005

Raichle, M. E. (2011). The restless brain. *Brain Connectivity, 1*(1), 3–9. https://doi.org/10.1089/brain.2011.0019

Raichle, M. E., MacLeod, A. M., Snyder, A. Z., Powers, W. J., Gusnard, D. A., & Shulman, G. L. (2001). A default mode of brain function. *Proceedings of the National Academy of Sciences, 98*(2), 676–682.

Raji, C. A., Tarzwell, R., Pavel, D., Schneider, H., Uszler, M., Thornton, J., . . . Henderson, T. (2014). Clinical utility of SPECT neuroimaging in the diagnosis and treatment of traumatic brain injury: A systematic review. *PLOS ONE, 9*(3), e91088. https://doi.org/10.1371/journal .pone.0091088

Ramalho, J., & Ramalho, M. (2017). Gadolinium deposition and chronic toxicity. *Magnetic Resonance Imaging Clinics of North America, 25*(4), 765–778. https://doi.org/10.1016/j.mric.2017.06.007

Reichenbach, J. R., Venkatesan, R., Schillinger, D. J., Kido, D. K., & Haacke, E. M. (1997). Small vessels in the human brain: MR venography with deoxyhemoglobin as an intrinsic contrast agent. *Radiology, 204*(1), 272–277. https://doi.org/10.1148/radiology.204.1.9205259

Ritaccio, A. L., Brunner, P., & Schalk, G. (2018). Electrical stimulation mapping of the brain: Basic principles and emerging alternatives. *Journal of Clinical Neurophysiology, 35*(2), 86–97. https://doi.org/10.1097/ WNP.0000000000000440

Rossi, S., Hallett, M., Rossini, P. M., & Pascual-Leone, A. (2009). Safety, ethical considerations, and application guidelines for the use of transcranial magnetic stimulation in clinical practice and research. *Clinical Neurophysiology, 90*(9), 2008–2039. https://doi.org/10.1016/j. clinph.2009.08.016

Ryvlin, P., & Rheims, S. (2008). Epilepsy surgery: Eligibility criteria and presurgical evaluation. *Dialogues in Clinical Neuroscience, 10*(1), 91–103.

Scheltens, P., Blennow, K., Breteler, M. M. B., de Strooper, B., Frisoni, G. B., Salloway, S., & Van der Flier, W. M. (2016). Alzheimer's disease. *The Lancet, 388*(10043), 505–517. https://doi.org/10.1016/S0140-6736(15)01124-1

Schwarz, D., Bendszus, M., & Breckwoldt, M. O. (2020). Clinical value of susceptibility weighted imaging of brain metastases. *Frontiers in Neurology, 11*. https://doi.org/10.3389/fneur.2020.00055

Shigematsu, T., Fujishima, I., & Ohno, K. (2013). Transcranial direct current stimulation improves swallowing function in stroke patients. *Neurorehabilitation and Neural Repair, 27*(4), 363–369. https://doi.org/10.1177/1545968312474116

Shukla, G., Alexander, G. S., Bakas, S., Nikam, R., Talekar, K., Palmer, J. D., & Shi, W. (2017). Advanced magnetic resonance imaging in glioblastoma: A review. *Chinese Clinical Oncology, 6*(4). https://doi.org/10.21037/cco.2017.06.28

Singer, W. (2018). Neuronal oscillations: Unavoidable and useful? *European Journal of Neuroscience, 48*(7), 2389–2398. https://doi.org/10.1111/ejn.13796

Slomka, P. J., Miller, R. J. H., Hu, L. H., Germano, G., & Berman, D. S. (2019). Solid-state detector SPECT myocardial perfusion imaging. *Journal of Nuclear Medicine, 60*(9), 1194–904. https://doi.org/10.2967/jnumed.118.220657

So, E. L., & Alwaki, A. (2018). A guide for cortical electrical stimulation mapping. *Journal of Clinical Neurophysiology, 35*(2), 98–105. https://doi.org/10.1097/WNP.0000000000000435

Sorensen, A. G., Buonanno, F. S., Gonzalez, R. G., Schwamm, L. H., Lev, M. H., Huang-Hellinger, F. R., . . . Koroshetz, W. J. (1996). Hyperacute stroke: Evaluation with combined multisection diffusion-weighted and hemodynamically weighted echo-planar MR imaging. *Radiology, 199*(2), 391–401. https://doi.org/10.1148/radiology.199.2.8668784

Syed, Y. Y., & Deeks, E. (2015). [18F] Florbetaben: A review in β-amyloid PET imaging in cognitive impairment. *CNS Drugs, 29*(7), 605–613. https://doi.org/10.1007/s40263-015-0258-7

Szelényi, A., Bello, L., Duffau, H., Fava, E., Feigl, G. C., Galanda, M., . . . Sala, F. (2010). Intraoperative electrical stimulation in awake craniotomy: Methodological aspects of current practice. *Neurosurgical Focus, 28*(2), E7. https://doi.org/10.3171/2009.12.FOCUS09237

Taplin, A. M., de Pesters, A., Brunner, P., Hermes, D., Dalfino, J. C., Adamo, M. A., . . . Schalk, G. (2016). Intraoperative mapping of expressive language cortex using passive real-time electrocorticography. *Epilepsy & Behavior Case Reports, 5*, 46–51. https://doi.org/10.1016/j.ebcr.2016.03.003

Thompson, A. J., Banwell, B. L., Barkhof, F., Carroll, W. M., Coetzee, T., Comi, G., . . . Cohen, J. A. (2018). Diagnosis of multiple sclerosis:

2017 revisions of the McDonald criteria. *The Lancet Neurology, 17*(2), 162–173. https://doi.org/10.1016/S1474-4422(17)30470-2

Vagal, A., Vossough, A., Lev, M. H., & Wintermark, M. (2016). Central nervous system infarction. In H. B. Newton (Ed.), *Handbook of neuro-oncology neuroimaging* (2nd ed., pp. 89–98). Elsevier. https://doi.org/10.1016/B978-0-12-800945-1.00011-2

Vakani, R., & Nair, D. R. (2019). Electrocorticography and functional mapping. In K. H. Levin & P. Chauvel (Eds.), *Handbook of clinical neurology* (Vol. 160, pp. 313–327). Elsevier. https://doi.org/10.1016/B978-0-444-64032-1.00020-5

Valkanova, V., & Ebmeier, K. P. (2014). Neuroimaging in dementia. *Maturitas, 79*(2), 202–208. https://doi.org/10.1016/j.maturitas.2014.02.016

Valotassiou, V., Malamitsi, J., Papatriantafyllou, J., Dardiotis, E., Tsougos, I., Psimadas, D., . . . Georgoulias, P. (2018). SPECT and PET imaging in Alzheimer's disease. *Annals of Nuclear Medicine, 32*(9), 583–593. https://doi.org/10.1007/s12149-018-1292-6

van den Berg, B., Walgaard, C., Drenthen, J., Fokke, C., Jacobs, B. C., & van Doorn, P. A. (2014). Guillain–Barré syndrome: Pathogenesis, diagnosis, treatment and prognosis. *Nature Reviews Neurology, 10*(8), 469–482. https://doi.org/10.1038/nrneurol.2014.121

Vilela, P. (2017). Acute stroke differential diagnosis: Stroke mimics. *European Journal of Radiology, 96*, 133–144. https://doi.org/10.1016/j.ejrad.2017.05.008

Whitwell, J. L. (2019). FTD spectrum: Neuroimaging across the FTD spectrum. In J. T. Becker & A. D. Cohen (Eds.), *Progress in molecular biology and translational science* (Vol. 165, pp. 187–223). Elsevier. https://doi.org/10.1016/bs.pmbts.2019.05.009

Wilkes, S., McCormack, E., Kenney, K., Stephens, B., Passo, R., Harburg, L., . . . Diaz-Arrastia, R. (2018). Evolution of traumatic parenchymal intracranial hematomas (ICHs): Comparison of hematoma and edema components. *Frontiers in Neurology, 9*. https://doi.org/10.3389/fneur.2018.00527

Willison, H. J., Jacobs, B. C., & van Doorn, P. A. (2016). Guillain-Barré syndrome. *The Lancet, 388*(10045), 717–727. https://doi.org/10.1016/S0140-6736(16)00339-1

Wintermark, M., Sanelli, P. C., Anzai, Y., Tsiouris, A. J., Whitlow, C. T., Druzgal, T. J., . . . Zeineh, M. (2015). Imaging evidence and recommendations for traumatic brain injury: Conventional neuroimaging techniques. *Journal of the American College of Radiology, 9*(2), e1–e14. https://doi.org/10.1016/j.jacr.2014.10.014

Wright, I. C., McGuire, P. K., Poline, J. B., Travere, J. M., Murray, R. M., Frith, C. D., . . . Friston, K. J. (1995). A voxel-based method for the statistical analysis of gray and white matter density applied to schizophrenia. *NeuroImage, 2*(4), 244–252. https://doi.org/10.1006/nimg.1995.1032

Yang, T., Hakimian, S., & Schwartz, T. H. (2014). Intraoperative electrocorticography (ECog): Indications, techniques, and utility in epilepsy surgery. *Epileptic Disorders, 16*(3), 271–279. https://doi.org/10.1684/epd.2014.0675

Zhang, X. Y., Yang, Z. L., Lu, G. M., Yang, G. F., & Zhang, L. J. (2017). PET/MR imaging: New frontier in Alzheimer's disease and other dementias. *Frontiers in Molecular Neuroscience, 10.* https://doi.org/10.3389/fnmol.2017.00343

Zhao, Q., Liu, M., Ha, L., Zhou, Y., & Alzheimer's Disease Neuroimaging Initiative. (2019). Quantitative 18F-AV1451 brain tau PET imaging in cognitively normal older adults, mild cognitive impairment, and Alzheimer's disease patients. *Frontiers in Neurology, 10.* https://doi.org/10.3389/fneur.2019.00486

Zukotynski, K., Kuo, P. H., Mikulis, D., Rosa-Neto, P., Strafella, A. P., Subramaniam, R. M., & Black, S. E. (2018). PET/CT of dementia. *American Journal of Roentgenology, 211*(2), 246–259. https://doi.org/10.2214/AJR.18.19822

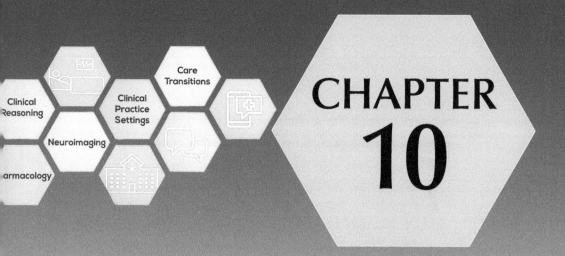

CHAPTER 10

The Role of Speech-Language Pathologists Across Systems— Case Studies in Care

Zachary Smith

Chapter Objectives

After reviewing the cases and reflecting on the questions listed below, readers should be able to:

- Consider clinical diagnoses to establish potential treatment plans across various care settings.
- Apply knowledge regarding interprofessional communication to support care transitions.

Chapter Overview

I n this chapter, six patients are introduced, each of whom have different medical conditions that necessitate care from a speech-language pathologist (SLP). As you read through the case examples, consider the following questions:

1. What are the primary goals of each of the SLPs involved in the patient's care?

2. How were the goals/assessment/treatment for each patient similar at each level of care? How did they differ?

3. In instances where they differed, what factors influenced the care the patient received from the SLP?

4. Brainstorm some speech-language pathology related care challenges you think each patient could experience when moving from one level of care to the next. What are some ideas you have to help prevent or reduce these challenges?

Case 1

Mx. Jaime Donovan is a nonbinary individual in their early thirties. They do not have significant past medical history. Jaime reported their interests as cooking and baking, being active in their community, and singing in their church choir. One winter, Jaime notices that they are having more difficulty both hitting and sustaining high notes during choir practice. Jaime initially attributes this to the cold weather and attempts some home remedies that have been previously successful, such as drinking warm lemon tea and keeping a humidifier close to their bed at night. After a month with no success, Jaime decides to get a referral to an otolaryngologist (ENT) to get a better understanding of their vocal difficulties. The ENT performs a laryngoscopy, during which they find a mass abutting the left arytenoid cartilage. A biopsy is recommended and completed, which shows a T3N1M0 squamous cell carcinoma. Jaime is recommended a debulking procedure to minimize the size of the mass, followed by a course of chemotherapy and radiation treatment to treat their newly diagnosed cancer.

debulking = taking part of tumor off

Jaime is admitted to their local hospital for completion of the debulking procedure, where they are planned to be kept for at least 3 nights for observation. It is during this admission that Jaime first meets an SLP for a clinical swallow evaluation. At that time, the SLP's clinical swallow evaluation is unrevealing, and Jaime is deemed appropriate to continue a regular diet and thin liquids. However, the SLP takes this opportunity to educate Jaime on the short- and long-term effects of their planned upcoming chemoradiation treatment, both in terms of vocal and swallow functions. Jaime is started on a home exercise program consisting of the effortful swallow, the Masako maneuver, and the chin tuck against resistance, which they are encouraged to complete daily. Jaime recuperates well following their debulking procedure and hospitalization and are discharged back home to prepare for their future treatments. Jaime establishes their first treatment appointment with their oncologist and begins treatment.

Undergoing both chemotherapy and radiation treatment has many effects on Jaime, though most notably they begin to not eat enough due to dysgeusia, nausea, and low appetite. As they are losing weight too rapidly, Jaime is recommended a percutaneous gastrostomy tube placement for supplemental tube feedings to ensure adequate nutritional support. This requires rehospitalization, and Jaime is again seen by the inpatient speech-language pathology team. Jaime is again recommended to continue completing their exercise program and to swallow whatever they can tolerate throughout their treatment course, to maintain adequate oropharyngeal function. They are sent home with visiting nursing assistance to optimally maintain their tube feeding regimen at home.

Ultimately, Jaime finishes their treatment regimen, begins to improve, and has their PEG tube removed. As they are now in the maintenance phase, Jaime is seen regularly by an outpatient SLP specializing in head and neck cancers. This is done to monitor oropharyngeal swallow function given the known later-term effects following radiation treatment. Jaime has been followed closely by SLPs over their continuum of care (Figure 10–1) and is motivated to continue these appointments, as continuing to eat by mouth is a high priority of theirs.

Case 2

Mr. Carlos Ruiz is a Spanish-speaking adult male in his fifties, who has a pertinent past medical history of hypertension, atrial fibrillation, and diabetes mellitus. He undergoes regular medical

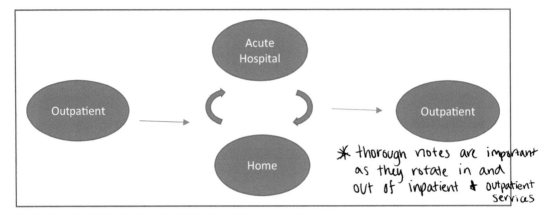

* thorough notes are important as they rotate in and out of inpatient & outpatient services

FIGURE 10–1. Head and neck cancer continuum.

checkups with his primary care physician, eats what he considers to be a healthy diet, and tries to exercise regularly. One night, Carlos is found down on the floor of his bedroom by his wife, Maria. She notices that Carlos has a right facial droop, is having difficulty moving the right side of his body, and is not making any sense when he speaks. Fearing that her husband is experiencing a stroke (cerebrovascular accident), Maria calls for emergency medical support, and Carlos is transferred to his local hospital for further care.

After presenting to the emergency department, Carlos is immediately sent for STAT head imaging, where he is found to have a large left-sided intraparenchymal hemorrhage. As Carlos can respond to simple yes/no questions, is following directions, and his vital signs remain otherwise stable, he is admitted to the neurologic/neurosurgical intensive care unit (ICU) for close monitoring. Once admitted to the ICU, Carlos undergoes a bedside swallow screening with nursing services, which he is found to "fail." As such, a consult order is placed for evaluation with an SLP. Following comprehensive evaluation with an SLP completed in conjunction with a certified medical interpreter, Carlos is found to have an oropharyngeal dysphagia characterized by overt sign (s/sx) of aspiration with both thin and mildly thick liquids, as well as a Broca's aphasia with co-occurring verbal apraxia. Carlos is sent for a videofluoroscopic swallowing study (VFSS), with recommendations for a soft and bite-sized diet with mildly thick liquids, and to utilize a chin-tuck posture during liquid intake. Following this assessment, Carlos is medically stabilized further and is recommended for an inpatient rehabilitation stay following evaluations with speech-language pathology, occupational therapy, and physical therapy. Case management (CM) services are consulted to assist with receiving authorization from Carlos' insurance plan to approve the transfer.

Following transfer, Carlos is excited for the opportunity to continue working toward getting well while undergoing 1 hour each of physical, occupational, and speech therapy while at rehab. Maria, however, has reported to Carlos' medical team that she is nervous about Carlos' anticipated 2- to 3-week stay, given that Carlos contributes much of their monthly mortgage payment, and their two teenage children are having trouble adjusting to their father's medical condition. As such, a social worker is consulted to assist the Ruiz family. Carlos continues to work with his SLP and makes tremendous progress in both swallowing and communication. At the time of discharge, Carlos has advanced to a regular diet and thin liquids without the need for strategies following a second VFSS and is communicating in three- to four-word utterances effectively. Following a meeting of his rehabilitation team, Carlos is found to be safe for a home transfer, as his family has been actively participating in his therapy sessions and knows how to assist him in the home. Carlos' SLP recommends he continues working with outpatient speech therapy services to continue making communicative progress.

Carlos establishes a referral for outpatient services and continues to work with his SLP on many different communicative methods. His SLP implements melodic intonation therapy, augmentative and alternative communication approaches, and other approaches to assist in grammatical structure and word finding. Carlos is (has been) diligent about working with his SLPs across medical settings (Figure 10–2), has great family support, and continues to make steady progress to being an effective total communicator via both verbal and nonverbal methods.

Case 3

Ms. Anna Deitrich is an adult female in her early thirties who has a pertinent past medical history of major depressive disorder and anxiety disorder. She is a highly active person and enjoys going to

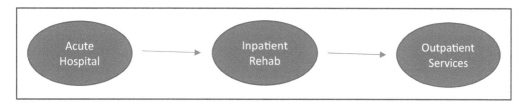

FIGURE 10–2. Stroke continuum.

the gym multiple days a week, spending time with her friends and her partner, and working as the head chef at a busy restaurant in the city in which she lives. One night after finishing her shift at work, Anna is driving home from work when she is involved in a high-speed motor collision, which results in her being ejected from her car, leading to a whole host of injuries. She is admitted to a local hospital as a Code Trauma, with primary injuries including a traumatic brain injury (TBI) with multiple areas of additional subarachnoid hemorrhages, multiple bilateral rib fractures, and a fracture of the left femur. Anna undergoes surgical correction of her femur fracture and is transferred to the ICU where she remains intubated and sedation. After some time, sedation is weaned, and Anna begins to wake, only to be found agitated and not easily redirectable. Following further evaluation with her physicians, they believe that Anna's underlying psychologic conditions have been exacerbated in the setting of her TBI. For this reason, psychiatry services are consulted, who recommend transfer to an inpatient psychiatric unit once Anna is medically stabilized.

After being transferred to an inpatient psychiatry unit associated with another nearby hospital, Anna continues to receive treatment from psychiatrists and various other physicians, and also begins working with physical therapists (PTs), occupational therapists (OTs), and SLPs. During her initial session with an SLP, Anna participates in comprehensive speech, language, cognitive-linguistic, and swallowing evaluations, following which she is found to have a functional oropharyngeal swallow with clearance for a regular diet with thin liquids, though she is found to have severe cognitive-linguistic deficits across multiple cognitive domains. She participates in daily treatment sessions working toward progressing her attention, sequencing skills, organizational skills, and other higher-level executive functioning skills. After a few weeks, Anna has made tremendous progress in both her psychiatric care as well as in physical therapy, occupational therapy, and speech-language pathology goals. She is cleared to discharge to an acute rehabilitation setting for an hour of skilled therapy services daily, with the intent of increasing her independence.

While at acute rehabilitation, Anna participates with physical therapy, occupational therapy, and speech-language pathology, and particularly enjoys working in co-treatment sessions in the mock kitchen, during which she practices skills necessary for her job as a chef. She develops many effective compensatory strategies for working in a high-stress environment, like the restaurant at which she is employed, and identifies triggers that may lead to increased agitation, which she attempts to avoid. Anna makes great further progress and is cleared to return home with her partner and to return to work on a trial basis of 1 day a week. She also continues to receive outpatient speech-language pathology services for ongoing cognitive-linguistic treatment and attends a weekly brain injury survivor group, co-led by an SLP and an OT. With the support of her partner, her friends, her survivor group members, and her therapists across medical settings (Figure 10–3), Anna continues to make strides toward returning to a life that closely mirrors her life before brain injury. She is now able to more independently regulate her emotional and cognitive state, advocate for herself in terms of adaptations she may require, and better understand when she needs to take physical, mental, or emotional breaks from her daily activities.

Case 4

Mr. Ranjit Shah is an adult male in his early eighties, who has a pertinent past medical history of coronary artery disease, atrial fibrillation, and supraventricular tachycardia, for which he receives regular medical evaluations by his cardiologist. During one of his appointments, Mr. Shah's coronary disease is found to have progressed, and he demonstrates up to 80% stenosis of multiple important arteries. He discusses his options with his cardiologist, who ultimately recommends cardiac surgical intervention. Specifically, Mr. Shah's cardiologist recommends a coronary artery bypass and graft (CABG), a procedure that diverts blood flow around Mr. Shah's blocked arteries. The cardiologist feels that this procedure will give Mr. Shah optimal outcomes, though the cardiologist discusses that there are some associated risks with the procedure, specifically related to Mr. Shah's advanced age. Mr. Shah considers

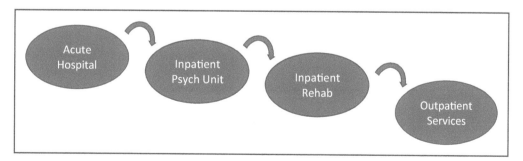

FIGURE 10–3. Traumatic brain injury continuum.

his options and ultimately consents to the procedure. Mr. Shah's surgery is scheduled for a few weeks following this appointment, and he is sent home to prepare.

The day of Mr. Shah's surgery arrives, and his cardiologist reviews the surgical plan once more. Mr. Shah will be placed under sedation and intubated upon arrival to the operating room, the surgery will be completed, and then Mr. Shah will be sent postoperatively to the postanesthesia care unit for monitoring after the surgery. Mr. Shah is brought to the operating room, though his surgery becomes complicated by unanticipated respiratory failure, for which the operation continues longer than anticipated, and Mr. Shah is transferred to a cardiac ICU for close monitoring with a CC team, registered nurses, and respiratory therapists. After a week on ventilator support, Mr. Shah shows improvement in his respiratory status, and he is successfully extubated. An SLP is consulted to complete a clinical swallow evaluation. During the evaluation, Mr. Shah is found to cough frequently on multiple PO consistencies and presents with a breathy, hypophonic vocal quality. The SLP recommends a consult to an otolaryngologist (ENT), who performs a fiberoptic endoscopy only to discover that Mr. Shah has a paralyzed left vocal fold stuck in a lateral position. ENT recommends a vocal fold augmentation to allow Mr. Shah to achieve better glottic closure for airway protection during swallowing as well as improved voicing. Following this procedure, Mr. Shah has improved vocal quality, though he feels he has not returned to his baseline. He also participates in a VFSS to further evaluate his risk for aspiration, following which he is cleared for a regular diet with thin liquids in a left head turn position to help improve airway protection. With further medical optimization, Mr. Shah is ultimately cleared for discharge home under 24-hour supervision from his children. He is recommended outpatient speech-language pathology services following discharge from the hospital, to continue working on both swallowing and voice functions.

Mr. Shah opts to have these services completed through the outpatient speech-language pathology department at the same hospital at which he had his surgery, as this will allow him to have follow-up appointments with his ENT on the same day. Mr. Shah works with his SLP on swallowing exercises and voice therapy and has begun to show spontaneous recovery of left vocal fold function during a repeat endoscopy with ENT. He participates in a repeat VFSS, which reveals that his swallowing has returned to baseline, and he is able to safely discontinue the use of the left head turn posture. After receiving care across multiple medical settings (Figure 10–4), with these improvements, Mr. Shah is ultimately and happily discharged from SLP services.

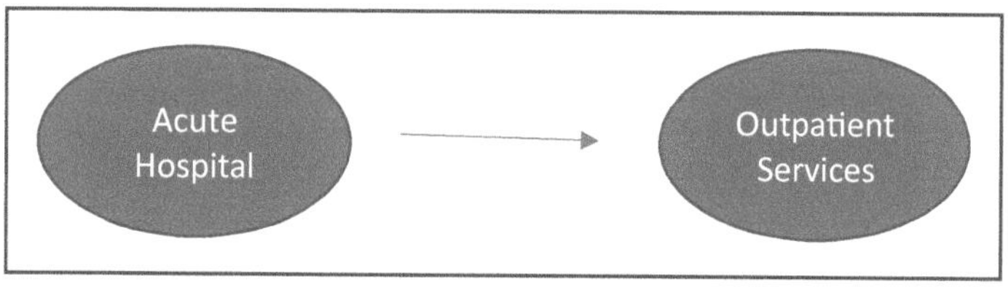

FIGURE 10–4. Cardiac surgery continuum.

Case 5

Mr. Jonathan Wu is an adult male in his late seventies. He has minimal past medical history including type 2 diabetes mellitus, which he independently manages with monitoring his blood glucose levels and injectable insulin as needed. Jonathan is very active in his community, with his activities including regularly attending events at his local senior center, being an active member in his church, and operating a community garden. While Jonathan normally has no difficulty participating in these activities, he has recently begun experiencing some shortness of breath with his more strenuous activities. Unfortunately, this shortness of breath progresses, and Jonathan is admitted to a hospital in respiratory failure. He is intubated shortly after admission and is primarily cared for by a critical care team, consisting of physicians of various specialties, nurses, respiratory therapists, social workers, and CM specialists. Jonathan's condition remains grossly stable though critical, for which he remains sedated and on ventilator support.

Due to difficulty weaning from the ventilator, Jonathan's family elects for him to undergo placement of a tracheostomy, as his physicians believe that this is a necessary first step to helping him recover. Following this procedure, Jonathan shows signs of improvement, and his physicians are slowly able to wean his sedation to the point that Jonathan is now alert and able to participate in his routine care, though remains delirious from prolonged use of sedation. He is then cleared for an evaluation with a SLP. Initially, the SLP works closely with RT to assess Jonathan's ability to tolerate an in-line speaking valve to restore his communication. Although Jonathan voices a high level of interest in resuming his ability to eat and drink, his physicians believe he is too medically frail to tolerate any aspiration, for which reason he is not cleared to receive PO trials with SLP. Instead, Jonathan's SLP trains him in some basic swallowing exercises to begin facilitating a return to PO intake once medically cleared, in addition to focusing on cognitive-linguistic treatment. Jonathan's medical condition improves, though he is still felt too medically frail for acute rehabilitation. Instead, Jonathan is recommended admittance to a long-term acute care hospital (**LTAC**), where he can continue his medical recovery under close supervision from his medical team.

Jonathan flourishes while at the LTAC and ultimately makes tremendous progress in swallowing, cognition, mobility, and ability to participate in activities of daily living under the care of the SLP, PT, and OT. He has weaned from the ventilator though continues to require respiratory support via his tracheostomy. Ultimately, once medically cleared, Jonathan is then sent to a further level of care, which takes place in a post-acute care rehabilitation setting. While there, Jonathan continues to make improvements in his overall medical condition and progresses to the point that he is decannulated and deemed medically fit to discharge home with supervision from his family.

Due to the medical complexities of his case, Jonathan has received care across multiple care settings (Figure 10–5) and is recommended to continue participating in outpatient speech, physical, and occupational therapy to continue making progress to returning to his preferred activities.

Case 6

Mrs. Roberta Jackson is an adult female in her mid-sixties, who has a pertinent past medical history of atrial fibrillation and chronic obstructive pulmonary disease. She lives happily in the suburbs with her wife of many years and has three adult children who live nearby. Over the course of a few months, Roberta notices that she seems to be tripping more frequently than average and seems to

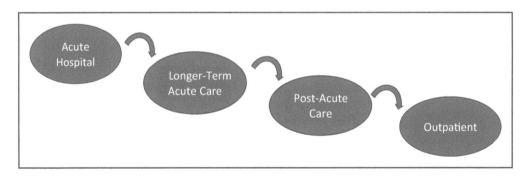

FIGURE 10–5. Respiratory failure continuum.

have some difficulty manipulating smaller objects, such as her keys. Ultimately this prompts Roberta to seek out an evaluation with her primary care physician, who then refers her to a neurologist. Unfortunately, after a series of neurologic evaluations, Roberta is diagnosed with spinal onset amyotrophic lateral sclerosis (ALS). Given the degenerative nature of her condition, Roberta is provided further referrals to a large variety of medical professionals for more targeted care.

One of Roberta's referrals is to an SLP at the ALS Clinic associated with her local hospital. During their first meeting, the SLP educates Roberta and her wife regarding expected progression of disease, particularly as it applies to communication and swallowing. Roberta is also introduced to the idea of voice banking as an ultimate means of alternative and augmentative communication. Roberta works with her SLP to establish an entire repertoire of messages for voice banking and works to establish mastery of her device. Roberta's wife and children are concurrently trained in device management, so they can assist Roberta as needed. Roberta establishes a schedule of appointments with her SLP every 6 months to monitor her throughout the progression of her disease.

As Roberta's disease progresses, she ultimately begins to experience difficulty with both breathing and swallowing and is admitted to her local hospital for respiratory failure. Given that her disease progression is expected to only worsen both processes, Roberta elects to undergo placement of a tracheostomy and feeding tube. She also participates in a modified barium swallow with the inpatient speech-language pathology team, following which she is cleared for a soft and bite-sized diet with mildly thick liquids. Roberta and her family then elect for her to return home, with follow-up scheduled at her ALS Clinic

In addition to receiving continued care from her SLP at the ALS Clinic, Roberta receives care with both physical and occupational therapy to better establish compensatory means for her to participate in daily activities and adaptive mobility methods to assist in her declining ability to move about her home. Roberta's SLP, PT, and OT work closely with other medical professionals to be a source of support as she continues to physically decline. Unfortunately, she experiences medical complications along the course of her disease, necessitating further hospitalizations related to various issues, including metabolic derangements, respiratory failure, and clogging of her feeding tube, among others. For this reason, Roberta receives support from both outpatient and inpatient speech-language pathology services (Figure 10–6), depending on her current needs.

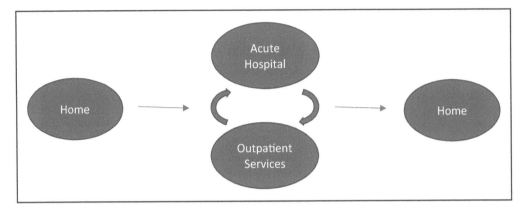

FIGURE 10–6. Amyotrophic lateral sclerosis continuum.

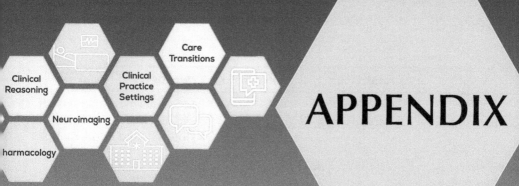

APPENDIX

Test	Specialty	Abbreviation	Purpose
Upper GI (barium swallow)	Gastroenterology, Otolaryngology	UGI	Uses fluoroscopy to evaluate the esophagus, stomach, and duodenum
Lower GI (barium enema)	Gastroenterology	LGI	Uses fluoroscopy to evaluate the rectum, the large intestine, and the lower part of the small intestine
Magnetic resonance imaging	Neurology, Gastroenterology, Pulmonology, Medicine, Oncology	MRI	Uses a combination of large magnets, radiofrequencies, and a computer to produce detailed images of organs and structures within various parts of the body including but not limited to the brain, oropharynx, chest, and abdominal regions
Radioisotope gastricemptying scan	Gastroenterology	Gastric emptying study	Uses radioactive substance to evaluate how quickly food empties the stomach
Ultrasound	Otolaryngology, Gastroenterology, Medicine	US	Uses high-frequency sound waves and a computer to create images of blood vessels, tissues, and organs
Modified barium swallow study/ videofluoroscopic evaluation of swallowing	Speech-Language Pathology	MBS/VFSS	Uses fluoroscopy to evaluate oropharyngeal swallowing function
Computer tomography	Neurology, Gastroenterology, Pulmonology, Medicine, Oncology	CT/CAT scan	Uses a combination of x-ray images and computer processing to evaluate blood vessels, bones, and soft tissues within the body including the brain, oropharynx, chest, and abdomen

Endoscopic Tests

Test	Specialty	Abbreviation	Purpose
Esophagogastro-duodenoscopy	Gastroenterology	EGD or Upper endoscopy	Uses a lighted endoscope guided through the throat, esophagus, and stomach to examine the inside of the esophagus, stomach, and duodenum
Fiberoptic laryngoscopy	Otolaryngology		Uses a lighted scope guided through the nose and into the throat or directly down into the throat to evaluate the pharynx and larynx
Fiberoptic endoscopic evaluation of swallowing	Speech-Language Pathology	FEES	Uses a lighted endoscope guided through the nose and into the throat or directly down into the throat to evaluate the pharynx and larynx
Laryngeal videoendoscopy/stroboscopy Videolaryngo-endoscopy	Otolaryngology/Speech-Language Pathology	LVES	Uses a lighted scope guided through the nose and into the throat or directly down into the throat to evaluate laryngeal function
Fiberoptic nasoendoscopy	Speech-Language Pathology	FNE	Uses a lighted scope guided through the nose to the nasopharynx to evaluate the velum
Bronchoscopy	Pulmonology		Uses a lighted scope guided through the nose or mouth to visualize the airway (vocal folds, trachea, lungs)

Procedure	Specialty	Abbreviation	Purpose
Esophageal manometry	Gastroenterology	Manometry	Uses a small tube guided into the nostril, throat, and esophagus to evaluate muscular activity in the pharynx and esophagus
Esophageal pH monitoring	Gastroenterology		Uses a small tube guided into the nostril, throat, and esophagus to evaluate acidity and reflux inside the esophagus
Gastric manometry	Gastroenterology		Uses a small tube guided into the stomach to evaluate muscular activity within the stomach
Laryngeal electromyography	Otolaryngology	EMG	Uses thin needles with electrodes to evaluate muscle activity in the throat
Laryngo-endoscopic videostroboscopy	Otolaryngology, Speech-Language Pathology	LVES	Uses a video camera with a strobe light to evaluate vocal cord function
Transesophageal echocardiogram	Cardiology	TEE	Uses a thin tube guided through your throat and esophagus as well as sound waves to evaluate heart function
Dialysis (hemodialysis and peritoneal dialysis)	Nephrology	HD/PD	Acts as an artificial kidney to cleanseblood either outside of the body and return it to the body (hemodialysis) or within the body (peritoneal dialysis)
Spirometry/ Pulmonary function test	Pulmonology, Respiratory Therapy	PFT	Measures the volume and force of air breathed in and out in one forced breath

Lab Values

Test	Abbreviation	Normative Values (Adults)	Purpose
Serum albumin	Alb	3.5–5.5 g/dL	Measure of the amount of albumin protein in the clear liquid portion of the blood (long-term)
Prealbumin	PAB	18–45 mg/dL	Measure of the amount of prealbumin protein and serves as a marker of nutrition (short term)
Red blood cell count	RBC	Men: 4.7–6.1 cells/mcL Women: 4.2–5.4 cells/mcL	Measure of how many red blood cells you have
Hemoglobin	Hgb	Men: 14–17 g/dL, Women: 12–16 g/dL	Measure of how much hemoglobin your red blood cells contain
Hematocrit	HCT	Men: 41%–51% Women: 36%–47%	Measure of how much of your blood is made up of red blood cells
White blood cell count	WBC	4.8–10.8 K/mm³	Measure of how many white blood cells you have
Absolute neutrophil count	ANC	>1,500/mm³	Measure of the number of neutrophils in the blood
Sodium	Sodium	135–145 mmol/L	Measure of the amount of sodium in your blood
Blood urea nitrogen	BUN	5–25 mg/dL	Measures the amount of urea nitrogen in your blood
Creatinine	Creat.	0.7–1.3 mg/dL	Measure of how well your kidneys are functioning
Ammonia	Ammonia	15–50 µmol/L	Measure of the amount of ammonia in your blood
Potassium	Potassium	3.5–5.0 mmol/L	Measure of the amount of potassium in your blood
Chloride	Chloride	98–107	Measure of the amount of chloride in your blood
Ionized calcium	Ionized calcium	4.4–5.4 mg/dL; 1.1–1.35 mmol/L	Measure of the amount of ionized calcium in your blood

Test	Abbreviation	Normative Values (Adults)	Purpose
Amylase	Amylase	<110 U/L (blood)	Measure of how much amylase is in your blood or urine to indicate gastrointestinal disease
Carbon dioxide	CO_2	23–28 mEq/L	Measure of how much carbon dioxide is in your serum
Thyroid-stimulating hormone	TSH	0.05–5.0 mcIU/mL	Measure of how much TSH is in your serum to indicate thyroid function
Ferritin	Ferritin	30–200 ng/mL (sex dependent)	Measure of how much iron is in your serum
Glucose	Glucose	70–105 mg/dL (after fasting)	Measure of how much glucose is in your plasma
Erythrocyte sedimentation rate (sed rate)	ESR	0–20 mm/hr (sex dependent)	Measure of how red blood cells "clump," indicative of inflammatory response
Low-density lipoprotein cholesterol	LDL	<100 mg/dL	Measure of cholesterol in your blood that can accumulate on blood vessel walls
High-density lipoprotein cholesterol	HDL	>60 mg/dL	Measure of cholesterol in your blood that can absorb cholesterol and return to liver
Triglycerides		<150 mg/dL	Measure of a particular type of fat in your blood
International normalized ratio	INR	2.0–3.0	Measure of the time for blood to clot
Lumbar puncture	LP	X	Measure of components of cerebrospinal fluid (CSF)
	CSF cell count	0–5 lymphocytes/mcL	Measure of number of cells in CSF
	CSF Glucose	40–80 mg/dL	Measure of glucose in CSF
	CSF MBS	<1.5 ng/mL	Measure of amount of protein in CSF
	CSF Protein total	15–60 mg/dL	Measure of amount of protein in CSF

Measure	Abbreviation	Normative Value (Adult)	Purpose
Respiratory Rate	RR	12–20	Measure of the number of breaths taken per minute
Oxygen Saturation	SpO_2	>93%	Measure of how much oxygen your blood is carrying as a percentage of the maximum it could carry
Heart Rate (pulse)	HR	60–100 beats/min	Measure of how many times your heart beats in a minute
Blood Pressure	BP	90/60–120/80 mm Hg	Measure of the amount of force with which your blood moves through your circulatory system
Forced Vital Capacity	FVC	80%–100%	Measure of the amount of air that you can forcefully exhale after breathing in as deeply as you can
Forced Expiratory Volume	FEV_1	80%–100%	Measure of how much air you can exhale forcefully from your lungs in 1 s

INDEX

Note: Page numbers in **bold** reference non-text material